Nutrition for Fitness

University of Toledo Special Edition

Marie A. Boyle
Sara Long Roth
Werner W.K. Hoeger
Sharon A. Hoeger
Judith E. Brown

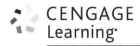

CENGAGE
Learning·

Australia • Brazil • Japan • Korea • Mexico • Singapore • Spain • United Kingdom • United States

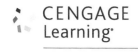
CENGAGE
Learning·

Nutrition for Fitness: University of Toledo Special Edition

Executive Editors:
 Maureen Staudt
 Michael Stranz

Senior Project Development Manager:
 Linda deStefano

Marketing Specialist:
 Courtney Sheldon

Senior Production/Manufacturing Manager:
 Donna M. Brown

Production Editorial Manager:
 Kim Fry

Sr. Rights Acquisition Account Manager:
 Todd Osborne

Sources:

Nutrition Now, 6th Edition
Judith E. Brown - University of Minnesota
© 2011 Cengage Learning. All rights reserved.

Fitness and Wellness, 10th Edition
Werner W.K. Hoeger - Boise State University
Sharon A. Hoeger
© 2013 Cengage Learning. All rights reserved.

Personal Nutrition, 8th Edition
Marie A. Boyle - College of St. Elizabeth
Sara Long Roth - Southern Illinois University
© 2013 Cengage Learning. All rights reserved.

For product information and technology assistance, contact us at
Cengage Learning Customer & Sales Support, 1-800-354-9706

For permission to use material from this text or product,
submit all requests online at **cengage.com/permissions**
Further permissions questions can be emailed to
permissionrequest@cengage.com

This book contains select works from existing Cengage Learning resources and was produced by Cengage Learning Custom Solutions for collegiate use. As such, those adopting and/or contributing to this work are responsible for editorial content accuracy, continuity and completeness.

Compilation © 2012 Cengage Learning
ISBN-13: 978-1-285-13563-2

ISBN-10: 1-285-13563-6

Cengage Learning
5191 Natorp Boulevard
Mason, Ohio 45040
USA
Cengage Learning is a leading provider of customized learning solutions with office locations around the globe, including Singapore, the United Kingdom, Australia, Mexico, Brazil, and Japan. Locate your local office at:
international.cengage.com/region.

Cengage Learning products are represented in Canada by Nelson Education, Ltd.
For your lifelong learning solutions, visit **www.cengage.com/custom.**
Visit our corporate website at **www.cengage.com.**

Printed in the United States of America

Brief Contents

Introduction to Physical Fitness and Wellness

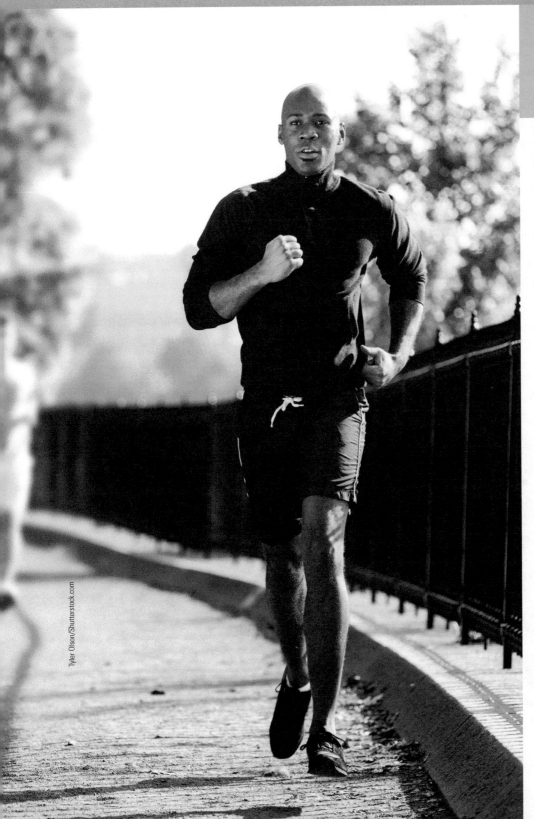

Tyler Olson/Shutterstock.com

"There is no drug in current or prospective use that holds as much promise for sustained health as a lifetime program of physical exercise."[1]

Objectives

- ▶ **Understand** the importance of lifetime fitness and wellness.
- ▶ **Learn** the recommended guidelines for weekly physical activity.
- ▶ **Define** physical fitness and list components of health-related and skill-related fitness.
- ▶ **Understand** the benefits of a comprehensive fitness and wellness program.
- ▶ **Learn** motivational and behavior modification techniques to enhance compliance with a healthy lifestyle program.
- ▶ **Learn** to write SMART goals to aid with the process of change.
- ▶ **Determine** whether medical clearance is required for safe participation in exercise.

CENGAGE brain .com

Visit **www.cengagebrain.com** to access course materials and companion resources for this text including quiz questions designed to check your understanding of the chapter contents, activities, labs, and more! See the preface on page xiii for more information.

1

Jordan's Experience

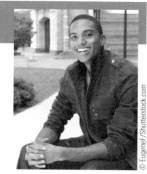

Last year as a freshman in college I was advised to enroll in a general ed fitness and wellness course. I played high school sports and thought I knew all there was to know about being fit and in shape. As the course started I realized I didn't really know how important it was to exercise regularly and take good care of myself. It quickly became my favorite class and I couldn't wait to try what I was learning. I started cardio and strength workouts according to an exercise prescription I wrote myself. I didn't even know there was such a thing as an "exercise prescription." I even stretched once in a while and started to eat better. As I became more fit, I started to feel better about myself, I lost weight, I toned up, I had so much more energy, and I actually started to enjoy exercise. It is fun to work out! I now know that how well I will live the rest of my life has a lot to do with wellness choices I make. My goal is to never stop exercising and take good care of myself.

Most people believe school will teach them how to make a better living. A fitness and wellness course will teach you how to live better—how to truly live your life to its fullest potential. Real success is about more than money: Making a good living will not help you unless you live a wellness lifestyle that will allow you to enjoy what you have. Your lifestyle is the most important factor affecting your personal well-being, but most people don't know how to make the right choices to live their best life.

The benefits of an active and healthy lifestyle have been clearly substantiated by scientific evidence linking increased physical activity and positive habits to better fitness, health, and improved quality of life. Even though a few individuals live long because of favorable genetic factors, for most people, the quality of life during middle age and the "golden years" is more often related to wise choices initiated during youth and continued throughout life.

Based on the abundance of scientific research on physical activity and exercise, a distinction has been established between **physical activity** and exercise. Physical activity is defined as bodily movement produced by skeletal muscles that requires the expenditure of energy and produces progressive health benefits. Examples of physical activity are walking to and from work and the store, taking the stairs instead of elevators and escalators, gardening, doing household chores, dancing, and washing the car by hand. Physical inactivity, by contrast, implies a predomi-

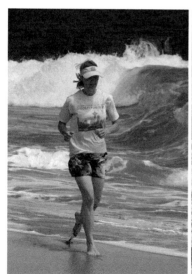 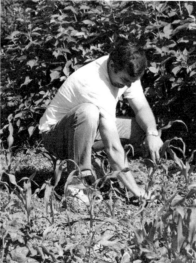 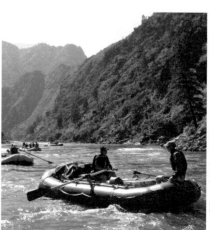

Physical activity and exercise lead to less disease, a longer life, and enhanced quality of life.

Figure 1.1 U.S. prevalence of recommended physical activity.*

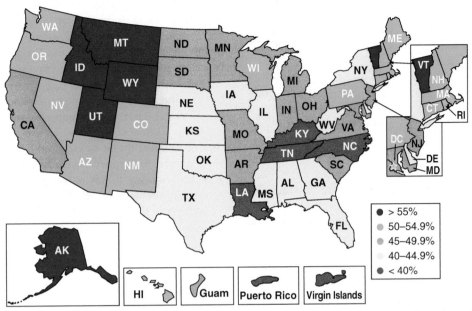

*Moderate-intensity physical activity at least 5 days a week for 30 minutes a day or vigorous-intensity physical activity 3 days a week for 20 minutes a day.

SOURCE: Centers for Disease Control and Prevention.

nantly sedentary lifestyle, characterized by excessive sitting throughout most days, a level of activity that is lower than that required to maintain good health.

Exercise is considered a type of physical activity that requires planned, structured, and repetitive bodily movement to improve or maintain one or more components of physical fitness. A regular weekly program of walking, jogging, cycling, aerobics, swimming, strength training, and stretching exercises are all examples of exercise.

Unfortunately, the current way of life in most developed nations does not provide the human body with sufficient physical exercise to maintain adequate health. Furthermore, many lifestyle patterns are such a serious threat to health that they actually speed up deterioration of the human body. In a few short years, lack of wellness leads to loss of vitality and gusto for life, as well as premature morbidity and mortality.

The typical North American is not a good role model in terms of physical fitness. Only about one-half of U.S. adults meet the minimal recommendation of 30 minutes of moderate physical activity at least 5 days per week.[2] Furthermore, data from the Centers for Disease Control and Prevention (CDC) indicate that 16 percent are completely inactive (that is, spending less than 10 minutes per week in

moderate- or vigorous-intensity physical activity). The prevalence of physical activity by state in the United States is displayed in Figure 1.1.

Even though most people in the United States believe a positive lifestyle has a great impact on health and longevity, most do not know how to implement a fitness and wellness program that will yield the desired results. Patty Neavill is an example of someone who frequently tried to change her life but was unable to do so because she did not know how to implement a sound exercise and weight control program. At age 24, Patty, a college sophomore, was discouraged with her weight, level of fitness, self-image, and quality of life in general.

She had struggled with weight most of her life. Like thousands of other people, she had made many unsuccessful attempts to lose weight. Patty put aside

Key Terms

Physical activity Bodily movement produced by skeletal muscles that requires energy expenditure and produces progressive health benefits.

Exercise A type of physical activity that requires planned, structured, and repetitive bodily movement done to improve or maintain one or more components of physical fitness.

her fears and decided to enroll in a fitness course. As part of the course requirement, she took a battery of fitness tests at the beginning of the semester. Patty's cardiorespiratory fitness and strength ratings were poor, her flexibility classification was average, she weighed more than 200 pounds, and she was 41 percent body fat.

Following the initial fitness assessment, Patty met with her course instructor, who prescribed an exercise and nutrition program such as the one presented in this book. Patty fully committed to carry out the prescription. She walked or jogged five times a week, worked out with weights twice a week, and played volleyball or basketball two to four times each week. Her daily caloric intake was set in the range of 1,500 to 1,700 calories. She took care to meet the minimum required amounts from the basic food groups each day, which contributed about 1,200 calories to her diet. The remainder of the calories came primarily from complex carbohydrates. At the end of the 16-week semester, Patty's cardiorespiratory fitness, strength, and flexibility ratings had all improved to the "good" category, she had lost 50 pounds, and her percent body fat had dropped to 22.5!

A thank-you note from Patty to the course instructor at the end of the semester read:

Thank you for making me a new person. I truly appreciate the time you spent with me. Without your kindness and motivation, I would have never made it. It's great to be fit and trim. I've never had this feeling before and I wish everyone could feel like this once in their life.

Thank you, Your trim Patty!

Patty never had been taught the principles governing a sound weight loss program. She needed this knowledge and, like most Americans who have never experienced the process of becoming physically fit, she needed to be in a structured exercise setting to truly feel the joy of fitness.

Of even greater significance, Patty maintained her aerobic and strength-training programs. A year after ending her calorie-restricted diet, her weight actually increased by 10 pounds—but her body fat decreased from 22.5 percent to 21.2 percent. As discussed in Chapter 8, the weight increase is related mostly to changes in lean tissue lost during the weight-reduction phase. Despite only a slight drop in weight during the second year following the calorie-restricted diet, Patty's 2-year follow-up revealed a further decrease in body fat, to 19.5 percent. Patty understands the new quality of life reaped through a sound fitness program.

Lifestyle, Health, and Quality of Life

Research findings have shown that physical inactivity and negative lifestyle habits pose a serious threat to health. Movement and physical activity are basic functions for which the human organism was created. Advances in modern technology, however, have all but eliminated the need for physical activity in daily life. Physical activity no longer is a natural part of our existence. This epidemic of physical inactivity is the second greatest threat to U.S. public health and has been termed **Sedentary Death Syndrome, or SeDS**. (The number-one threat is tobacco use—the largest cause of preventable deaths.)

Today we live in an automated society. Most of the activities that used to require strenuous physical exertion can be accomplished by machines with the simple pull of a handle or push of a button. If people go to a store that is only a couple of blocks away, most drive their automobiles and then spend a couple of minutes driving around the parking lot to find a spot 10 yards closer to the store's entrance. During a visit to a multilevel shopping mall, nearly everyone chooses to ride the escalators instead of taking the stairs.

Automobiles, elevators, escalators, cell phones, intercoms, remote controls, electric garage door openers—all are modern-day commodities that minimize the amount of movement and effort required of the human body.

One of the most significant detrimental effects of modern-day technology has been an increase in

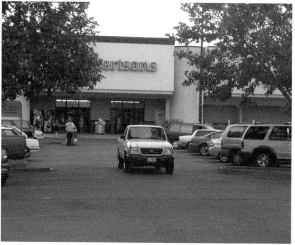

The epitome of physical inactivity is to drive around a parking lot for several minutes in search of a parking spot 10 to 20 yards closer to the store's entrance.

© Fitness & Wellness, Inc.

chronic diseases related to a lack of physical activity. These include hypertension (high blood pressure), heart disease, diabetes, chronic low back pain, and obesity, among others. They sometimes are referred to as **hypokinetic diseases**. ("Hypo" means low or little, and "kinetic" implies motion.) Lack of adequate physical activity is a fact of modern life that most people can avoid no longer. According to the World Health Organization (WHO), chronic diseases account for almost 60 percent of all deaths worldwide and 43 percent of the global burden of disease.[3] If we want to enjoy contemporary commodities and still expect to live life to its fullest, a personalized lifetime exercise program must become a part of our daily lives.

With the developments in technology, three additional factors have changed our lives significantly and have had a negative effect on human health: nutrition, stress, and environment. Fatty foods, sweets, alcohol, tobacco, excessive stress, and environmental hazards (such as wastes, noise, and air pollution) have detrimental effects on people's health.

The leading causes of death in the United States today (see Figure 1.2) are lifestyle-related. About 53 percent of all deaths in the United States are caused by cardiovascular disease and cancer.[4] Almost 80 percent of these deaths could be prevented by adhering to a healthy lifestyle. The third leading cause of death—chronic lower respiratory (lung) disease—is related largely to tobacco use. Accidents are the fourth leading cause of death. Even though not all accidents are preventable, many are. Fatal accidents often are related to abusing drugs and not wearing seat belts.

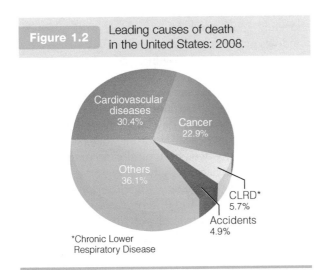

| Figure 1.2 | Leading causes of death in the United States: 2008. |

*Chronic Lower Respiratory Disease

SOURCE: U.S. Department of Health and Human Services, Centers for Disease Control and Prevention, National Center for Health Statistics, National Vital Statistics reports, *Deaths: Preliminary Data for 2008*, 59:2 (December 9, 2010).

According to Dr. David Satcher, former U.S. surgeon general, more than 50 percent of the people who die in the United States each year die because of what they do. Estimates indicate that more than half of disease is lifestyle-related, a fifth is attributed to environmental factors, and a tenth is influenced by the health care the individual receives. Only 16 percent is related to genetic factors. Thus, the individual controls as much as 84 percent of disease and quality of life. The data also indicate that 83 percent of deaths that occur before age 65 are preventable. In essence, most people in the United States are threatened by the very lives they lead today.[5]

Based on the most recent data available, the average **life expectancy** in the United States is now 75.7 years for men and 80.8 years for women. Based on the WHO data, the United States ranks 38th in the world for life expectancy (see Figure 1.3). Between 2000 and 2010, U.S. male life expectancy slipped from 18th to 24th in the world and female life expectancy from 28th to 35th. Japan ranks first in the world with an overall life expectancy of 82.6 years.

Several factors may account for the current U.S. life expectancy ranking: the extremely poor health of some groups (such as Native Americans, rural African Americans, and the inner-city poor), the obesity epidemic, the low level of daily physical activity, the high incidence of tobacco use and coronary heart disease, and fairly high levels of violence (notably homicides).

Although life expectancy in the United States gradually increased by 30 years over the last century, scientists from the National Institute of Aging believe that in the coming decades the average lifespan may decrease by as much as 5 years. This decrease in life expectancy will be related primarily to the growing epidemic of obesity. About 34 percent of the adult population in the United States is obese. Additional information on the obesity epidemic and its detrimental health consequences is given in Chapter 5.

Key Terms

Sedentary Death Syndrome (SeDS) Deaths that are attributed to a lack of regular physical activity.

Chronic diseases Illnesses that develop and last over a long time.

Hypokinetic diseases Diseases related to a lack of physical activity.

Life expectancy Number of years a person is expected to live based on the person's birth year.

Figure 1.3   Life expectancy at birth for selected countries: 2005–2010 projections.

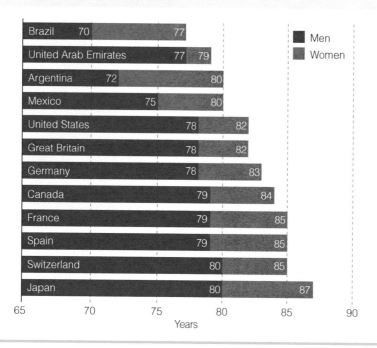

United Nations, *Social Indicators: Indicators on Health,* http://unstats.un.org/unsd/demographic/products/socind/health.htm (downloaded March 31, 2011).

Importance of Increased Physical Activity

The U.S. surgeon general has stated that poor health as a result of lack of physical activity is a serious public health problem that must be met head-on at once. Regular moderate physical activity provides substantial benefits in health and well-being for the vast majority of people who are not physically active. For those who are already moderately active, even greater health benefits can be achieved by increasing the level of physical activity.

Among the benefits of regular physical activity and exercise are significantly reduced risks for developing or dying from heart disease, stroke, type 2 diabetes, colon and breast cancers, high blood pressure, and osteoporotic fractures.[6] Regular physical activity also is important for the health of muscles, bones, and joints, and it seems to reduce symptoms of depression and anxiety, improve mood, and enhance one's ability to perform daily tasks throughout life. It also can help control health care costs and maintain a high quality of life into old age.

Moderate physical activity has been defined as any activity that requires an energy expenditure of 150 calories per day, or 1,000 calories per week. The general health recommendation is that people strive to accumulate at least 30 minutes of physical activity a minimum of five days per week. Whereas 30 minutes of continuous activity is preferred, on days when time is limited, three activity sessions of at least 10 minutes each provide about half the aerobic benefits. Examples of moderate physical activity are walking, cycling, playing basketball or volleyball, swimming, water aerobics, dancing fast, pushing a stroller, raking leaves, shoveling snow, washing or waxing a car, washing windows or floors, and even gardening.

Because of the ever-growing epidemic of obesity in the United States, however, the Institute of Medicine of the National Academy of Sciences increased the recommendation to 60 minutes of moderate-intensity physical activity every day.[7] This recommendation was based on evidence indicating that people who maintain healthy weight typically accumulate one hour of daily physical activity.

Subsequently, the Dietary Guidelines for Americans recommend that up to 60 minutes of moderate- to vigorous-intensity physical activity per day may be necessary to prevent weight gain, and between 60 and 90 minutes of moderate-intensity physical activity daily is recommended to sustain weight loss for previously overweight people.[8]

In sum, although health benefits are derived with 30 minutes per day, people with a tendency to gain weight need to be physically active daily for an hour to an hour and a half to prevent weight gain. And 60 to 90 minutes of activity per day provides additional health benefits, including a lower risk for cardiovascular disease and diabetes.

2008 Federal Guidelines for Physical Activity

Because of the importance of physical activity to our health, in October 2008 the U.S. Department of Health and Human Services issued Federal Physical Activity Guidelines for Americans for the first time. These guidelines complement the Dietary Guidelines for Americans and further substantiate previous recommendations issued by the American College of Sports Medicine (ACSM) and the American Heart Association (AHA) in 2007[9] and the U.S. surgeon general in 1996.[10] The federal guidelines provide science-based guidance on the importance of being physically active and eating a healthy diet to promote health and reduce the risk of chronic diseases. The federal guidelines include the following recommendations[11]:

Adults between 18 and 64 years of age
- Adults should do 2 hours and 30 minutes a week of **moderate-intensity aerobic (cardiorespiratory) physical activity**, 1 hour and 15 minutes (75 minutes) a week of **vigorous-intensity aerobic physical activity**, or an equivalent combination of moderate- and vigorous-intensity aerobic physical activity (also see Chapter 8). When combining moderate- and vigorous-intensity activities, a person could participate in moderate-intensity activity twice a week for 30 minutes and high-intensity activity for 20 minutes on another two days. Aerobic activity should be performed in episodes of at least 10 minutes long each, preferably spread throughout the week.
- *Additional health benefits* are provided by increasing to 5 hours (300 minutes) a week of moderate-intensity aerobic physical activity, 2 hours and 30 minutes a week of vigorous-intensity physical activity, or an equivalent combination of both.
- Adults should also do muscle-strengthening activities that involve all major muscle groups, performed on 2 or more days per week.

Older adults (ages 65 and older)
- Older adults should follow the adult guidelines. If this is not possible due to limiting chronic conditions, older adults should be as physically active as their abilities allow. They should avoid inactivity. Older adults should do exercises that maintain or improve balance if they are at risk of falling.

Children 6 years of age and older and adolescents
- Children and adolescents should do 1 hour (60 minutes) or more of physical activity every day.
- Most of the 1 hour or more a day should be either moderate- or vigorous-intensity aerobic physical activity.
- As part of their daily physical activity, children and adolescents should do vigorous-intensity activity on at least 3 days per week. They also should do muscle-strengthening and bone-strengthening activities on at least 3 days per week.

Pregnant and postpartum women
- Healthy women who are not already doing vigorous-intensity physical activity should get at least 2 hours and 30 minutes (150 minutes) of moderate-intensity aerobic activity a week. Preferably, this activity should be spread throughout the week. Women who regularly engage in vigorous-intensity aerobic activity or high amounts of activity can continue their activity provided that their condition remains unchanged and they talk to their health care provider about their activity level throughout their pregnancy.

The 2007 ACSM and AHA joint statement on physical activity recommendations for healthy adults states that a greater amount of physical activity that exceeds the minimum recommendations given above for adults between 18 and 64 years of age provides even greater benefits. Such an exercise prescription is recommended for individuals who wish to further improve personal fitness, reduce the risk for chronic disease and disabilities, prevent pre-

Key Terms

Moderate-intensity aerobic physical activity Defined as the equivalent of a brisk walk that noticeably increases the heart rate.

Vigorous-intensity aerobic physical activity Defined as an activity similar to jogging that causes rapid breathing and a substantial increase in heart rate.

mature mortality, or prevent unhealthy weight gain.[12]

The ACSM/AHA report also states that only 49 percent of the U.S. adult population meets the basic moderate-intensity physical activity recommendations. College graduates are more likely to adhere to the recommendations (about 53 percent of them), followed by individuals with some college education, then high school graduates; the least likely to meet the recommendations are those with less than a high school diploma (37.8 percent).

In conjunction with the above report, the ACSM and the American Medical Association (AMA) have launched a nationwide *Exercise is Medicine* program.[13] The goal of this initiative is to help improve the health and wellness of the nation through exercise prescriptions from physicians and health care providers: "Exercise is medicine and it's free." All physicians should be prescribing exercise to all patients and participate in exercise themselves. Exercise is considered to be the much-needed vaccine of our time to prevent chronic diseases. Physical activity and exercise are powerful tools for both the treatment and prevention of chronic diseases and premature death.

Critical Thinking

Do you consciously incorporate physical activity into your daily lifestyle? • Can you provide examples? • Do you think you get sufficient daily physical activity to maintain good health?

Wellness

After the initial fitness boom swept across the United States in the 1970s, it became clear that improving physical fitness alone was not always enough to lower the risk for disease and ensure better health. For example, individuals who run 3 miles a day, lift weights regularly, participate in stretching exercises, and watch their body weight can be classified as having good or excellent fitness. If these same people, however, have high blood pressure, smoke, are under constant stress, consume too much alcohol, and eat too many fatty and processed foods, they are exposing themselves to **risk factors** for disease of which they may not be aware.

Good health no longer is viewed as simply the absence of disease. The notion of good health has evolved notably in the last few years and continues to change as scientists learn more about lifestyle factors that bring on illness and affect wellness. Once

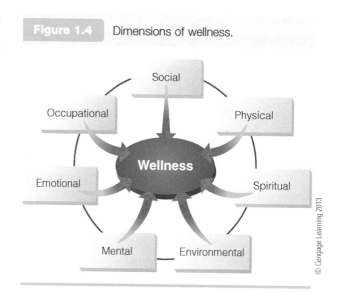

Figure 1.4   Dimensions of wellness.

© Cengage Learning 2013

the idea took hold that fitness by itself would not necessarily decrease the risk for disease and ensure better health, the wellness concept developed in the 1980s.

Wellness is an all-inclusive umbrella covering a variety of health-related factors. A wellness lifestyle requires the implementation of positive programs to change behavior and thereby improve health and quality of life, prolong life, and achieve total well-being. To enjoy a wellness lifestyle, a person has to practice behaviors that will lead to positive outcomes in seven dimensions of wellness: physical, emotional, intellectual, social, environmental, spiritual, and occupational (Figure 1.4). These dimensions are interrelated; one frequently affects the others. For example, a person who is "emotionally down" often has no desire to exercise, study, go to work, socialize with friends, or attend church.

The concept behind the seven dimensions of wellness shows that high-level wellness clearly goes beyond optimum fitness and the absence of disease. Wellness incorporates fitness, proper nutrition, stress management, disease prevention, social support, self-worth, nurturance (a sense of being needed), spirituality, personal safety, substance control and not smoking, regular physical examinations, health education, and environmental support.

For a wellness way of life, individuals must be physically fit and manifest no signs of disease, and they also must avoid all risk factors for disease (such as physical inactivity, hypertension, abnormal cholesterol levels, cigarette smoking, excessive stress, faulty nutrition, or careless sex). Even though an individual tested in a fitness center might demonstrate adequate or even excellent fitness, indulgence in unhealthy life-style behaviors will increase the risk for chronic diseases and decrease the person's well-being. Additional information on wellness and how to implement a wellness program is given in Chapter 8.

Unhealthy behaviors contribute to the staggering U.S. health care costs. Risk factors for disease carry a heavy price tag. Health care costs in the United States rose from $12 billion in 1950 to $2.3 trillion in 2008, or about 16 percent of the gross domestic product (GDP). In 1980, health care costs represented 8.8 percent of the GNP, and they are projected to reach about 20 percent by the year 2015. Based on estimates, 1 percent of Americans account for 30 percent of these costs. Half of the people use up about 97 percent of the health care dollars.

In terms of yearly health care costs per person, the United States spends more per person than any other industrialized nation. U.S. health care costs per capita are above $7,000 per year. Overall, the U.S. health care system ranks only 37th in the world.

One of the reasons for the low overall ranking is the overemphasis on state-of-the-art cures instead of prevention programs. The United States is the best place in the world to treat people once they are sick, but the system does a poor job of keeping people healthy in the first place.

Physical Fitness

Individuals are physically fit when they can meet both the ordinary and the unusual demands of daily life safely and effectively without being overly fatigued and still have energy left for leisure and recreational activities. **Physical fitness** can be classified into health-related and skill-related fitness.

Health-Related Fitness

Health-related fitness has four components: cardiorespiratory endurance, muscular strength and endurance, muscular flexibility, and body composition (see Figure 1.5).

1. *Cardiorespiratory endurance:* the ability of the heart, lungs, and blood vessels to supply oxygen to the cells to meet the demands of prolonged physical activity (also referred to as aerobic exercise).
2. *Muscular strength and endurance:* the ability of the muscles to generate force.

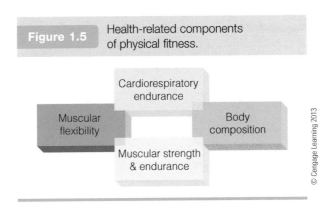

Figure 1.5 Health-related components of physical fitness.

Cardiorespiratory endurance

Muscular flexibility

Body composition

Muscular strength & endurance

© Cengage Learning 2013

3. *Muscular flexibility:* the achievable range of motion at a joint or group of joints without causing injury.
4. *Body composition:* the amount of lean body mass and adipose tissue (fat mass) in the human body.

Skill-Related Fitness

Fitness in motor skills is essential in activities such as basketball, racquetball, golf, hiking, soccer, and water skiing. Good skill-related fitness also enhances overall quality of life by helping people cope more effectively in emergency situations (see Chapter 2). The components of **skill-related fitness** are agility, balance, coordination, power, reaction time, and speed (see Figure 1.6).

1. *Agility:* the ability to change body position and direction quickly and efficiently. Agility is important in sports such as basketball, soccer, and racquetball, in which the participant must change direction rapidly and at the same time maintain proper body control.

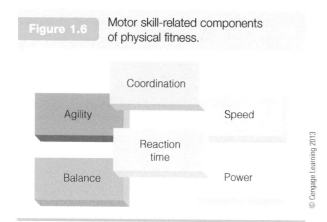

Figure 1.6 Motor skill-related components of physical fitness.

© Cengage Learning 2013

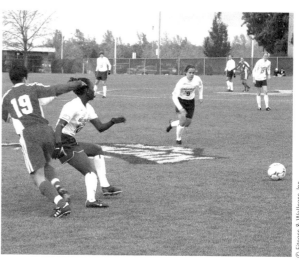

© Fitness & Wellness, Inc.

Good skill-related fitness enhances success in sports performance.

2. *Balance:* the ability to maintain the body in equilibrium. Balance is vital in activities such as gymnastics, diving, ice skating, skiing, and even football and wrestling, in which the athlete attempts to upset the opponent's equilibrium.

3. *Coordination:* integration of the nervous system and the muscular system to produce correct, graceful, and harmonious body movements. This component is important in a wide variety of motor activities such as golf, baseball, karate, soccer, and racquetball, in which hand-eye or foot-eye movements, or both, must be integrated.

4. *Power:* the ability to produce maximum force in the shortest time. The two components of power are muscle speed and force (strength). An effective combination of these two components allows a person to produce explosive movements such as required in jumping; putting the shot; and spiking, throwing, and hitting a ball.

5. *Reaction time:* the time required to initiate a response to a given stimulus. Good reaction time is important for starts in track and swimming; for quick reactions when playing tennis at the net; and in sports such as ping-pong, boxing, and karate.

6. *Speed:* the ability to propel the body or a part of the body rapidly from one point to another. Examples of activities that require good speed for success are soccer, basketball, stealing a base in baseball, and sprints in track.

In terms of preventive medicine, the main emphasis of fitness programs should be on the health-related components. Skill-related fitness is crucial for success in sports and athletics, and it also con-

tributes to wellness. Improving skill-related fitness affords an individual more enjoyment and success in lifetime sports, and regular participation in skill-related fitness activities also helps develop health-related fitness. Further, total fitness is achieved by taking part in specific programs to improve health-related and skill-related components alike.

Benefits of Physical Fitness

The benefits to be enjoyed from participating in a regular fitness program are many. In addition to a longer life (see Figures 1.7 and 1.8), the greatest benefit of all is that physically fit people who lead a positive lifestyle have a healthier and better quality of life. These people live life to its fullest and have fewer health problems than inactive individuals who also indulge in negative lifestyle habits. Compiling an all-inclusive list of the benefits to be reaped through participation in a fitness program is a challenge, but the list provided in Table 1.1 summarizes many of these benefits.

In addition to the benefits listed in Table 1.1, **epidemiological** research studies linking physical activity habits and mortality rates have shown lower premature mortality rates in physically active people. Pioneer work in this area demonstrated that, as the amount of weekly physical activity increased, the risk of cardiovascular deaths decreased.[14] In this study, conducted among 16,936 Harvard alumni, the greatest decrease in cardiovascular deaths was observed in alumni who burned more than 2,000 calories per week through physical activity.

| Figure 1.7 | Death rates by physical fitness levels. |

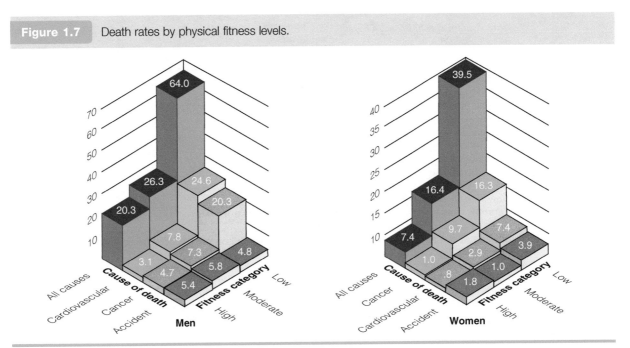

Numbers on top of the bars are all-cause death rates per 10,000 person-years of follow-up for each cell: 1 person-year indicates one person who was followed up 1 year later.

SOURCE: Based on data from S. N. Blair, H. W. Kohl III, R. S. Paffenbarger, Jr., D. G. Clark, K. H. Cooper, and L. W. Gibbons, "Physical Fitness and All-Cause Morality: A Prospective Study of Healthy Men and Women," *Journal of the American Medical Association* 262 (1989): 2395–2401.

A landmark study subsequently upheld the findings of the Harvard alumni study.[15] Based on data from 13,344 individuals who were followed over an average of 8 years, the results confirmed that the level of cardiorespiratory fitness is related to mortality from all causes. These findings showed a graded and consistent inverse relationship between physical fitness and mortality, regardless of age and other risk factors.

In essence, the higher the level of cardiorespiratory fitness, the longer the life (see Figure 1.7). The death rate from all causes for the low-fit men was 3.4 times higher than for the high-fit men. For the low-fit women, the death rate was 4.6 times higher than for the high-fit women. The study also reported a greatly reduced rate of premature deaths, even at moderate fitness levels, which most adults can achieve easily. People gain further protection when they combine higher fitness levels with reduction in other risk factors such as hypertension, elevated cholesterol, cigarette smoking, and excessive body fat.

Additional research that looked at changes in fitness and mortality found a substantial (44 percent) reduction in mortality risk when the study participants abandoned a sedentary lifestyle and became moderately fit (see Figure 1.8).[16] The lowest death

| Figure 1.8 | Effects of fitness changes on mortality rates. |

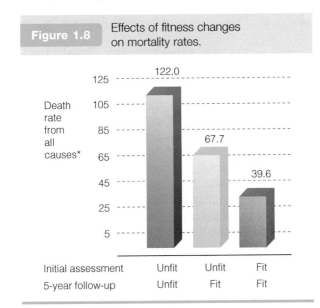

| Initial assessment | Unfit | Unfit | Fit |
| 5-year follow-up | Unfit | Fit | Fit |

*Death rates per 10,000 man-years observation.

SOURCE: S. N. Blair et al., "Changes in Physical Fitness and All-Cause Morality: A Prospective Study of Healthy Men and Women," *Journal of the American Medical Association* 273 (1995): 1193–1198.

| Key Terms |

Epidemiological The study of epidemic diseases.

Table 1.1	Long-term (chronic) benefits of exercise

Regular participation in exercise

- improves and strengthens the cardiorespiratory system.
- maintains better muscle tone, muscular strength, and endurance.
- improves muscular flexibility.
- enhances athletic performance.
- helps maintain recommended body weight.
- helps preserve lean body tissue.
- increases resting metabolic rate.
- improves the body's ability to use fat during physical activity.
- improves posture and physical appearance.
- improves functioning of the immune system.
- lowers the risk for chronic diseases and illness (including heart disease, stroke, and certain cancers).
- decreases the mortality rate from chronic diseases.
- thins the blood so it doesn't clot as readily (thereby decreasing the risk for coronary heart disease and strokes).
- helps the body manage cholesterol levels more effectively.
- prevents or delays the development of high blood pressure and lowers blood pressure in people with hypertension.
- helps prevent and control type 2 diabetes.
- helps achieve peak bone mass in young adults and maintain bone mass later in life, thereby decreasing the risk for osteoporosis.
- helps people sleep better.
- helps prevent chronic back pain.
- relieves tension and helps in coping with life stresses.
- raises levels of energy and job productivity.
- extends longevity and slows the aging process.
- improves and helps maintain cognitive function.
- promotes psychological well-being, including higher morale, self-image, and self-esteem.
- reduces feelings of depression and anxiety.
- encourages positive lifestyle changes (improving nutrition, quitting smoking, controlling alcohol and drug use).
- speeds recovery time following physical exertion.
- speeds recovery following injury or disease.
- regulates and improves overall body functions.
- improves physical stamina and counteracts chronic fatigue.
- reduces disability and helps to maintain independent living, especially in older adults.
- enhances quality of life: People feel better and live a healthier and happier life.

rate was found in people who were fit and remained fit, and the highest rate was found in men who remained unfit.

Further research in this area substantiated the previous findings and also indicated that primarily vigorous activities are associated with greater longevity.[17,18] Vigorous activity was defined as activity that requires a **MET** level equal to or greater than 6 METs (see Chapter 2, Table 2.1, page 43). This level represents exercising at an energy level of 6 times the resting energy requirement. Examples of vigorous activities used in the previous study include brisk walking, jogging, swimming laps, squash, racquetball, tennis, and shoveling snow. Results also indicated that vigorous exercise is as important as maintaining recommended weight and not smoking.

While it is clear that moderate-intensity exercise does provide substantial health benefits, the research data shows a dose-response relationship between physical activity and health. That is, greater health and fitness benefits occur at higher duration and/or intensity of physical activity.

Vigorous activities are preferable to the extent of one's capabilities because they are most clearly associated with better health and longer life. Compared to prolonged moderate-intensity activity, vigorous-intensity has been shown to provide the best improvements in aerobic capacity, coronary heart disease risk reduction, blood pressure, blood glucose control, and overall cardiovascular health.[19,20]

A word of caution, however, is in order. Vigorous exercise should be reserved for healthy individuals who have been cleared to do so (see Activity 1.2) and who have been participating regularly in at least moderate-intensity activities.

While most of the chronic (long-term) benefits of exercise are well-established, what many people fail to realize is that there are *immediate benefits* derived by participating in just one single bout of exercise. Most of these benefits dissipate within 48 to 72 hours fol-

Table 1.2	Immediate (acute) benefits of exercise.

You can expect a number of benefits as a result of a single exercise session. Some of these benefits last up to 72 hours following your workout. Exercise

- increases head rate, stroke volume, cardiac output, pulmonary ventilation, and oxygen uptake.
- begins to strengthen the heart, lungs, and muscles.
- enhances metabolic rate or energy production (burning calories for fuel) during exercise and recovery—for every 100 calories you burn during exercise you can expect to burn another 15 during recovery.
- uses blood glucose and muscle glycogen.
- improves insulin sensitivity (decreasing type 2 diabetes risk).
- immediately enhances the body's ability to burn fat.
- lowers blood lipids.
- improves joint flexibility.
- reduces low-grade (hidden) inflammation (see page 217 in Chapter 8).
- increases endorphins (hormones), naturally occurring opioids that are responsible for exercise-induced euphoria.
- increases fat storage *in muscle,* which can then be burned for energy.
- improves endothelial function (endothelial cells line the entire vascular system providing a barrier between the vessel lumen and surrounding tissue—endothelial dysfunction contributes to several disease processes, including tissue inflammation and subsequent atherosclerosis).
- enhances mood and self-worth.
- provides a sense of achievement and satisfaction.
- decreases blood pressure the first few hours following exercise.
- decreases arthritic pain.
- leads to muscle relaxation.
- decreases stress.
- improves brain function.
- promotes better sleep (unless exercise is performed too close to bedtime).
- improves digestion.
- boosts energy levels.
- improves resistance to infections.

lowing exercise. The acute (immediate) benefits, summarized in Table 1.2, are so striking that they prompted Dr. William L. Haskell of Stanford University to state: *"Most of the health benefits of exercise are relatively short term, so people should think of exercise as a medication and take it on a daily basis."* Of course, as you regularly exercise a minimum of 30 minutes five times per week, you will realize the impressive long-term benefits listed in Table 1.1.

National Health Objectives for the Year 2020

Every 10 years, the U.S. Department of Health and Human Services releases a list of objectives for preventing disease and promoting health. Since 1979, the "Healthy People" initiative has set and monitored national health objectives to meet a broad range of health needs, encourage collaborations across sectors, guide individuals toward making informed health decisions, and measure the impact of our prevention activity. Currently Healthy People is leading the way to achieve increased quality and years of healthy life and seek to eliminate health disparities among all groups of people. The objectives address three important points[21]:

1. *Personal responsibility for health behavior.* Individuals need to become ever more health conscious. Responsible and informed behaviors are the keys to good health.

2. *Health benefits for all people and all communities.* Lower socioeconomic conditions and poor health often are interrelated. Extending the benefits of good health to all people is crucial to the health of the nation.

3. *Health promotion and disease prevention.* A shift from treatment to preventive techniques will drasti-

Key Terms

MET Short for metabolic equivalent, represents the rate of energy expenditure while sitting quietly at rest. This energy expenditure is approximately 3.5 milliliters of oxygen per kilogram of body weight per minute (mL/kg/min) or 1.2 calories per minute for a 70-kilogram person. A 3-MET activity requires three times the energy expenditure of sitting quietly at rest.

Figure 1.9	Selected national health objectives for the year 2020.

- Increase the proportion of persons with health insurance, a usual primary care provider, and coverage for clinical preventive services.
- Ensure that all people, including those with illnesses and chronic disability, participate daily in meaningful and freely chosen recreation, leisure, and physical activity, which directly influences well-being and quality of life.
- Reduce the proportion of adults who engage in no leisure-time physical activity.
- Increase the proportion of adolescents and adults who meet current Federal physical activity guidelines.
- Increase the proportion of adults who are at a healthy weight, and reduce the proportion of children, adolescents, and adults who are overweight or obese.
- Reduce coronary heart disease and stroke deaths.
- Reduce the mean total blood cholesterol levels among adults and the proportion of persons in the population with hypertension.
- Increase the proportion of adults aged 20 years and older who are aware of, and respond to, early warning symptoms and signs of a heart attack and stroke.
- Reduce the overall cancer death rate and provide counseling about cancer prevention.
- Reduce the diabetes death rate and the annual number of new cases of diagnosed diabetes in the population.

- Reduce infections caused by key pathogens commonly transmitted through food.
- Increase the proportion of sexually active persons who use condoms.
- Reduce the rate of HIV transmission among adults and adolescents, and reduce the number of deaths resulting from HIV infection.
- Increase the proportion of substance-abuse treatment facilities that offer HIV/AIDS education, counseling, and support.
- Increase school-based health promotion programs available to youth between the ages of 14 and 22 to decrease the rate of sexually transmitted diseases and teen pregnancy and to increase the proportion of adolescents who abstain from sexual intercourse or use condoms if sexually active.
- Reduce tobacco use by adults and adolescents and reduce the initiation among children, adolescents, and young adults.
- Reduce average annual alcohol consumption and increase the proportion of adolescents who disapprove of substance abuse.
- Increase the proportion, among persons who need alcohol and/or illicit drug treatment, of those who receive specialized treatment for abuse or dependence.
- Reduce drug-induced deaths.

© Cengage Learning 2013

cally cut health care costs and help all Americans achieve a better quality of life.

Developing these health objectives involves more than 10,000 people representing 300 national organizations, including the Institute of Medicine of the National Academy of Sciences, all state health departments, and the federal Office of Disease Prevention and Health Promotion. Figure 1.9 summarizes the key 2020 objectives. Living the fitness and wellness principles provided in this book will enhance the quality of your life and also will allow you to be an active participant in achieving the Healthy People 2020 Objectives.

The Path to Fitness and Wellness

Current scientific data and the fitness movement that began more than three decades ago in the United States have led many people to see the advantages of participating in fitness programs that will improve and maintain health. Because fitness and wellness needs vary from one person to another, exercise and wellness prescriptions must be personalized for best results. This book provides the necessary guidelines for developing a lifetime program to improve fitness and promote preventive health care and personal

wellness. As you study the book and complete the assignments in each chapter, you will learn to

- Determine whether medical clearance is required for you to participate safely in exercise.
- Assess your overall level of physical fitness, including cardiorespiratory endurance, muscular strength and endurance, muscular flexibility, and body composition.
- Prescribe personal programs for total fitness development.
- Learn behavior modification techniques that will allow you to change unhealthy lifestyle patterns.
- Develop sound diet and weight-control programs.
- Implement a healthy lifestyle program that includes prevention of cardiovascular diseases and cancer, stress management, and smoking cessation, if applicable.
- Discern myths from facts pertaining to exercise and health-related concepts.

Behavior Modification

Scientific evidence of the benefits derived from living a healthy lifestyle continues to mount each day. Although the data are impressive, most people still don't adhere to a healthy lifestyle. To understand why this is so, one has to examine what motivates people

Behavior Modification

Healthy Lifestyle Habits

Research indicates that adherence to the following 12 lifestyle habits will significantly improve health and extend life:

1. Participate in a lifetime physical activity program.
2. Do not smoke cigarettes.
3. Eat right.
4. Avoid snacking.
5. Maintain recommended body weight through adequate nutrition and exercise.
6. Sleep 7 to 8 hours each night.
7. Lower your stress levels.
8. Drink alcohol moderately or not at all.
9. Surround yourself with healthy friendships.
10. Seek to live and work in a healthy environment.
11. Use the mind: Keep your brain engaged throughout life to maintain cognitive function.
12. Take personal safety measures to lessen the risk for avoidable accidents.

Try It Look at the list above and indicate which habits are already a part of your lifestyle. What changes could you make to incorporate additional healthy habits into your daily life?

and what actions are required to make permanent changes in behavior, called **behavior modification**.

Let's look at an all-too-common occurrence on college campuses. Most students understand that they should be exercising. They contemplate enrolling in a fitness course. The motivating factor might be enhanced physical appearance, health benefits, or simply fulfillment of a college requirement. They sign up for the course, participate for a few months, finish the course—and stop exercising! Various excuses are offered: too busy, no one to exercise with, already have the grade, inconvenient open-gym hours, or job conflicts. A few months later, they realize once again that exercise is vital and repeat the cycle (see Figure 1.10).

The information in this book will be of little value to you if you are unable to abandon negative habits and adopt and maintain new, healthy behaviors. Before looking at the physical fitness and wellness guidelines, you need to take a critical look at your behaviors and lifestyle—and most likely make some permanent changes to promote your overall health and wellness.

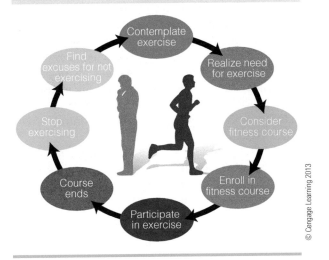

Figure 1.10   Exercise–exercise dropout cycle.

Contemplate exercise · Realize need for exercise · Consider fitness course · Enroll in fitness course · Participate in exercise · Course ends · Stop exercising · Find excuses for not exercising

© Cengage Learning 2013

Changing Behavior

The very first step in addressing behavioral change is to recognize that indeed a problem exists. Five general categories of behaviors are addressed in the process of willful change:

1. Stopping a negative behavior
2. Preventing relapse of a negative behavior
3. Developing a positive behavior
4. Strengthening a positive behavior
5. Maintaining a positive behavior

Changing chronic, unhealthy behaviors to stable, healthy behaviors is often challenging. Change usually does not happen all at once but, rather, is a lengthy process with several stages.

The simplest model of change is the two-stage model of unhealthy behavior and healthy behavior. This model states that either you do it or you don't. Most people who use this model attempt self-change but end up asking themselves why they're unsuccessful: They just can't do it (start and adhere to exercise or quit smoking, for example). Their intention to change may be good, but to accomplish it, they need knowledge about how to achieve change. The following discussion may help.

Key Terms

Behavior modification The process used to permanently change negative behaviors in favor of positive behaviors that will lead to better health and well-being.

To aid in this process, psychologists James Prochaska, John Norcross, and Carlo DiClemente developed a behavioral change model.[22] The model's five stages are important to understanding the process of willful change. The stages of change describe underlying processes that people go through to change most problem behaviors and adopt healthy behaviors. Most frequently, the model is used to change health-related behaviors such as physical inactivity, smoking, nutrition, weight control, stress, and alcohol abuse.

The five stages of change are precontemplation, contemplation, preparation, action, and maintenance. A sixth stage of change, termination/adoption, was subsequently added to this model.

After years of study, researchers found that applying specific behavior-change techniques during each stage of the model increases the rate of success for change. Understanding each stage of this model will help you determine where you are in relation to your personal healthy-lifestyle behaviors. It also will help you identify techniques to make successful changes.

Precontemplation

People in the **precontemplation stage** are not considering or do not want to change a specific behavior. They typically deny having a problem and presently do not intend to change. These people are usually unaware or underaware of the problem. Other people around them, including family, friends, health care practitioners, and coworkers, however, identify the problem quite clearly.

Precontemplators do not care about the problem behavior and might even avoid information and materials that address the issue. They avoid free screenings and workshops that could help identify and change the problem, even if they receive financial incentives for attending. Frequently these people actively resist change and seem resigned to accept the unhealthy behavior as their "fate."

Precontemplators are the most difficult people to reach for behavioral change. They often think that change isn't even a possibility. Educating them about the problem behavior is critical to helping them start contemplating the process of change. It is said that knowledge is power, and the challenge is to find ways to help them realize that they will be ultimately responsible for the consequences of their behavior. Sometimes they initiate change only when under pressure from others.

Contemplation

In the **contemplation stage**, people acknowledge that they have a problem and begin to think seriously about overcoming it. Although they are not quite ready for change yet, they are weighing the pros and cons. People may remain in this stage for years, but in their mind they are planning to take some action within the next 6 months or so. Education and peer support are valuable during this stage.

Preparation

In the **preparation stage**, people are seriously considering and planning to change a behavior within the next month. They are taking initial steps for change and may even try it for a short while, such as stopping smoking for a day or exercising a few times during this month. In this stage, people define a general goal for behavior change (say, to quit smoking by the last day of the month) and write specific objectives to accomplish this goal (see the discussion on SMART goals, pages 20–22). Continued peer and environmental support are recommended during the preparation phase.

Action

The **action stage** requires the most commitment of time and energy by the individual. Here people are actively doing things to change or modify the problem behavior or to adopt a new health behavior. The action stage requires that the person follow the specific guidelines set forth for that specific behavior. For example, a person has actually stopped smoking completely, is exercising aerobically three times per week according to exercise prescription guidelines (see Chapter 3), or is maintaining a healthy diet.

Relapse, in which the individual regresses to a previous stage, is common during this stage. Once people maintain the action stage for 6 consecutive months, they move into the maintenance stage.

Maintenance

During the **maintenance stage**, the person continues to adhere to the behavior change for up to 5 years. The maintenance phase requires continuously adhering to the specific guidelines that govern the target behavior (for example, complete smoking cessation, aerobic exercise three times per week, or proper stress management techniques). At this time, a person works to reinforce the gains made through the various stages of change and strives to prevent lapses and relapses.

Figure 1.11	Identifying your current stage of change.

Please indicate which response most accurately describes your current _____
behavior (in the blank space identify the behavior: smoking, physical activity, stress, nutrition, weight control, etc.).
Next, select the statement below (select only one) that best represents your current behavior pattern. To select the most
appropriate statement, fill in the blank for one of the first three statements if your current behavior is a problem behavior. (For example, you might say, "I currently smoke, and I do *not* intend to change in the foreseeable future," or "I currently *do not* exercise, but I am contemplating changing in the next 6 months.") If you have already started to make changes, fill in the blank in one of the last three statements. (In this case, you might say: "I currently *eat a low-fat diet,* but I have done so only within the last 6 months," or "I currently *practice adequate stress management techniques,* and I have done so for more than 6 months.") As you can see, you may use this form to identify your stage of change for any type of health-related behavior.

1. I currently _____, and I do not intend to change in the foreseeable future.

2. I currently _____, but I am contemplating changing in the next 6 months.

3. I currently _____ regularly but intend to change in the next month.

4. I currently _____, but I have done so only within the last 6 months.

5. I currently _____, and I have done so for more than 6 months.

6. I currently _____, and I have done so for more than 5 years.

STAGES OF CHANGE

1 =	Precontemplation	4 =	Action
2 =	Contemplation	5 =	Maintenance
3 =	Preparation	6 =	Termination/Adoption

Termination/Adoption

Once a person has maintained a behavior more than 5 years, he or she enters the **termination/adoption stage** without fear of relapse. In the case of negative behaviors that have been terminated, this stage of change is referred to as termination. If the person has adopted a positive behavior for more than 5 years, this stage is designated the adoption stage. Many experts believe that after this period of time, any former addictions, problems, or lack of compliance with healthy behaviors no longer present an obstacle in the quest for wellness. The change has become a part of one's lifestyle. This phase is the ultimate goal for everyone who seeks a healthier lifestyle.

Use the form provided in Figure 1.11 to determine where you stand in respect to behaviors that you want to change or new ones that you wish to adopt. As you fill out this form, you will realize that you are at different stages for different behaviors. For instance, you may be in the termination stage for aerobic exercise and smoking, in the action stage for

Key Terms

Precontemplation stage Stage of change in which people are unwilling to change their behavior.

Contemplation stage Stage of change in which people are considering changing behavior in the next 6 months.

Preparation stage Stage of change in which people are getting ready to make a change within the coming month.

Action stage Stage of change in which people are actively changing a negative behavior or adopting a new, healthy behavior.

Relapse Slipping or falling back into unhealthy behavior(s) or failing to maintain healthy behaviors.

Maintenance stage Stage of change in which people maintain behavioral change for up to 5 years.

Termination/adoption stage Stage of change in which people have eliminated an undesirable behavior or maintained a positive behavior for more than 5 years.

strength training, but only in the contemplation stage for a healthy diet. Realizing where you are at with respect to different behaviors will help you design a better action plan for a healthy lifestyle.

Using the form provided in Activity 1.1, pages 24–25, select two or three behaviors that you have targeted for the next 3 months. Developing new behavioral patterns takes time, and trying to work on too many components at once most likely will lower your chances for success. Start with components in which you think you will have a high chance for success.

Critical Thinking

What factors do you think keep you from participating in a regular exercise program? • How about factors that keep you from managing your daily caloric intake?

Motivation and Locus of Control

Motivation often explains why some people succeed and others do not. Although motivation comes from within, external factors are what trigger the inner desire to accomplish a given task. These external factors, then, control behavior.

Understanding **locus of control** is helpful to the study of motivation. People who believe they have control over events in their lives are said to have an internal locus of control. People with an external locus of control, by contrast, believe that what happens to them is a result of chance or environmental factors and is unrelated to their behavior. The latter group often has difficulty getting out of the precontemplation or contemplation stages.

People with an internal locus of control are apt to be healthier and have an easier time initiating and adhering to a wellness program than those who perceive that they have little control and think of themselves as powerless and vulnerable. The latter people also are at greater risk for illness. When illness does strike, restoring a sense of control is vital to regaining health.

Few people have either a completely external or a completely internal locus of control. They fall somewhere along a continuum. The more external, the greater is the challenge in changing and adhering to exercise and other healthy lifestyle behaviors. Fortunately, a person can develop a more internal locus of control. Understanding that most events in life are not determined genetically or environmentally helps people pursue goals and gain control

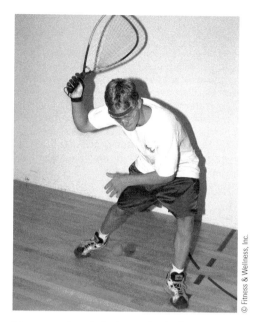

Many people refrain from physical activity because they lack the necessary skills to enjoy and reap the benefits of regular participation.

over their lives. Three impediments, however, can keep people from entering the preparation or action stages: problems of competence, confidence, and motivation.

1. *Problems of competence.* Lacking the skills to get a given task done leads to less competence. If your friends play basketball regularly but you don't know how to play, you might not be inclined to participate. The solution to this problem of competence is to master the skills you need for participation. Most people are not born with all-inclusive natural abilities, including playing sports.

A college professor continuously watched a group of students play an entertaining game of basketball every Friday at noon. Having no basketball skills, he was reluctant to play (contemplation stage). Eventually, however, the desire to join in the fun was strong enough that he enrolled in a beginning course at the college so he would learn to play the game (preparation stage). To his surprise, most of the students were impressed that he was willing to do this. Now, with greater competence, he is able to join in on Friday's "pick-up games" (action phase).

Another alternative is to select an activity in which you are skilled. It may not be basketball, but it well could be aerobics. And don't be afraid to try new activities. Similarly, if your body weight is a problem, you could learn to cook low-fat meals. Try different recipes until you find foods you like.

Patty's story at the beginning of this chapter exemplifies a lack of competence. Patty was motivated and knew she could do it, but she lacked the skills to reach her goal. All along, Patty was fluctuating between the contemplation and action stages. Once she mastered the skills, she was able to achieve and maintain her goal.

2. *Problems of confidence.* Problems with confidence arise when you have the skills but you don't believe you can get it done. Fear and feelings of inadequacy often interfere with the ability to perform the task.

Don't talk yourself out of something until you have given it a fair try. If the skills are there, the sky is the limit. Initially, try to visualize yourself doing the task and getting it done. Repeat this several times, then actually give it a try. You will surprise yourself.

Sometimes, lack of confidence sets in when the task seems to be insurmountable. In these situations, dividing a goal into smaller, realistic objectives helps to accomplish the task. You may know how to swim, but the goal of swimming a continuous mile could take you several weeks to accomplish. Set up your training program so you swim a little farther each day until you are able to swim the entire mile. If you don't meet your objective on a given day, try it again, reevaluate, cut back a little, and, most important, don't give up.

3. *Problems of motivation.* With problems of motivation, both the competence and the confidence are there, but individuals are unwilling to change because the reasons for change are not important to them. For example, a person begins contemplating a smoking cessation program when the reasons for quitting outweigh the reasons for smoking.

The lack of knowledge and lack of goals are the primary causes of unwillingness to change (precontemplators). Knowledge often determines goals, and goals determine motivation. How badly you want something dictates how hard you'll work at it. Many people are unaware of the magnitude of the benefits of a wellness program. When it comes to a healthy lifestyle, however, there may not be a second chance. A stroke, a heart attack, or cancer can have irreparable or fatal consequences. Greater understanding of what leads to disease may be all that is needed to initiate change.

Also, feeling physically fit is difficult to explain unless you have experienced it yourself. What Patty expressed to her instructor—fitness, self-esteem, confidence, health, and quality of life—cannot be conveyed to someone who is constrained by sedentary living. In a way, wellness is like reaching the top of a mountain. The quiet, the clean air, the lush vegetation, the flowing water in the river, the wildlife, and the majestic valley below are difficult to explain to someone who has spent a lifetime within city limits.

Behavior Modification Principles

Over the course of many years, we all develop habits that we would like to change at some point. The adage "old habits die hard" comes to mind. Acquiring positive behaviors that will lead to better health and well-being requires continuous effort. When wellness is concerned, the sooner we implement a healthy lifestyle program, the greater are the health benefits and quality of life that lie ahead. Adopting the following behavior modification principles can help change behavior.

Self-Analysis

The first step in modifying behavior is a decisive desire to do so. If you have no interest in changing a behavior, you won't do it (precontemplator). A person who has no intention of quitting smoking will not quit, regardless of what anyone says or how strong the evidence is against it. As part of your self-analysis, you may want to prepare a list of reasons for continuing or discontinuing the behavior. When the reasons for changing outweigh the reasons for not changing, you are ready for the next step (contemplation stage).

Behavior Analysis

Now you have to determine the frequency, circumstances, and consequences of the behavior to be altered or implemented. If the desired outcome is to consume less fat, you first must find out what foods in your diet are high in fat, when you eat them, and when you don't eat them (preparation stage). Knowing when you don't eat fatty foods points to circumstances under which you exert control of your diet and will help as you set goals.

Key Terms

Motivation The desire and will to do something.
Locus of control The extent to which a person believes he or she can influence the external environment.

Goal Setting

A goal motivates change in behavior. The stronger the goal, or desire, the more motivated you will be either to change unwanted behaviors or to implement new healthy behaviors. The final topic of this chapter, SMART goals, will help you write goals and prepare an action plan to achieve those goals. This will aid with behavior modification.

Social Support

Surrounding yourself with people who will work toward a common goal with you or will encourage you along the way will be helpful. Attempting to quit smoking, for instance, is easier when the person is around others who are trying to quit as well. The person also may get help from friends who have quit already. Peer support is a strong incentive for behavior change. During this process, people who will not be supportive should be avoided. Friends who have no desire to quit smoking may tempt the person to smoke and encourage relapse. People who achieved the same goal earlier might not be supportive either. For instance, someone might say, "I can do six consecutive miles." The response should be, "I'm proud that I can jog three consecutive miles."

Monitoring

During the action and maintenance stages, continuous behavior monitoring increases awareness of the desired outcome. Sometimes this principle in itself is sufficient to cause change. For example, keeping track of daily food intake reveals sources of fat in the diet. This can help a person cut down gradually or completely eliminate some high-fat foods before consuming them. If the goal is to increase daily intake of fruits and vegetables, keeping track of the number of servings eaten each day raises awareness and may help increase their intake.

A Positive Outlook

Having a positive outlook means taking an optimistic approach from the beginning and believing in yourself. Following the guidelines in this chapter will help you pace yourself so you can work toward

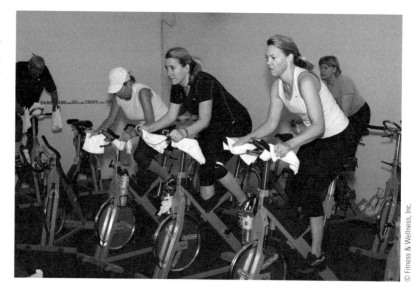

Social support enhances regular participation and the process of behavior modification.

change. Also, you may become motivated by looking at the outcomes—how much healthier you will be, how much better you will look, or how much farther you can jog.

Reinforcement

People tend to repeat behaviors that are rewarded and disregard those that are not rewarded or are punished. If you have successfully cut down your fat intake during the week, reward yourself by going to a show or buying a new pair of shoes. Do not reinforce yourself with destructive behaviors such as eating a high-fat dinner. If you fail to change a desired behavior (or to implement a new one), you may want to put off buying those new shoes. When a positive behavior becomes habitual, give yourself an even better reward. Treat yourself to a weekend away from home, buy a new bike, or get that tennis racket you always wanted.

SMART Goals

Only a well-conceived action plan will help you attain goals. Determining what you want to accomplish is the starting point, but to reach your goal you need to write **SMART** goals. The SMART acronym means that goals are Specific, Measurable, Acceptable, Realistic, and Time-specific.

1. *Specific.* When writing goals, state exactly and in a positive manner what you would like to accom-

plish. For example, if you are overweight at 150 pounds and at 27 percent body fat, simply stating "I will lose weight" is not a specific goal. Instead, re-write your goal to state "I will reduce my body fat to 20 percent body fat (137 pounds) in 12 weeks."

Be sure to write down your goals. An unwritten goal is simply a wish. A written goal, in essence, becomes a contract with yourself. Show this goal to a friend or an instructor and have him or her witness the contract you made with yourself by signing alongside your signature.

Once you have identified and written down a specific goal, write the specific **objectives** that will help you reach that goal. These objectives are the necessary steps required to reach your goal. For ex-ample, a goal might be to achieve recommended body weight. Several specific objectives could be to

(a) lose an average of 1 pound (or 1 fat per-centage point) per week.
(b) monitor body weight before breakfast every morning.
(c) assess body composition every 3 weeks.
(d) limit fat intake to less than 25 percent of total daily caloric intake.
(e) eliminate all pastries from the diet during this time.
(f) walk/jog in the proper target zone for 60 minutes, six times per week.

2. *Measurable.* Whenever possible, goals and objec-tives should be measurable. For example, "I will lose weight" is not measurable, but "I will reduce body fat to 20 percent" is measurable. Also note that all of the sample specific objectives (a) through (f) in item 1 above are measurable. For instance, you can figure out easily whether you are losing a pound or a per-centage point per week; you can conduct a nutrient analysis to assess your average fat intake; or you can monitor your weekly exercise sessions to make sure you are meeting this specific objective.

3. *Acceptable.* Goals that you set for yourself are more motivational than goals that someone else sets for you. These goals will motivate and challenge you and should be consistent with other goals that you have. As you set an acceptable goal, ask yourself: Do I have the time, commitment, and necessary skills to accomplish this goal? If not, you need to restate your goal so that it is acceptable to you.

In instances where successful completion of a goal involves others, such as an athletic team or an organization, an acceptable goal must be compatible with those of the other people involved. If a team's practice schedule is set Monday through Friday

from 4:00 to 6:00 p.m., it is unacceptable for you to train only three times per week or at a different time of the day.

Acceptable goals are also embraced with positive thoughts. Visualize and believe in your success. As difficult as some tasks may seem, where there's a will, there's a way. A plan of action, prepared ac-cording to the guidelines in this chapter, will help you achieve your goals.

4. *Realistic.* Goals should be within reach. If you cur-rently weigh 190 pounds and your target weight (at 20 percent body fat) is 140 pounds, setting a goal to lose 50 pounds in a month would be unsound, if not impossible. Such a goal does not allow for the imple-mentation of adequate behavior modification tech-niques or ensure weight maintenance at the target weight. Unattainable goals only set you up for fail-ure, discouragement, and loss of interest.

On the other hand, do not write goals that are too easy to achieve and do not challenge you. If a goal is too easy, you may lose interest and stop working toward it.

At times, problems arise even with realistic goals. Try to anticipate potential difficulties as much as possible, and plan for ways to deal with them. If your goal is to jog for 30 minutes on six consecutive days, what are the alternatives if the weather turns bad? Possible solutions are to jog in the rain, find an indoor track, jog at a different time of day when the weather is better, or participate in a different aerobic activity such as stationary cy-cling, swimming, or step aerobics.

Monitoring your progress as you move toward a goal also reinforces behavior. Keeping an exercise log or doing a body composition assessment peri-odically enables you to determine your progress at any given time.

5. *Time-specific.* A goal always should have a specific date set for completion. The above example to reach 20 percent body fat in 12 weeks is time-specific. The chosen date should be realistic but not too distant in the future. Allow yourself enough time to achieve the goal, but not too much time, as this could affect

Key Terms

Goal The ultimate aim toward which effort is directed.
SMART An acronym for Specific, Measurable, Attainable, Realistic, and Time-specific goals.
Objectives Steps required to reach a goal.

your performance. With a deadline, a task is much easier to work toward.

Goal Evaluation

In addition to the SMART guidelines provided above, you should conduct periodic evaluations of your goals. Reevaluations are vital for success. You may find that after you have fully committed and put all your effort into a goal, that goal may be unreachable. If so, reassess the goal.

Recognize that you will face obstacles and that you will not always meet your goals. Use your setbacks and learn from them. Rewrite your goal and create a plan that will help you get around self-defeating behaviors in the future. Once you achieve a goal, set a new one to improve upon or maintain what you have achieved. Goals keep you motivated.

In addition to previously discussed guidelines, throughout this book you will find information on behavioral change. For example, Chapter 3 includes the Exercise Readiness Questionnaire, tips to start and adhere to an exercise program, and how to set your fitness goals; Chapter 2 offers tips to enhance your aerobic workout; Chapter 8 gives suggestions on how to adhere to a lifetime weight management program; Chapter 7 sets forth stress management techniques; and Chapter 8 outlines a six-step smoking cessation plan.

A Word of Caution Before You Start Exercise

Even though exercise testing and participation is relatively safe for most apparently healthy individuals, a small but real risk exists for exercise-induced abnormalities in people with a history of cardiovascular problems and those who are at higher risk for disease. These people should be screened before initiating or increasing the intensity of an exercise program.

Before you engage in an exercise program or participate in any exercise testing, as a minimum you should fill out the Physical Activity Readiness Questionnaire (PAR-Q & YOU) found in Activity 1.2. A "yes" answer to any of these questions may signal the need for a physician's approval before you participate. If you don't have any "yes" responses, you may proceed to Chapter 2 to assess your current level of fitness.

Assess Your Behavior

CENGAGENOW™ Log on to www.cengagebrain.com to access CengageNOW and the Behavior Change Planner where you can take a wellness inventory to assess the behaviors that might benefit most from healthy change.

1. Are you aware of lifestyle factors that may negatively impact your health?

2. Do you accumulate at least 30 minutes of moderate-intensity physical activity five days per week?

3. Do you participate in vigorous-intensity physical activity a minimum of two times per week?

4. Do you make a constant and deliberate effort to stay healthy and achieve the highest potential for well-being?

Assess Your Knowledge

CENGAGENOW Evaluate how well you understand the concepts presented in this chapter using the chapter-specific quizzing available in the online materials at www.cengagebrain.com.

1. Bodily movement produced by skeletal muscles is called
   a. physical activity.
   b. kinesiology.
   c. exercise.
   d. aerobic exercise.
   e. muscle strength.

2. The 2008 Federal Guidelines for Physical Activity state that adults between 18 and 64 years of age should
   a. do 2 hours and 30 minutes a week of moderate-intensity aerobic physical activity.
   b. do 1 hour and 15 minutes (75 minutes) a week of vigorous-intensity aerobic physical activity.
   c. do an equivalent combination of moderate- and vigorous-intensity aerobic physical activity listed under choices a and b above.
   d. do muscle-strengthening activities that involve all major muscle groups on two or more days per week.
   e. All of the above choices are correct.

3. The leading cause of death in the United States is
   a. cancer.
   b. accidents.
   c. chronic lower respiratory disease.
   d. diseases of the cardiovascular system.
   e. drug-related illness.

4. The constant and deliberate effort to stay healthy and achieve the highest potential for well-being is defined as
   a. health.
   b. physical fitness.
   c. wellness.
   d. health-related fitness.
   e. metabolic fitness.

5. Which of the following is not a component of health-related fitness?
   a. cardiorespiratory endurance
   b. body composition
   c. agility
   d. muscular strength and endurance
   e. muscular flexibility

6. Research on the effects of fitness on mortality indicates that the largest drop in premature mortality is seen between
   a. the average and excellent fitness groups.
   b. the least fit and moderately fit groups.
   c. the good and high fitness groups.
   d. the moderately fit and good fitness groups.
   e. The drop is similar between all fitness groups.

7. What is the greatest benefit of being physically fit?
   a. absence of disease
   b. a higher quality of life
   c. improved sports performance
   d. better personal appearance
   e. maintenance of ideal body weight

8. Which of the following is a stage in the behavioral modification model?
   a. recognition
   b. motivation
   c. relapse
   d. preparation
   e. goal setting

9. A precontemplator is a person who
   a. has no desire to change a behavior.
   b. is looking to make a change in the next six months.
   c. is preparing for change in the next 30 days.
   d. willingly adopts healthy behaviors.
   e. is talking to a therapist to overcome a problem behavior.

10. A SMART goal is effective when it is
    a. realistic.
    b. measurable.
    c. specific.
    d. acceptable.
    e. All are correct choices.

Correct answers can be found on page 307.

Behavior Modification: Stages of Change

Name _____   Date _____

Course _____   Section _____

Instructions

Please indicate which response most accurately describes your stage of change for three different behaviors (in the blank space identify the behavior: smoking, physical activity, stress, nutrition, weight control, etc.). Next, select the statement (select only one) that best represents your current behavior pattern. To select the most appropriate statement, fill in the blank for one of the first three statements if your current behavior is a problem behavior. (For example, you might say, "I currrently smoke and I do *not* intend to change in the foreseeable future." *or* "I currently *do not* exercise but I am contemplating changing in the next 6 months."

If you have already started to make changes, fill in the blank in one of the last three statements. (In this case, you might say: "I currently eat a *low-fat* diet but I have done so only within the last 6 months," or "I currently *practice adequate stress management techniques* and I have done so for more than 6 months.") You may use this technique to identify your stage of change for any type of health-related behavior.

Now write SMART goals (see pages 20–22) and identify three behavior modification principles (pages 19–20) that will aid you with the process of change.

Behavior 1: _____

1. I currently _____, and I do not intend to change in the foreseeable future.

2. I currently _____, but I am contemplating changing in the next 6 months.

3. I currently _____ regularly but intend to change in the next month.

4. I currently _____, but I have done so only within the last 6 months.

5. I currently _____, and I have done so for more than 6 months.

6. I currently _____, and I have done so for more than 5 years.

Stage of change: (see Figure 1.11, page 17). _____

Specific goal and date to be accomplished: _____

Principles of behavior modification to be used: _____

Behavior 2: _____

1. I currently _____, and I do not intend to change in the foreseeable future.

2. I currently _____, but I am contemplating changing in the next 6 months.

3. I currently _____ regularly but intend to change in the next month.

4. I currently _____, but I have done so only within the last 6 months.

5. I currently _____, and I have done so for more than 6 months.

6. I currently _____, and I have done so for more than 5 years.

Stage of change: (see Figure 1.11, page 17). _____

Specific goal and date to be accomplished: _____

Principles of behavior modification to be used: _____

Behavior Modification: Stages of Change (continued)

Behavior 3: _____

1. I currently _____, and I do not intend to change in the foreseeable future.

2. I currently _____, but I am contemplating changing in the next 6 months.

3. I currently _____ regularly but intend to change in the next month.

4. I currently _____, but I have done so only within the last 6 months.

5. I currently _____, and I have done so for more than 6 months.

6. I currently _____, and I have done so for more than 5 years.

Stage of change: (see Figure 1.11, page 17). _____

Specific goal and date to be accomplished: _____

Principles of behavior modification to be used: _____

Stages of Change

1 = Precontemplation   4 = Action
2 = Contemplation   5 = Maintenance
3 = Preparation   6 = Termination/Adoption

Self-Reflection

In your own words, indicate barriers (what may keep you from changing) that you may encounter during the process of change and how can you best prepare to overcome these barriers.

_____

_____

_____

_____

_____

_____

_____

_____

_____

Physical Activity Readiness Questionnaire (PAR-Q)

Name _____ Date _____ Grade _____

Instructor _____ Course _____ Section _____

I.

Physical Activity Readiness
Questionnaire — PAR-Q
(revised 2002)

PAR-Q & YOU
(A Questionnaire for People Aged 15 to 69)

Regular physical activity is fun and healthy, and increasingly more people are starting to become more active every day. Being more active is very safe for most people. However, some people should check with their doctor before they start becoming much more physically active.
If you are planning to become much more physically active than you are now, start by answering the seven questions in the box below. If you are between the ages of 15 and 69, the PAR-Q will tell you if you should check with your doctor before you start. If you are over 69 years of age, and you are not used to being very active, check with your doctor.
Common sense is your best guide when you answer these questions. Please read the questions carefully and answer each one honestly: check YES or NO.

YES	NO	
☐	☐	1. Has your doctor ever said that you have a heart condition <u>and</u> that you should only do physical activity recommended by a doctor?
☐	☐	2. Do you feel pain in your chest when you do physical activity?
☐	☐	3. In the past month, have you had chest pain when you were not doing physical activity?
☐	☐	4. Do you lose your balance because of dizziness or do you ever lose consciousness?
☐	☐	5. Do you have a bone or joint problem (for example, back, knee, or hip) that could be made worse by a change in your physical activity?
☐	☐	6. Is your doctor currently prescribing drugs (for example, water pills) for your blood pressure or heart condition?
☐	☐	7. Do you know of <u>any other reason</u> why you should not do physical activity?

If you answered

YES to one or more questions

Talk with your doctor by phone or in person BEFORE you start becoming much more physically active or BEFORE you have a fitness appraisal. Tell your doctor about the PAR-Q and which questions you answered YES.
- You may be able to do any activity you want—as long as you start slowly and build up gradually. Or, you may need to restrict your activities to those which are safe for you. Talk with your doctor about the kinds of activities you wish to participate in and follow his/her advice.
- Find out which community programs are safe and helpful for you.

NO to all questions

If you answered NO honestly to all PAR-Q questions, you can be reasonably sure that you can:
- start becoming much more physically active—begin slowly and build up gradually. This is the safest and easiest way to go.
- take part in a fitness appraisal—this is an excellent way to determine your basic fitness so that you can plan the best way for you to live actively. It is also highly recommended that you have your blood pressure evaluated. If your reading is over 144/94, talk with your doctor before you start becoming much more physically active.

→

DELAY BECOMING MUCH MORE ACTIVE:
- if you are not feeling well because of a temporary illness such as a cold or a fever—wait until you feel better; or
- if you are or may be pregnant—talk to your doctor before you start becoming more active.

PLEASE NOTE: If your health changes so that you then answer YES to any of the above questions, tell your fitness or health professional. Ask whether you should change your physical activity plan.

<u>Informed Use of the PAR-Q</u>: The Canadian Society for Exercise Physiology, Health Canada, and their agents assume no liability for persons who undertake physical activity, and if in doubt after completing this questionnaire, consult your doctor prior to physical activity.

No changes permitted. You are encouraged to photocopy the PAR-Q but only if you use the entire form.

NOTE: If the PAR-Q is being given to a person before he or she participates in a physical activity program or a fitness appraisal, this section may be used for legal or administrative purposes.

"I have read, understood and completed this questionnaire. Any questions I had were answered to my full satisfaction."

NAME _____

SIGNATURE _____ DATE _____

SIGNATURE OF PARENT _____ WITNESS _____
or GUARDIAN (for participants under the age of majority)

Note: This physical activity clearance is valid for a maximum of 12 months from the date it is completed and becomes invalid if your condition changes so that you would answer YES to any of the seven questions.

 © Canadian Society for Exercise Physiology   Supported by: [🍁] Health   Santé
                                                                          Canada Canada

Source: Physical Activity Readiness Questionnaire (PAR-Q) © 2002. Used with permission from the Canadian Society for Exercise Physiology, www.csep.ca.

Physical Activity Readiness Questionnaire (PAR-Q) (continued)

II. Do you feel that it is safe for you to proceed with an exercise program? Explain any concerns or limitations that you may have regarding your safe participation in a comprehensive exercise program to improve cardiorespiratory endurance, muscular strength and endurance, and muscular flexibility.

_____

_____

_____

_____

_____

_____

_____

_____

_____

_____

III. In a few words, describe your previous experiences with sports participation, whether you have taken part in a structured exercise program, and express your own feelings about exercise participation.

_____

_____

_____

_____

_____

_____

_____

_____

_____

_____

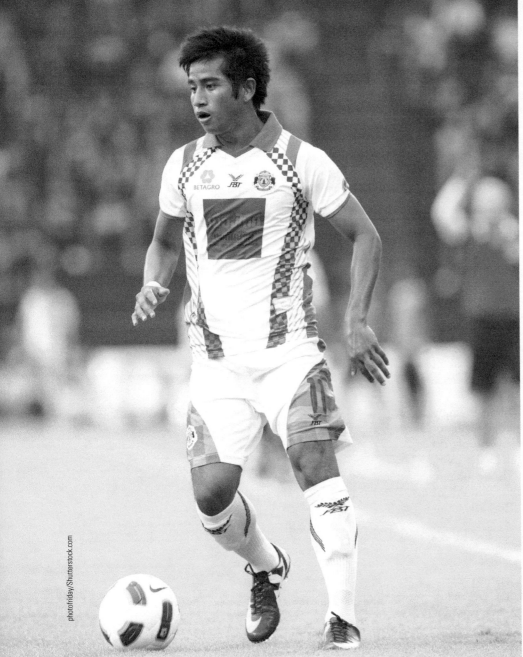

Evaluating Fitness Activities

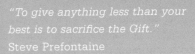

2

"To give anything less than your best is to sacrifice the Gift."
Steve Prefontaine

Objectives

▶ **Learn** the benefits and advantages of selected aerobic activities.

▶ **Learn** to rate the fitness benefits of aerobic activities.

▶ **Evaluate** the contributions of skill-related fitness activities.

▶ **Understand** the sequence of a standard aerobic workout.

▶ **Learn** ways to enhance your aerobic workouts.

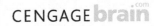

Visit **www.cengagebrain.com** to access course materials and companion resources for this text including quiz questions designed to check your understanding of the chapter contents, activities, labs, and more! See the preface on page xiii for more information.

29

Sunithas' Exercise Routine

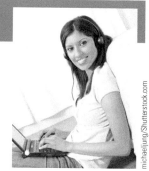

The extent of my exercise program was all jogging. I like to jog because I ran track my first year in high school. Always running, however, was sometimes boring and I wasn't enjoying it as much as when I ran track with friends. Sometimes I dreaded going out because I wasn't motivated to go by myself or it was either too cold or too hot to exercise. After enrolling in a college fitness and wellness course, we were required to try a minimum of five aerobic activities. I quickly learned that there was more to "exercise life" than running all the time. I really enjoyed Spinning, swimming, and elliptical training. Doing different activities took away the monotony of my exercise routine and I found out that exercise is much more fun this way. I also discovered that I am exercising longer and more often than before. I really do feel that cross-training is the way to go if one feels stale or bored of the same exercise routine all the time.

One of the fun aspects of exercise is the sheer variety of activities promoting fitness that are available to you. You can select one or a combination of activities for your program—your choice should be based on personal enjoyment, convenience, and availability. A summary of the most popular physical activities in the United States and the percentage of adults who participate in them are presented in Figure 2.1.

Aerobic Activities

Most people who exercise pick and adhere to a single mode, such as walking, swimming, or jogging. Yet no single activity develops total fitness. Many activities contribute to cardiorespiratory development, but the extent of contribution to other fitness components is limited and varies among the activities. For total fitness, aerobic activities should be supplemented with strength and flexibility exercises. Cross-training can add enjoyment to the program, decrease the risk of incurring injuries from overuse, and keep exercise from becoming monotonous.

Exercise sessions should be convenient. To enjoy exercise, you should select a time when you will not be rushed and a location that is nearby. People do not enjoy driving across town to get to the gym, health club, track, or pool. If parking is a problem, you may get discouraged quickly and quit. All of these factors can supply excuses not to stick to an exercise program.

Walking

The most natural, easiest, safest, and least expensive form of aerobic exercise is walking. For years, many fitness practitioners believed that walking was not vigorous enough to improve cardiorespiratory functioning, but brisk walking at speeds of 4 miles per hour or faster does improve cardiorespiratory fitness. From a health fitness viewpoint, a regular walking program can prolong life significantly (see the discussion of cardiovascular diseases in Chapter 8). Although walking obviously takes longer than jogging, the caloric cost of brisk walking is only about 10 percent lower than jogging the same distance.

Walking is perhaps the best activity to start a conditioning program for the cardiorespiratory system.

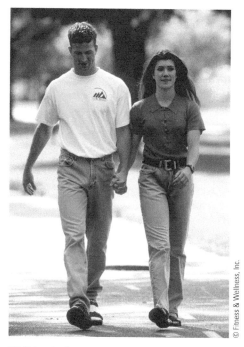

Walking is the most natural aerobic physical activity.

Figure 2.1	Most popular adult physical activities in the United States.

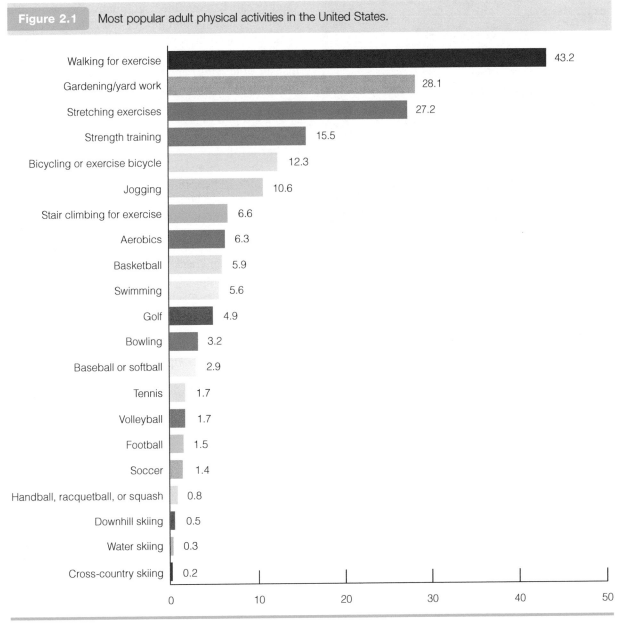

SOURCE: Centers for Disease Control and Prevention, Atlanta.

Inactive people should start with 1-mile walks four or five times per week. Walk times can be increased gradually by 5 minutes each week. Following 3 to 4 weeks of conditioning, a person should be able to walk 2 miles at a 4-mile-per-hour pace, five times per week. Greater aerobic benefits accrue from walking longer and swinging the arms faster than normal. Light hand weights, a backpack (4 to 6 pounds), or tension belts that add load to the upper body (arms) also add to the intensity of walking. Because of the additional load on the cardiorespiratory system, extra weights or loads are not recommended for people who have or are at risk for cardiovascular disease.

Walking in chest-deep water is an excellent form of aerobic activity, particularly for people who have leg and back problems. Because of the buoyancy of water, individuals submerged in water to armpit level weigh only about 10 percent to 20 percent of their weight outside the water. The resistance the water creates as a person walks in the pool adds to the intensity of the activity and provides a good cardiorespiratory workout.

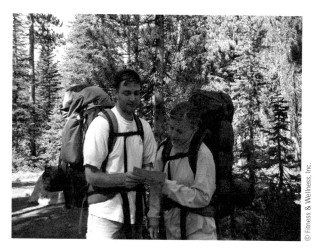

An 8-hour hike can burn as many calories as a 20-mile walk or jog.

Hiking

Hiking is an excellent activity for the entire family, especially during the summer and on summer vacations. Many people feel guilty if they are unable to continue their exercise routine during vacations. The intensity of hiking over uneven terrain is greater than walking. An 8-hour hike can burn as many calories as a 20-mile walk or jog.

Another benefit of hiking is the relaxing effects of beautiful scenery. This is an ideal activity for highly stressed people who live near woods and hills. A rough day at the office can fade quickly in the peacefulness and beauty of the outdoors.

Jogging

Next to walking, jogging is one of the most accessible forms of exercise. A person can find places to jog almost everywhere. The lone requirement to prevent injuries is a good pair of jogging shoes.

The popularity of jogging in the United States started shortly after publication of Dr. Kenneth Cooper's first *Aerobics* book in 1968. Jim Fixx's *Complete Book of Running*, listed for 11 weeks in 1977 as No. 1 on the best-selling list, further contributed to the phenomenal growth of jogging as a fitness activity in the United States.

Jogging three to five times a week is one of the fastest ways to improve cardiorespiratory fitness. The risk of injury, however—especially in beginners—is higher with jogging than walking. For proper conditioning, jogging programs should start with 1 to 2 weeks of walking. As fitness improves, walking and jogging can be combined, gradually increasing the jogging segment until it fills the full 20 to 30 minutes.

A word of caution when it comes to jogging: The risk of injury increases greatly as speed (running instead of jogging) and mileage go up. Jogging approximately 15 miles per week is sufficient to reach an excellent level of cardiorespiratory fitness.

A good pair of shoes is a must for joggers. Many foot, knee, and leg problems originate from improperly fitted or worn-out shoes. A good pair of shoes should offer lateral stability and not lean to either side when placed on a flat surface. The shoe also should bend at the ball of the foot, not at midfoot. Worn-out shoes should be replaced. After 500 miles of use, jogging shoes lose about a third of their shock absorption capabilities. If you suddenly have problems, check your shoes first. It may be time for a new pair.

For safety reasons, joggers (and walkers) should follow these precautions:

1. Stay away from high-speed roads.

2. Do not wear headphones so that you can be aware of your surroundings. Using a headphone may keep you from hearing a car horn, a voice, or a potential attacker.

3. Go against the traffic so that you can spot and avoid all oncoming traffic.

4. Do not wear dark clothes. Reflective clothing or fluorescent material worn on different parts of the body is highly recommended. A flashlight, particularly an LED light, not only alerts drivers of your presence but also helps illuminate the street. Motorists can see a light from a greater distance than they can spot the reflective material.

5. Wear a billed cap and clear glasses in the dark. The billed cap will hit a branch or other object before such hits your head. Clear glasses can protect your eyes from unseen objects or insects.

6. Run behind vehicles at intersections. Drivers often look only in the direction of oncoming traffic and do not look in the opposite direction before proceeding onto the street.

7. Select different routes. A potential attacker may lie in wait if you are predictable in your running route. Running with a partner is also preferable because there is always strength in numbers. And do not wear your hair in a ponytail because it provides an easy grip for a potential attacker.

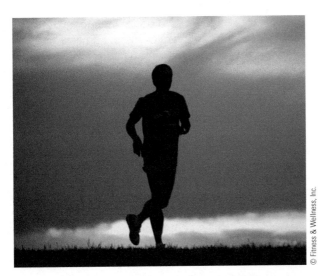

Jogging is one the most popular forms of aerobic exercise.

8. Avoid walking or jogging in unfamiliar areas. When visiting a new area, always inquire as to safe areas to walk or jog.

Deep-Water Jogging

An alternative form of jogging, especially for injured people, those with chronic back problems, and overweight individuals, is deep-water jogging—jogging in place while treading water. Deep-water jogging is almost as strenuous as jogging on land. In deep-water jogging, the jogging motions used on land are accentuated by pumping the arms and legs hard through a full range of motion. The participant usually wears a flotation vest to help maintain the body in an upright position. Many elite athletes train frequently in water to lessen the wear and tear on the body caused by long-distance running. These athletes have been able to maintain high oxygen uptake values through rigorous water jogging programs.

Aerobics

Aerobics is a very popular fitness activity for women in the United States. Routines consist of a combination of stepping, walking, jogging, skipping, kicking, and arm swinging movements performed to music. It is a fun way to exercise and promote cardiorespiratory development at the same time.

High-impact aerobics (HIA) is the traditional form of aerobics. The movements exert a great

amount of vertical force on the feet as they contact the floor. Proper leg conditioning through other forms of weight-bearing aerobic exercises (brisk walking and jogging), as well as strength training, is recommended prior to participating in HIA.

HIA is an intense activity, and it produces the highest rate of aerobics injuries. Shin splints, stress fractures, low back pain, and tendinitis are all too common in HIA enthusiasts. These injuries are caused by the constant impact of the feet on firm surfaces. As a result, several alternative forms of aerobics have been developed.

In **low-impact aerobics (LIA)**, the impact is reduced because each foot contacts the surface separately, but the recommended intensity of exercise is more difficult to maintain than with HIA. To help elevate the exercise heart rate, all arm movements and weight-bearing actions that lower the center of gravity should be accentuated. Sustained movement throughout the program is also crucial to keep the heart rate in the target cardiorespiratory zone.

Step aerobics (SA) is an activity in which participants step up and down from a bench. Benches range in height from 2 to 10 inches. SA adds another dimension to the aerobics program. As noted previously, variety adds enjoyment to aerobic workouts. SA is considered a high-intensity but low-impact activity. The intensity of the activity can be controlled easily by the height of the bench. Aerobic benches or plates can be stacked together safely to adjust the height of the steps. Beginners are encouraged to use the lowest stepping height and then advance gradually to a higher bench. This will decrease the risk for injury. Even though one foot is always in contact with the floor or bench during step aerobics, this activity is not recommended for individuals with ankle, knee, or hip problems.

Key Terms

Aerobics A series of exercise routines that include a combination of stepping, walking, jogging, skipping, kicking, and arm swinging movements performed to music.

High-impact aerobics (HIA) Exercises incorporating movements in which both feet are off the ground at the same time momentarily.

Low-impact aerobics (LIA) Exercises in which at least one foot is in contact with the ground or floor at all times.

Step aerobics (SA) A form of exercise that combines stepping up and down from a bench with arm movements.

Other forms of aerobics include a combination of HIA and LIA, as well as **moderate-impact aerobics (MIA)**. MIA incorporates **plyometric training**. This type of training is used frequently by jumpers (high, long, and triple jumpers) and athletes in sports that require quick jumping ability, such as basketball and gymnastics. With MIA, one foot is in contact with the ground most of the time. Participants, however, continuously try to recover from all lower-body flexion actions. This is done by extending the hip, knee, and ankle joints quickly without allowing the foot (or feet) to leave the ground. These quick movements make the exercise intensity of MIA quite high.

An extremely popular dance fitness program that was created in Colombia by Alberto "Beto" Perez in the mid '90s is **zumba**. Zumba combines Latin and international music (cumbia, salsa, merengue, reggaeton, tango, and rock and roll among others) with dance to develop fitness and make exercise fun. The zumba motto has become "Ditch the workout, join the party!" Several types of zumba have been developed, including traditional zumba, zumba gold, zumba toning, aqua zumba, zumbatomic, and zumba marumba.

Swimming

Swimming, another excellent form of aerobic exercise, uses many of the major muscle groups in the body. This provides a good training stimulus for the heart and lungs. Swimming is a great exercise option for individuals who cannot jog or walk for extended periods.

Compared to other activities, the risk of injuries from swimming is low. The aquatic medium helps to support the body, taking pressure off bones and joints in the lower extremities and the back.

Maximal heart rates during swimming are approximately 10 to 13 beats per minute (bpm) lower than during running. The horizontal position of the body is thought to aid blood flow distribution throughout the body, decreasing the demand on the cardiorespiratory system. Cool water temperatures and direct contact with the water seem to help dissipate body heat more efficiently, further decreasing the strain on the heart.

Some exercise specialists recommend that this difference in maximal heart rate (10 to 13 bpm) be subtracted prior to determining cardiorespiratory training intensities. For example, the estimated maximal swimming heart rate for a 20-year-old would be approximately 180 bpm [$207 - (.7 \times 20) - 13$]. Studies are inconclusive as to whether this decrease

in heart rate in water also occurs at submaximal intensities below 70 percent of maximal heart rate.[1]

To produce better training benefits during swimming, swimmers should minimize gliding periods such as those in the breaststroke and sidestroke. Achieving proper training intensities with these strokes is difficult. The forward crawl is recommended for better aerobic results.

Overweight individuals have to swim fast enough to achieve an adequate training intensity. Excessive body fat makes the body more buoyant, and often the tendency is to float along. This may be good for reducing stress and relaxing, but it does not greatly increase caloric expenditure to aid with weight loss. Walking or jogging in waist- or armpit-deep water is a better choice for overweight individuals who cannot walk or jog on land for an extended period of time.

With reference to the principle of specificity of training, cardiorespiratory improvements from swimming cannot be measured adequately with a land-based walk/jog test. This is because most of the work with swimming is done by the upper body musculature.

Although the heart's ability to pump more blood improves significantly with any type of aerobic activity, the primary increase in the ability of cells to utilize oxygen (VO$_2$, or oxygen uptake) with swimming occurs in the upper body and not the lower extremities. Therefore, fitness improvements with swimming are best assessed by comparing changes in distance a person swims in a given time, say, 12 minutes.

Critical Thinking

Participation in sports is a good predictor of adherence to exercise later in life. • What previous experiences have you had with participation in sports? • Were these experiences positive, and what effect do they have on your current physical activity patterns?

Water Aerobics

Water aerobics is fun and safe for people of all ages. Besides developing fitness, it provides an opportunity for socialization and fun in a comfortable, refreshing setting.

Water aerobics incorporates a combination of rhythmic arm and leg actions performed in a vertical position while submerged in waist- to armpit-deep water. The vigorous limb movements against the water's resistance during water aerobics provide the training stimuli for cardiorespiratory development.

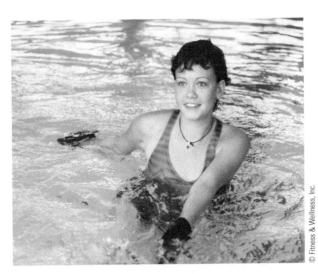

© Fitness & Wellness, Inc.

Water aerobics offers fitness and fun in an environment relatively low in risk for injury.

The popularity of water aerobics as an exercise modality to develop the cardiorespiratory system can be attributed to several factors:

1. Water buoyancy reduces weight-bearing stress on joints and thereby lessens the risk for injuries.
2. Water aerobics is a more feasible type of exercise for overweight individuals and those with arthritic conditions who may not be able to participate in weight-bearing activities such as walking, jogging, and aerobics.
3. Water aerobics is an excellent exercise modality to improve functional fitness in older adults (see Chapter 9, pages 259–261).
4. Heat dissipation in water is beneficial to obese participants, who seem to undergo a higher heat strain than average-weight individuals.
5. Water aerobics is available to swimmers and nonswimmers alike.

The exercises used during water aerobics are designed to elevate the heart rate, which contributes to cardiorespiratory development. In addition, the aquatic medium provides increased resistance for strength improvement with virtually no impact. Because of this resistance to movement, strength gains with water aerobics seem to be better than with land-based aerobic activities.

Another benefit is the reduction of pain and fear of injuries common to many people who initiate exercise programs. Water aerobics provides a relatively safe environment for injury-free participation in exercise. The cushioned environment of the water allows patients recovering from leg and back injuries, individuals with joint problems, injured athletes,

pregnant women, and obese people to benefit from water aerobics.

As in swimming, maximal heart rates achieved during water aerobics are lower than during running. The difference between water aerobics and running is about 10 bpm.[2] Further, research comparing physiologic differences between self-paced treadmill running and self-paced water aerobics exercise showed that even though individuals work at a lower heart rate intensity in water, the oxygen uptake level was the same for both treadmill and water exercise modalities.[3] Apparently healthy people, therefore, can sustain land-based exercise intensities during a water aerobics workout and experience fitness benefits similar to or greater than those acquired during land aerobics.[4]

Cycling

Most people learn cycling in their youth. Because it is a non-weight-bearing activity, cycling is a good exercise modality for people with lower-body or lower back injuries. Cycling helps to develop the cardiorespiratory system, as well as muscular strength and endurance in the lower extremities.

Because cycling is a non-weight-bearing activity, raising the heart rate to the proper training intensity is more difficult. As the amount of muscle mass involved during aerobic exercise decreases, so does the demand placed on the cardiorespiratory system. The thigh muscles do most of the work in cycling, making it harder to achieve and maintain a high cardiorespiratory training intensity.

Maintaining a continuous pedaling motion and eliminating coasting periods helps the participant achieve a faster heart rate. Exercising for longer periods also helps to compensate for the lower heart rate intensity during cycling. Comparing cycling to jogging, similar aerobic benefits take roughly three times the distance at twice the speed of jogging. Cycling, however, puts less stress on muscles and joints than

---

Key Terms

Moderate-impact aerobics (MIA) Aerobics that include plyometric training.

Plyometric training A form of exercise that requires forceful jumps or springing off the ground immediately after landing from a previous jump.

Zumba An aerobics program that combines Latin and international music with dance to develop fitness and make exercise fun.

jogging does, making the former a good exercise modality for people who cannot walk or jog.

The height of the bike seat should be adjusted so the knee is flexed at about 30 degrees when the foot is at the bottom of the pedaling cycle. The body should not sway from side to side as the person rides. The cycling cadence also is important for maximal efficiency. Bike tension or gears should be set at a moderate level so the rider can achieve about 60 to 100 revolutions per minute.

Safety is a key issue in road cycling. More than a million bicycle injuries occur each year. Proper equipment and common sense are necessary. A well-designed and well-maintained bike is easier to maneuver. Toe clips are recommended to keep feet from sliding and to maintain equal upward and downward force on the pedals.

Skill is important in both road and mountain cycling. Cyclists must be in control of the bicycle at all times. They have to be able to maneuver the bike in traffic, maintain balance at slow speeds, switch gears, apply the brakes, watch for pedestrians and stoplights, ride through congested areas, and overcome a variety of obstacles in the mountains. Stationary cycling, in contrast, does not require special skills. Nearly everyone can do it.

Bike riders must follow the same rules as motorists. Many accidents happen because cyclists run traffic lights and stop signs. Some further suggestions are as follows:

1. Select the right bike. Frame size is important. The size is determined by standing flatfooted while straddling the bike. Regular bikes (road bikes) should have a 1- to 2-inch clearance between the groin and the top tube of the frame. On mountain bikes, the clearance should be about 3 inches. The recommended height of the handlebars is about 1 inch below the top of the seat. Upright handlebars are available for individuals with neck or back problems. Hard, narrow seats on road or racing bikes tend to be especially uncomfortable for women. To avoid saddle soreness, use wider and more cushioned seats such as gel-filled saddles.

2. Use bike hand signals to let the traffic around you know of your intended actions.

3. Don't ride side by side with another rider; single file is safer.

4. Be aware of turning vehicles and cars backing out of alleys and parking lots; always yield to motorists in these situations.

Tips for People Who Have Been Inactive for a While

- Take the sensible approach by starting slowly.
- Begin by choosing moderate-intensity activities you enjoy the most. By choosing activities you enjoy, you'll be more likely to stick with them.
- Gradually build up the time spent exercising by adding a few minutes every few days or so until you can comfortably perform a minimum recommended amount of exercise (20 minutes per day).
- As the minimum amount becomes easier, gradually increase either the length of time exercising or the intensity of the activity, or both.
- Vary your activities, both for interest and to broaden the range of benefits.
- Explore new physical activities.
- Reward and acknowledge your efforts.

SOURCE: Adapted from Centers for Disease Control and Prevention, Atlanta.

Try It Fill out the cardiorespiratory exercise prescription in Activity 2.3. In your Online Journal or class notebook, describe how well you implement the above suggestions.

5. Be on the lookout for storm drains, railroad tracks, and cattle guards, which can cause unpleasant surprises. Front wheels can get caught and riders may be thrown from the bike if these hazards are not crossed at the proper angle (preferably 90 degrees).

6. Wear a good helmet, certified by the Snell Memorial Foundation or the American National Standards Institute. Many serious accidents and even deaths have been prevented by the use of helmets. Fashion, aesthetics, comfort, or price should not be a factor when selecting and using a helmet for road cycling. Health and life are too precious to give up because of vanity and thriftiness.

7. Wear appropriate clothes and shoes. Clothing should be bright, very visible, lightweight, and not restrict movement. Cycling shorts are recommended to prevent skin irritation. For greater comfort, the shorts have extra padding sewn into the seat and crotch areas. They do not tend to wrinkle, and they

wick away perspiration from the skin. Shorts should be long enough to keep the skin from rubbing against the seat. Experienced cyclists also wear special shoes with a cleat that snaps directly onto the pedal.

8. Take extra warm clothing in a backpack during the winter months in case you have a breakdown and have to walk a long distance for assistance.

9. Watch out for ice in cold weather. If you see ice on car windows, expect ice on the road. Be especially careful on and under bridges because they tend to have ice even when the roads elsewhere are dry.

10. Use the brightest bicycle lights you can when riding in the dark, and always keep the batteries well charged. For additional safety, wear reflectors on the upper torso, arms, and legs so passing motorists are alerted to you. Stay on streets that have good lighting and plenty of room on the side of the road, even if that means riding an extra few minutes to get to your destination.

11. Take a cell phone if you have one, and let someone else know where you are going and when to expect you back.

Before buying a stationary bike, though, be sure to try the activity for a few days. If you enjoy it, you may want to purchase one. Invest with caution. If you opt to buy a lower-priced model, you may be disappointed. Good stationary bikes have comfortable seats, are stable, and provide a smooth and uniform pedaling motion. A sticky bike that is hard to pedal leads to discouragement and ends up being stored in the corner of a basement.

Spinning

Spinning is a low-impact activity typically performed under the direction of a certified instructor in a room or studio with dim lights, motivational music, and the noise of many bikes working together. This exercise modality gained immediate popularity upon its introduction in the mid-1990s.

Spinning, sometimes referred to as "studio" or "indoor cycling," is performed on specially designed Spinner bikes that include racing handlebars, pedals with clips, adjustable seats, and a resistance knob to control the intensity of the workout. Use of an exercise heart rate monitor is also encouraged to monitor the intensity of the various stages of the workout.

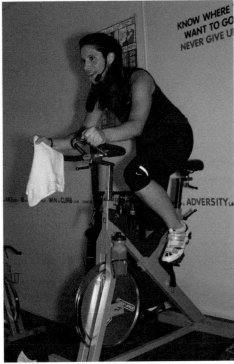

Spinning is a vigorous-intensity aerobic activity performed on specially designed spinner bikes.

Spinning programs typically combine five basic movements and five workout stages with the understanding that participants' exercise needs and goals vary. Following are the five exercise movements:

1. Seated flat—pedaling in the basic seated bike position
2. Seated hill climb—pedaling in the basic seated position but with increased resistance applied
3. Standing running—pedaling while standing up
4. Standing hill climb—pedaling standing up but with a more challenging resistance level
5. Jumping—surging out of the saddle using either controlled movements and a constant speed or at a fast pace, as during a breakaway in a bike race

The five workout stages, also known as energy zones, are used to simulate actual cycling training and racing. The workouts are divided into endurance, all-terrain, strength, recovery, and advanced training. Cadence, exercise movements, and exercise heart rate dictate the differences between the various zones. Workouts are planned according to each person's fitness level and selected percentages of maximal heart rate during each stage. These workouts provide a challenging program for people of all ages and fitness levels. The social aspect of this activity makes Spinning appealing to many exercisers.

Cross-Training

Cross-training combines two or more activities. This type of training is designed to enhance fitness, provide needed rest for tired muscles, decrease injuries, and eliminate the monotony and burnout of single-activity programs. Cross-training may combine aerobic and nonaerobic activities such as moderate jogging, speed training, and strength training.

Cross-training can produce better workouts than a single activity. For example, jogging develops the lower body and swimming builds the upper body. Rowing contributes to upper-body development and cycling builds the legs. Combining activities such as these provides good overall conditioning and at the same time helps to improve or maintain fitness. Cross-training also offers an opportunity to develop skill and have fun with differing activities.

Speed training often is coupled with cross-training. Faster performance times in aerobic activities (running, cycling) are generated with speed or **interval training**. People who want to improve their running times often run shorter intervals at faster speeds than the actual racing pace. For example, a person wanting to run a 6-minute mile may run four 440-yard intervals at a speed of 1 minute and 20 seconds per interval. A 440-yard walk/jog can become a recovery interval between fast runs.

Strength training is used commonly with cross-training. It helps to condition muscles, tendons, and ligaments. Improved strength enhances overall performance in many activities and sports. For example, although road cyclists in one study who trained with weights showed no improvement in aerobic capacity, the cyclists' riding time to exhaustion improved 33 percent when exercising at 75 percent of their maximal capacity.[5]

Rope Skipping

Rope skipping not only contributes to cardiorespiratory fitness but also helps to increase reaction time, coordination, agility, dynamic balance, and muscular strength in the lower extremities. At first, rope skipping may appear to be a highly strenuous form of aerobic exercise. As skill improves, however, the energy demands decrease considerably.

As with high-impact aerobics, a major concern of rope skipping is the stress placed on the lower extremities. Skipping with one foot at a time decreases

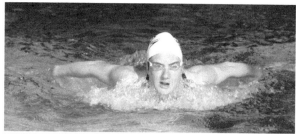

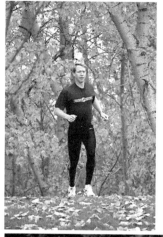

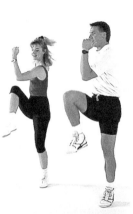

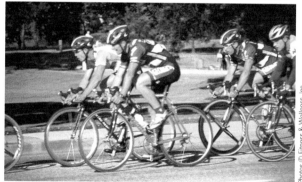

Cross-training enhances fitness, decreases the rate of injuries, and eliminates the monotony of single-activity programs.

the impact somewhat, but it does not eliminate the risk of injuries. Fitness experts recommend that skipping be used sparingly, primarily as a supplement to an aerobic exercise program.

Cross-Country Skiing

Many people consider cross-country skiing the ultimate aerobic exercise because it requires vigorous lower- and upper-body movements. The large amount of muscle mass involved in cross-country skiing makes the intensity of the activity high, yet it places little strain on muscles and joints. One of the highest maximal oxygen uptakes ever mea-

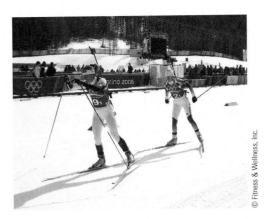

Cross-country skiing requires more oxygen and energy than most other aerobic activities.

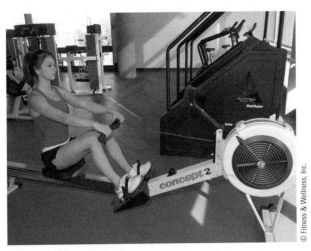

In addition to aerobic development, rowing also contributes to good strength development.

sured (85 mL/kg/min) was found in an elite cross-country skier.

In addition to being an excellent aerobic activity, cross-country skiing is soothing. Skiing through the beauty of the snow-covered countryside can be highly enjoyable. Although the need for snow is an obvious limitation, simulation equipment for year-round cross-country training is available at many sporting goods stores.

Some skill is necessary to be proficient at cross-country skiing. Poorly skilled individuals are not able to elevate the heart rate enough to cause adequate aerobic development. Individuals contemplating this activity should seek instruction to be able to fully enjoy and reap the rewards of cross-country skiing.

In-Line Skating

In-line skating has its origin in ice skating. Because warm-weather ice skating was not feasible, blades were replaced by wheels for summertime participation. The in-line concept took hold in the United States in 1980, when hockey skates were adapted for road skating.

In-line skating is an excellent activity to develop cardiorespiratory fitness and lower-body strength. Intensity of the activity is regulated by how hard you blade. The key to effective cardiorespiratory training is to maintain a constant and rhythmic pattern, using arms and legs, and minimizing the gliding phase. Because this is a weight-bearing activity, in-line skaters also develop superior leg strength.

Instruction is necessary to achieve a minimum level of proficiency in this sport. In-line skaters commonly encounter hazards—potholes, cracks, rocks, gravel, sticks, oil, street curbs, and driveways. Unskilled skaters are more prone to falls and injuries.

Good equipment will make the activity safer and more enjoyable. An adequate blade should provide strong ankle support; soft and flexible boots do not provide enough support. Small wheels offer more stability, and larger wheels enable greater speed. Blades should be purchased from stores that understand the sport and can provide sound advice according to your skill level and needs.

Protective equipment is a must for in-line skating. As in road cycling, a good helmet that meets the safety standards set by the Snell Memorial Foundation or the American National Standards Institute is important to protect yourself in case of a fall. Wrist guards and knee and elbow pads also are recommended because the kneecaps and the elbows are easily injured in a fall. Nighttime skaters should wear light-colored clothing and reflective tape.

Rowing

Rowing is a low-impact activity that provides a complete body workout. It mobilizes most major muscle groups, including those in the arms, legs, hips, abdomen, trunk, and shoulders. Rowing is a good form of aerobic exercise, and because of the nature of the activity (constant pushing and pulling against resistance), it also promotes strength development.

Key Terms

Interval training A repeated series of exercise work bouts (intervals) interspersed with low-intensity or rest intervals.

To accommodate different fitness levels, workloads can be regulated on most rowing machines. Stationary rowing, however, is not among the most popular forms of aerobic exercise. As with stationary bicycles, people should try the activity for a few weeks before purchasing a unit.

Elliptical Training/Stair Climbing

If sustained for at least 20 minutes, elliptical training and stair climbing are very efficient forms of aerobic exercise. Precisely because of the high intensity of stair climbing, many people stay away from stairs and instead take escalators and elevators. Many people dislike living in two-story homes because they have to climb the stairs frequently.

Elliptical training and stair climbing are relatively safe exercise modalities. Because the feet never leave the climbing surface, they are considered low-impact activities. Joints and ligaments are not strained while climbing. The intensity of exercise is controlled easily because the equipment can be programmed to regulate the workload.

Racquet Sports

In racquet sports such as tennis, racquetball, squash, and badminton, the aerobic benefits are dictated by players' skill, the intensity of the game, and the length of time spent playing. Skill is necessary to participate effectively in these sports and also is crucial to sustain continuous play. Frequent pauses during play do not allow people to maintain the heart rate in the appropriate target zone to stimulate cardiorespiratory development.

Many people who participate in racquet sports do so for enjoyment, social fulfillment, and relaxation. For cardiorespiratory fitness development, these people supplement the sport with other forms of aerobic exercise such as jogging, cycling, or swimming.

If a racquet sport is the main form of aerobic exercise, participants need to try to run hard, fast, and as constantly as possible during play. They should not have to spend much time retrieving balls (or, in badminton, the bird or shuttlecock). Similar to low-impact aerobics, all movements should be accentuated by reaching out and bending more than usual, for better cardiorespiratory development.

> **Critical Thinking**
>
> In your own experience with personal fitness programs throughout the years, what factors have motivated you and helped you the most to stay with a program? • What factors have kept you from being physically active, and what can you do to change these factors?

High-Intensity Interval Training

A type of training that is becoming very popular lately is **high-intensity interval training (HIIT)**. This aerobic/anaerobic training modality (80 to 90 percent of maximal capacity) had primarily been used by athletes, but it is now used by fitness participants seeking better, faster, and more effective development. Following an appropriate warm-up, HIIT includes high- to very high-intensity intervals that are interspersed with a low- to moderate-intensity recovery phase. Typically, a 1:3, 1:2, or 1:1 work-to-recovery ratio is used; the more intense the interval, the longer the recovery period. HIIT can be performed with a variety of activities, including running, cycling, elliptical training, stair climbing, and swimming. You may use the same activity for your entire HIIT, or you may use a combination of activities.

Research indicates that additional health and fitness benefits are reaped as the intensity of exercise increases. HIIT produces the greatest improvements in aerobic capacity (VO_{2max}) and increases the capability to exercise at a higher percentage of that capacity (anaerobic threshold), thus allowing the participant to burn more calories during the exercise session.

The data also show that HIIT increases the capacity for fat oxidation during exercise. Although the fuel used during high-intensity intervals is primarily glucose (carbohydrates), molecular changes occur in the muscle that increase the body's capability for fatty acid oxidation (fat burning).

Furthermore, following light- to moderate-intensity aerobic activity, resting metabolism returns to normal in about 90 minutes. Depending on the volume of training (intensity and number of intervals performed), with HIIT it takes 24 to 72 hours for the body to return to its "normal" resting metabolic rate. Thus, a greater amount of calories (primarily from fat) are burned up to three days following HIIT. While the extra calories burned during recovery can

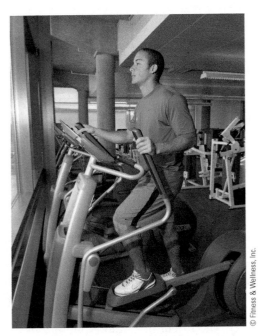

Elliptical training provides a rigorous aerobic workout.

make a difference in the long run, keep in mind that the most significant factor is the number of calories burned during the actual HIIT session. The extra calories burned during recovery are minimal compared to those used during training.

Four training variables impact HIIT. The acronym *DIRT* is frequently used to denote these variables:

D = Distance of each speed interval
I = Interval or length of recovery between speed intervals
R = Repetitions or number of speed intervals to be performed
T = Time of each speed interval

Using these four variables, a person can practically design an unlimited number of HIIT sessions.

The intervals consist of a 1:4 down to a 1:1 work-to-recovery ratio. The more intense the speed interval, the longer the required recovery interval. For aerobic intervals (lasting longer than 3 minutes), 1:2, 1:1, or even lower ratios are used. For intense anaerobic speed intervals (30 seconds to 3 minutes), recovery intervals that last two to four times as long (1:2 to 1:4) as the work period are required.

A 1:3 ratio, for example, indicates that you'll work at a fairly high intensity for, say, 30 seconds and then spend 90 seconds on light- to moderate-intensity recovery. Be sure to keep moving during the recov-

ery phase. Perform four or five intervals at first, then gradually progress to 10 intervals. As your fitness improves, you can lengthen the high-intensity proportion of the intervals progressively to 1 minute and/or decrease the total recovery time.

The following are sample programs performed using HIIT:

Five-Minute Very Hard-Intensity Aerobic Intervals

Exercise at a "very hard" rate (about 90 percent of maximal capacity) for 5 minutes, followed by 5 to 10 minutes of recovery at a "light" to "moderate" intensity. Start with one interval and work up to three by the third to fifth training session. Initially, use a 1:2 work-to-recovery ratio. Gradually decrease the recovery to a 1:1 ratio.

Step-Wise Intensity Interval Training

Using 3- to 5-minute intervals, start at a "light" intensity rate and progressively step up to the "very hard" intensity level (light, moderate, somewhat hard, vigorous, hard, and very hard). Start with 3-minute intervals and as you become more fit, increase to 5 minutes each. As time allows, and you develop greater fitness, you can add a step-down approach by stepping down to hard, vigorous, somewhat hard, moderate, and light.

Fartlek Training

The word fartlek means "speed play" in Swedish. It is an unstructured form of interval training where intensity (speed) and distance of each interval are varied as the participant wishes. There is no set structure and the individual alternates intensity (from "somewhat hard" to "very hard") and the length of each speed interval, along with the recovery intervals ("light" to "moderate") and length thereof. Total duration of fartlek training is between 20 and 60 minutes.

Key Terms

High-intensity interval training (HIIT) A training program consisting of high- to very high-intensity intervals (80 to 90 percent of maximal capacity) that are interspersed with low- to moderate-intensity recovery intervals.

Tempo Training

Although no formal intervals are conducted with tempo training, the intensity of training qualifies it as a HIIT program. Tempo runs involve continuous training between "vigorous" (70 percent) and "hard" (80 percent) for 20 to 60 minutes at a time.

All-out or Supramaximal Interval Training

All-out interval training involves 10 to 20 supramaximal or "sprint" intervals lasting 30 to 60 seconds each. Depending on the level of conditioning and the length of the speed interval, 2 to 5 minutes of recovery at a "light" to "moderate" level are allowed.

Cardio/Resistance Training Program

You may use a combination of aerobic and resistance training for HIIT. Following a brief aerobic and strength training warm-up, select about eight resistance training exercises that you can alternate with treadmill running, cycling, elliptical training, or rowing. Perform one set of 8 to 20 RM (based on personal preference) on each exercise followed by 90 seconds of aerobic work after each set. You can pace the aerobic intensity according to the preceding strength-training set. For example, you may choose a "light" intensity aerobic interval following a 10 RM for the leg press exercise and a "vigorous" aerobic interval after a 10 RM arm curl set. Allow no greater recovery time (2 to 5 seconds) between exercise modes than what it takes to walk from the strength-training exercise to the aerobic station (and vice versa).

Fitness Boot Camp

A relatively new vigorous-intensity outdoor/indoor group exercise program, **fitness boot camp** combines traditional calisthenics, running, interval training, strength training (using body weight exercises such as push-ups, lunges, pull-ups, burpees, squats), plyometrics, and competitive games to develop cardiorespiratory fitness, muscular strength, and muscular flexibility and to lose body fat. This program is based on military-style training and also aims at developing camaraderie and team effort. The program (camp) typically lasts 4 to 8 weeks. Fitness boot camps are challenging, and the group dynamic truly helps to motivate participants.

Rating the Fitness Benefits of Aerobic Activities

The fitness contributions of the aerobic activities discussed in this chapter vary according to the specific activity and the individual. As noted previously, the health-related components of physical fitness are cardiorespiratory endurance, muscular strength and endurance, muscular flexibility, and body composition. Although accurately assessing the contributions to each fitness component is difficult, a summary of likely benefits of these activities is provided in Table 2.1. Instead of a single rating or number, ranges are given for some of the categories because the benefits derived are based on the person's effort while participating in the activity.

Regular participation in aerobic activities provides notable health benefits, including an increase in cardiorespiratory endurance, quality of life, and longevity. The extent of cardiorespiratory development (improvement in VO_{2max}) depends on the intensity, duration, and frequency of the activity. The nature of the activity often dictates potential aerobic development. For example, jogging is much more strenuous than walking.

The effort during exercise also influences the amount of physiological development. The training benefits of just going through the motions of a low-impact aerobics routine are less than those of accentuating all motions (see earlier discussion of low-impact aerobics). Table 2.1 includes a starting fitness level for each aerobic activity. Beginners should start with low-intensity activities that have a minimum risk for injuries. In some cases, such as in high-impact aerobics and rope skipping, the risk of injuries remains high despite adequate conditioning. These activities should be used only to supplement training and are not recommended for beginners or as the sole mode of exercise.

Physicians who work with cardiac patients frequently use METs to measure activity levels. One **MET** represents the body's energy requirement at

| Table 2.1 | Ratings of Selected Aerobic Activities |

Activity	Recommended Starting Fitness Level[1]	Injury Risk[2]	Potential Cardiorespiratory Endurance Development (VO_{2MAX})[3,4]	Upper Body Strength Development[3]	Lower Body Strength Development[3]	Upper Body Flexibility Development[3]	Lower Body Flexibility Development[3]	Weight Management[3]	MET Level[4,5,6]	Caloric Expenditure (cal/hour)[4,6]
Aerobics										
High-Impact Aerobics	A	H	3–4	2	4	3	2	4	6–12	450–900
Moderate-Impact Aerobics	I	M	2–4	2	3	3	2	3	6–12	450–900
Low-Impact Aerobics	B	L	2–4	2	3	3	2	3	5–10	375–750
Step Aerobics	I	M	2–4	2	3–4	3	2	3–4	5–12	375–900
Cross-Country Skiing	B	M	4–5	4	4	2	2	4–5	10–16	750–1,200
Cross-Training	I	M	3–5	2–3	3–4	2–3	1–2	3–5	6–15	450–1,125
Cycling										
Road	I	M	2–5	1	4	1	1	3	6–12	450–900
Stationary	B	L	2–4	1	4	1	1	3	6–10	450–750
Hiking	B	L	2–4	1	3	1	1	3	6–10	450–750
In-Line Skating	I	M	2–4	2	4	2	2	3	6–15	450–1,125
Jogging	I	M	3–5	1	3	1	1	5	8–15	600–1,125
Jogging, Deep Water	A	L	3–5	2	2	1	1	5	8–15	600–1,125
Racquet Sports	I	M	2–4	3	3	3	2	3	6–10	450–750
Rope Skipping	I	H	3–5	2	4	1	2	3–5	8–15	600–1,125
Rowing	B	L	3–5	4	2	3	1	4	8–14	600–1,050
Spinning	I	L	4–5	1	4	1	1	4	8–15	600–1,125
Stair Climbing	B	L	3–5	1	4	1	1	4–5	8–15	600–1,125
Swimming (front crawl)	B	L	3–5	4	2	3	1	3	6–12	450–900
Walking	B	L	1–2	1	2	1	1	3	4–6	300–450
Walking, Water, Chest-Deep	I	L	2–4	2	3	1	1	3	6–10	450–750
Water Aerobics	B	L	2–4	3	3	3	2	3	6–12	450–900

[1]B = Beginner, I = Intermediate, A = Advanced

[2]L = Low, M = Moderate, H = High

[3]1 = Low, 2 = Fair, 3 = Average, 4 = Good, 5 = Excellent

[4]Varies according to the person's effort (intensity) during exercise.

[5]1 MET represents the rate of energy expenditure at rest (3.5 mL/kg/min). Each additional MET is a multiple of the resting value. For example, 5 METs represents an energy expenditure equivalent to five times the resting value, or about 17.5 mL/kg/min.

[6]Varies according to body weight.

rest, or the equivalent of a VO_2 of 3.5 mL/kg/min. A 10-MET activity requires a tenfold increase in the resting energy requirement, or approximately 35 mL/kg/min. MET levels for a given activity vary according to the individual's effort. The harder a person exercises, the higher the MET level. The MET ranges for the various activities are included in Table 2.1.

The various aerobic activities' effectiveness in aiding weight management also is indicated in Table 2.1. As a rule, the greater the muscle mass involved during exercise, the better the results. Rhythmic and continuous activities that involve considerable muscle mass are most effective in burning calories.

Higher-intensity activities burn more calories as well. Increasing exercise time will compensate for lower intensities. If carried out long enough (60 to 90 minutes, five to six times per week), even brisk walking can be a good exercise mode to lose weight. Additional information on a comprehensive weight management program is given in Chapter 6.

Skill-Related Fitness

Skill-related fitness is needed for success in athletics and effective performance of lifetime sports and activities. The components of skill-related fitness, defined in Chapter 1, are agility, balance, coordination, power, speed, and reaction time. All of these are important, to varying degrees, in sports and athletics.

For example, outstanding gymnasts must achieve good skill-related fitness in all components. Significant agility is necessary to perform a double back somersault with a full twist—a skill in which the athlete must rotate simultaneously around one axis and twist around a different one. Static balance is essential for maintaining a handstand or a scale. Dynamic balance is needed to perform many of the gymnastics routines (for example, balance beam, parallel bars, pommel horse).

Coordination is important to successfully integrate into one routine various skills requiring varying degrees of difficulty. Power and speed are needed to propel the body into the air, such as when tumbling or vaulting. Quick reaction time is necessary in determining when to end rotation upon a visual clue, such as spotting the floor on a dismount.

As with the health-related fitness components, the principle of specificity of training applies to skill-related components. According to this principle, the training program must be specific to the type of skill the individual is trying to achieve.

Development of agility, balance, coordination, and reaction time is highly task-specific. To attain a certain skill, the individual must practice the same task many times. There is little crossover learning effect from one skill to another.

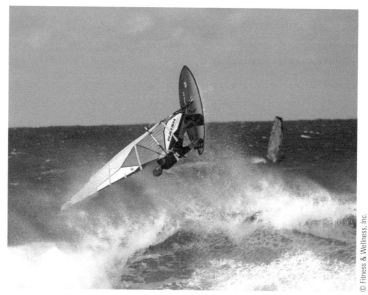

A high degree of skill-related fitness is required to participate in elite-level windsurfing.

For instance, proper practice of a handstand (balance) eventually will lead to successful performance of that skill, but complete mastery of the skill does not ensure that the person will immediately be able to transfer this mastery to other static balance positions in gymnastics. Power and speed may be improved with a specific strength-training program or frequent repetition of the specific task to be improved, or both.

The rate of learning in skill-related fitness varies from person to person, mainly because these components seem to be determined to a large extent by hereditary factors. Individuals with good skill-related fitness tend to do better and learn faster when performing a wide variety of skills. Nevertheless, few individuals enjoy complete success in all skill-related components. Furthermore, though skill-related fitness can be enhanced with practice, improvements in reaction time and speed are limited and seem to be related primarily to genetic endowment.

Although we do not know how much skill-related fitness is desirable, everyone should attempt to develop and maintain a better-than-average level. This type of fitness is crucial for athletes and also is important in leading a better and happier life. Improving skill-related fitness affords an individual more enjoyment and success in a wider variety of lifetime sports (for instance, basketball, tennis, and racquetball) and also can help a person cope more effectively in emergency situations. For example:

1. Good reaction time, balance, coordination, and agility can help you avoid a fall or break a fall and thereby minimize injury.

2. The ability to generate maximum force in a short time (power) may be crucial to ameliorate injury or even preserve life in a situation in which you may be called upon to move a person out of danger or lift a heavy object that has fallen.

3. In our society, with an expanding average life-span, maintaining speed can be especially important for older adults. Many of them and, for that matter, many unfit and overweight young people no longer have the speed they need to cross an intersection safely before the light changes for oncoming traffic.

Regular participation in a health-related fitness program can heighten performance of skill-related components, and vice versa. For example, significantly overweight people do not have good agility or speed. Because participating in aerobic and strength-training programs helps take off body fat, an overweight individual who loses weight through an exercise program may also improve agility and speed. A sound flexibility program decreases resistance to motion around body joints, which may increase agility, balance, and overall coordination. Improvements in strength definitely help develop power.

Similar to the fitness benefits of the aerobic activities discussed previously in this chapter and given in Table 2.1, the contributions of skill-related activities also vary among activities and individuals. The extent to which an activity helps develop each skill-related component varies by the effort the individual makes and, most important, by proper execution (technique) of the skill (correct coaching is highly recommended) and the individual's potential based on genetic endowment. A summary of potential contributions to skill-related fitness for selected activities is provided in Table 2.2.

Team Sports

Choosing activities that you enjoy will greatly enhance your adherence to exercise. People tend to repeat things they enjoy doing. Enjoyment by itself is a reward. Therefore, combining individual activities (such as jogging or swimming) with team sports can deepen your commitment to fitness.

Table 2.2	Contributions of Selected Activities to Skill-Related Components					
Activity	**Agility**	**Balance**	**Coordination**	**Power**	**Reaction Time**	**Speed**
Alpine Skiing	4	5	4	2	3	2
Archery	1	2	4	2	3	1
Badminton	4	3	4	2	4	3
Baseball	3	2	4	4	5	4
Basketball	4	3	4	3	4	3
Bowling	2	2	4	1	1	1
Cross-Country Skiing	3	4	3	2	2	1
Football	4	4	4	4	4	3
Golf	1	2	5	3	1	3
Gymnastics	5	5	5	4	3	3
Ice Skating	5	5	5	3	3	3
In-Line Skating	4	4	4	3	2	4
Judo/Karate	5	5	5	4	5	4
Racquetball	5	4	4	4	5	4
Soccer	5	3	5	5	3	4
Table Tennis	5	3	5	3	5	3
Tennis	4	3	5	3	5	3
Volleyball	4	3	5	4	5	3
Water Skiing	3	4	3	2	2	1
Wrestling	5	5	5	4	5	4

1 = Low, 2 = Fair, 3 = Average, 4 = Good, 5 = Excellent

© Cengage Learning 2013

People with good skill-related fitness usually participate in lifetime sports and games, which in turn helps develop health-related fitness. Individuals who enjoyed basketball or soccer in their youth tend to stick to those activities later in life. The availability of teams and community leagues may be all that is needed to stop contemplating and start participating. The social element of team sports provides added incentive to participate. Team sports offer an opportunity to interact with people who share a common interest. Being a member of a team creates responsibility—another incentive to exercise because you are expected to be there. Furthermore, team sports foster lifetime friendships, strengthening the social and emotional dimensions of wellness.

For those who were not able to participate in youth sports, it's never too late to start (see the discussion of behavior modification and motivation in

Chapter 1). Don't be afraid to select a new activity, even if that means learning new skills. The fitness and social rewards will be ample.

Tips to Enhance Your Aerobic Workout

A typical aerobic workout is divided into three parts (see Figure 2.2):

1. A 5- to 10-minute warm-up phase during which the heart rate is increased gradually to the target zone
2. The actual aerobic workout, during which the heart rate is maintained in the target zone for 20 to 60 minutes
3. A 10-minute aerobic cool-down, when the heart rate is lowered gradually toward the resting level

To monitor the target training zone, you will have to check your exercise heart rate. As described in Chapter 2, the pulse can be checked on the radial or the carotid artery. When you check the heart rate, begin with zero and count the number of beats in a 10-second period, then multiply by 6 to get the per-minute pulse rate. You should take your exercise heart rate for 10 seconds rather than a full minute because the heart rate begins to slow down 15 seconds after you stop exercising.

Feeling the pulse while exercising is difficult. Therefore, participants should stop during exercise to check the pulse. If the heart rate is too low, increase the intensity of the exercise. If the rate is too high, slow down. You may want to practice taking your pulse several times during the day to become familiar with the technique. Inexpensive heart rate monitors can also be obtained at sporting goods stores or through the Internet. These monitors increase the accuracy of monitoring the heart rate during exercise.

For the first few weeks of your program, you should monitor your heart rate several times during the exercise session. As you become familiar with your body's response to exercise, you may have to monitor the heart rate only twice—once at 5 to 7 minutes into the exercise session and a second time near the end of the workout.

Another technique sometimes used to determine your exercise intensity is simply to talk during exercise and then take your pulse immediately after that. Learning to associate the amount of difficulty when talking with the actual exercise heart rate will allow you to develop a sense of how hard you are working. Generally, if you can talk easily, you are not working hard enough. If you can talk but are slightly breathless, you should be close to the target range. If you cannot talk at all, you are working too hard.

Figure 2.2   Typical aerobic workout pattern.

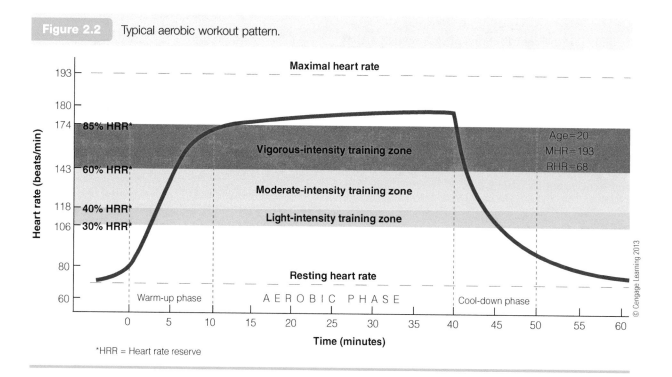

If you have difficulty keeping up with your exercise program, you may need to reconsider your goals and start much more slowly. Behavior modification is a process. From a physiological and psychological point of view, initially, you may not be able to carry out an exercise session for a full 20 to 30 minutes. For the first 2 to 3 weeks, therefore, you may just want to take a few 10-minute daily walks. As your body adapts physically and mentally, you may increase the length and intensity of the exercise sessions gradually.

Most important, learn to listen to your body. At times you will feel unusually fatigued or have much discomfort. Pain is the body's way of letting you know that something is wrong. If you have pain or undue discomfort during or after exercise, you need to slow down or discontinue your exercise program and notify the course instructor. The instructor may be able to pinpoint the reason for the discomfort or recommend that you consult your physician. You also will be able to prevent potential injuries by paying attention to pain signals and making adjustments accordingly.

Assess Your Behavior

CENGAGENOW™ Log on to www.cengagebrain.com to access CengageNOW and the Behavior Change Planner where you can take a wellness inventory to assess the behaviors that might benefit most from healthy change.

1. Are you able to incorporate a variety of activities into your exercise program?

2. Do you participate in recreational sports as a means to further enhance fitness and add enjoyment to your exercise program?

3. Do you have an alternate plan in case of inclement weather (rain/cold) or injury that would keep you from your regular training program (jogging, cycling)?

Assess Your Knowledge

CENGAGENOW™ Evaluate how well you understand the concepts presented in this chapter using the chapter-specific quizzing available in the online materials at www.cengagebrain.com.

1. Using a combination of aerobic activities to develop overall fitness is known as
   a. health-related fitness.
   b. circuit training.
   c. plyometric exercises.
   d. cross-training.
   e. skill-related fitness.

2. The best aerobic activity choice for individuals with leg or back injuries is
   a. walking in chest-deep water.
   b. jogging.
   c. step aerobics.
   d. rope skipping.
   e. cross-country skiing.

3. The approximate jogging mileage to reach the excellent cardiorespiratory fitness classification is
   a. 5 miles.
   b. 10 miles.
   c. 15 miles.
   d. 25 miles.
   e. 50 miles.

4. To help elevate the exercise heart rate during low-impact aerobics, a person should
   a. accentuate arm movements.
   b. sustain movement throughout the program.
   c. accentuate weight-bearing actions.
   d. All of the above are correct choices.
   e. None of the above choices is correct.

5. Achieved maximal heart rates during swimming are approximately _____ beats per minute (bpm) lower than during running.
   a. 2–4
   b. 5–9
   c. 10–13
   d. 14–20
   e. 20–25

6. Which of the following is not a basic movement in spinning?
   a. seated running
   b. standing hill climb
   c. seated flat
   d. jumping
   e. All of the above are exercise movements in spinning.

7. Cross-country skiing
   a. is a high-impact activity.
   b. is primarily an anaerobic activity.
   c. places great strain on muscles and joints.
   d. is a low-intensity activity.
   e. All are incorrect choices.

8. A MET represents
   a. the symbol used to indicate that the exercise goal has been met.
   b. a unit of measure that is used to express the value achieved during the Metabolic Exercise Test.
   c. the Maximal Exercise Time achieved.
   d. the rate of energy expenditure at rest.
   e. All choices are incorrect.

9. Which of the following is not a component of skill-related fitness?
   a. mobility
   b. coordination
   c. reaction time
   d. agility
   e. All are skill-related components.

10. When checking exercise heart rate, one should
    a. continue to exercise at the prescribed rate while checking the heart rate.
    b. stop exercising and take the pulse for no longer than 15 seconds.
    c. exercise at a low-to-moderate intensity.
    d. stop exercise and take the heart rate for a full minute.
    e. All choices are valid ways to check exercise heart rate.

Correct answers can be found on page 307.

My Personal Fitness Program

Name _____   Date _____

Course _____   Section _____

I. In the spaces below, provide a list of five activities in which you have participated during the last 6 months. In addition to fitness activities (jogging, aerobics, swimming, strength training), you may list other activities in which you frequently participate that require physical effort (for example, walking, cycling, sweeping, vacuuming, gardening).

   According to your own effort of participation, rate each activity for its health-related and motor skill-related benefits (1 = low, 2 = fair, 3 = average, 4 = good, 5 = excellent). Also indicate the frequency and duration of participation (list times per week, month, or 6 months) and add comments regarding your personal feelings related to your participation in the respective activity (liked it, was fun, too hard, got hurt, need more skill, could do it forever, etc.).

	Cardiorespiratory Endurance	Muscular Strength	Muscular Flexibility	Weight Management	Agility	Balance	Coordination	Power	Reaction Time	Speed
1.										

Comments

2.										

Comments

3.										

Comments

4.										

Comments

My Personal Fitness Program (continued)

	Cardiorespiratory Endurance	Muscular Strength	Muscular Flexibility	Weight Management	Agility	Balance	Coordination	Power	Reaction Time	Speed
5.										

Comments

II. On a separate sheet of paper, keep a 7-day log of all physical activities that you perform. On a daily basis, keep a record of the exact minutes throughout the day that you are active and rate each activity according to its intensity (moderate- or vigorous-intensity). Total your minutes for each day and compute a daily average for all activities. Attach the log to this activity and then answer the following questions:

A. Did you exercise aerobically at least 3 times per week for 20 to 30 minutes each session?

_____ Yes _____ No

B. Did you accumulate an average of 60 minutes of daily physical activity?

_____ Yes _____ No

C. What percentage of your total physical activity was moderate intensity,

_____ %

and what percentage was vigorous intensity?

_____ %

III. According to items I and II above, evaluate your current level of physical activity. State how you feel about your results and indicate if your program is primarily conducive to health fitness or physical fitness (or neither). Do you deem any changes necessary to meet previously stated goals (see Activity 3.4, page 100)?

_____

_____

_____

_____

_____

_____

_____

_____

_____

The Pursuit of a Healthy Diet

Ask Yourself . . .

Which of the following statements about nutrition are true, and which are false? For each false statement, what is true?

1. It is wise to eat the same foods every day.
2. Milk is such a perfect food that it alone can provide all the nutrients a person needs.
3. Cookies cannot be included in a healthful diet.
4. When it comes to nutrients, more is always better.
5. A person's energy needs are based on his or her age, gender, and physical activity levels.
6. From a nutritional standpoint, there is nothing wrong with grazing on snacks all day, provided the snacks meet nutrient needs without supplying too many calories.
7. If you don't meet your recommended intake for a nutrient every day, you will end up with a deficiency of that nutrient.
8. If a food label claims that a product is low in fat, you can believe it.
9. Most dietitians encourage people to think of their diets in terms of the four basic food groups.
10. According to the government, people should try to eat at least 2 cups of fruit and 2½ cups of vegetables—totaling 9 servings—a day.

Answers found on the following page.

Contents

For most people, eating is so habitual that they give hardly any thought to the foods they choose to eat. Yet, as Chapter 1 emphasized, the foods you select can have a profound effect on the quality, and possibly even the length, of your life. Given all the statistics and government mandates presented so far, however, designing a healthful diet may seem like a complicated matter involving a rigid regimen that excludes certain foods from the diet. Fortunately, that's not the case. The government, as well as many major health organizations, has devised dietary guidelines and tools (such as food labels) to help you choose the most healthful diet. This chapter provides an overview of some of the best guides and tools and shows you how to use them.

As you read the following pages, keep in mind that one of the biggest misconceptions about planning a healthful diet is believing that some foods (say, carrots and celery sticks) are "good," whereas others, like cookies and candy, are "bad." People who categorize foods this way often feel guilty every time they "splurge" on a so-called bad food.

If the doctors of today will not become the nutritionists of tomorrow, the nutritionists of today will become the doctors of tomorrow.

THOMAS EDISON (1847–1931, AMERICAN INVENTOR)

The overall diet is what really counts. A diet consisting of nothing but carrot sticks is just as unhealthful as one made up of only candy bars. The trick is choosing a healthful balance of foods. The ideal diet contains primarily foods that supply adequate nutrients, fiber, and calories without an excess of fat, sugar, sodium, or alcohol.

The Nutrients in Foods

Almost any food you eat is mostly water, and some foods are as high as 99 percent water. The bulk of the solid materials consists of carbohydrate, fat, and protein. If you could remove these materials, you would be left with a tiny residue of minerals, vitamins, and other materials. Water, carbohydrate, fat, protein, vitamins, and some of the minerals are **nutrients**. Some of the other materials are not nutrients. The six classes of nutrients are carbohydrate, fat, protein, vitamins, minerals, and water.

A complete chemical analysis of your body would show that it is made of similar materials in roughly the same proportions as most foods. For example, if you weigh 150 pounds (and if that is a desirable weight for you), your body contains about 90 pounds of water and about 30 pounds of fat. The other 30 pounds consist mostly of protein, carbohydrate, and the major minerals of your bones—calcium and phosphorus. Vitamins, other minerals, and incidental extras constitute only a fraction of a pound.

Scientists use the term **essential nutrient** to describe the nutrients that the body must obtain from food. About 40 nutrients are known to be *essential*; that is, they are compounds that the body cannot make for itself but are indispensable to life processes. How can you be sure you're getting all the nutrients you need? The rest of this chapter, along with the diet-planning tools presented in Chapter 2, will help you design a diet that supports good health.

The Energy-Yielding Nutrients   Upon being broken down in the body, or digested, three of the nutrients—carbohydrate, protein, and fat—yield the **energy** that the body uses to fuel its various activities. In contrast, vitamins, minerals, and water, once broken down in the body, do not yield energy but perform other tasks, such as maintenance and repair. Each gram of carbohydrate and protein consumed supplies your body with 4 calories, and each gram of fat provides 9 calories (see Figure 3-1). Only one other substance that people consume supplies calories, and that is alcohol, which provides 7 calories per gram. Alcohol is not

The six classes of nutrients:

- carbohydrate
- fat
- protein
- vitamins
- minerals
- water

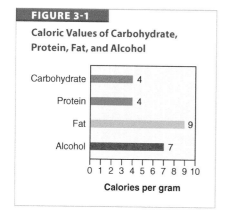

FIGURE 3-1

Caloric Values of Carbohydrate, Protein, Fat, and Alcohol

The energy-yielding nutrients:

- carbohydrate
- fat
- protein

nutrients substances obtained from food and used in the body to promote growth, maintenance, and repair. The nutrients include carbohydrate, fat, protein, vitamins, minerals, and water.

essential nutrient a nutrient that must be obtained from food because the body cannot make it for itself.

energy the capacity to do work, such as moving or heating something.

calorie the unit used to measure energy.

ASK YOURSELF ANSWERS: **1.** False. It is unwise to eat the same foods day in and day out; your diet will lack variety and probably will not supply all the nutrients your body needs. **2.** False. Milk rates as an excellent source of nutrients such as calcium and protein, but it contains only very small amounts of iron and several other essential nutrients. **3.** False. Any food can fit into a healthful eating plan. It's the total diet, not individual foods, that can be either good or bad for health. **4.** False. Too much or too little of a nutrient is often equally harmful. **5.** True. **6.** True. **7.** False. Even if you don't meet your recommended intake for a nutrient, you still may be consuming a sufficient amount of the nutrient. **8.** True. **9.** False. Dietitians today encourage people to think about eating from the five food groups in the MyPlate Food Guide. **10.** True.

considered a nutrient, however, because it does not help maintain or repair body tissues the way nutrients do.

The body uses energy from carbohydrate, fat, and protein to do work or generate heat. This energy is measured in **calories**—familiar to almost everyone as markers of how "fattening" foods are. If your body doesn't use (release) the energy you obtained from a food soon after you've eaten it, it stores that energy, usually as body fat, for later use. If a person eats excess amounts of protein, fat, or carbohydrate fairly regularly, the stored fat builds up over time and leads to obesity. Too much of any food, whether lean meat (a protein-rich food), potatoes (a high-carbohydrate food), or butter (a fatty food), can contribute excess calories that result in overweight.

Vitamins, Minerals, and Water   Unlike carbohydrate, fat, and protein, **vitamins** and **minerals** do not supply energy, or calories. Instead, they regulate the release of energy and other aspects of **metabolism**. As Table 3-1 shows, there are 13 vitamins, each with its special role to play. Vitamins are divided into two classes: water-soluble (the B vitamins and vitamin C) and fat-soluble (vitamins A, D, E, and K). This distinction has many implications for the kinds of foods that provide the different vitamins and how the body uses them, as you will see in Chapter 7.

The minerals also perform important functions. Some, such as calcium, make up the structure of bones and teeth. Others, including sodium, float about in the body's fluids, where they help regulate crucial bodily functions, such as heartbeat and muscle contractions.

Often neglected but equally vital, **water** is the medium in which all the body's processes take place. Some 60 percent of your body's weight consists of water, which carries materials to and from cells and provides the warm, nutrient-rich bath in which cells thrive. Water also transports hormonal messages from place to place. When energy-yielding nutrients release energy, they break down into water and other simple compounds. Without water, you could live only a few days.

Each day your body loses water in the form of sweat and urine. Therefore, you must replace large amounts of it—on the order of two to three quarts a day. To be sure, you don't need to *drink* that much water daily, because the foods and other beverages you consume do supply some of the water you need.

vitamins organic, or carbon-containing, essential nutrients that are vital to life but needed only in relatively minute amounts (*vita* = life; *amine* = containing nitrogen).

minerals inorganic compounds, some of which are essential nutrients.

metabolism collective term for all the chemical and physical reactions occurring in living cells, including the reactions by which the body obtains and uses energy from foods.

water provides the medium for life processes.

TABLE 3-1	The Vitamins and Minerals						
	The Vitamins				**The Minerals**		
The water-soluble vitamins:			**The fat-soluble vitamins:**	**The major minerals:**		**The trace minerals:**	
B vitamins			Vitamin A	Calcium	Potassium	Chromium	Manganese
Thiamin	Vitamin B$_{12}$		Vitamin D	Chloride	Sodium	Copper	Molybdenum
Riboflavin	Folate		Vitamin E	Magnesium	Sulfur	Fluoride	Selenium
Niacin	Biotin		Vitamin K	Phosphorus		Iodine	Zinc
Vitamin B$_6$	Pantothenic acid					Iron	
Vitamin C							

Note: A number of trace minerals are currently under study to determine possible dietary requirements for humans. These include arsenic, boron, cadmium, cobalt, lead, lithium, nickel, silicon, tin, and vanadium.

The ABCs of Eating for Health

When you plan a diet for yourself, try to make sure it has the following characteristics:

- **Adequacy** (to provide enough of the essential nutrients, fiber, and energy—in the form of calories)

- **Balance** (to avoid overemphasis on any food type or nutrient at the expense of another)

- **Calorie control** (to supply the amount of energy you need to maintain a healthy weight—not more, not less)

- **Moderation** (to avoid excess amounts of unwanted constituents, such as solid fats and added sugars)

- **Variety** (to consume different foods rather than eating the same meals day after day)

Equally important, be sure that your diet suits you—that it consists of foods that fit your personality, family and cultural traditions, lifestyle, and budget. At best, your diet can be a source of both pleasure and good health.

Adequacy   Any nutrient can be used to demonstrate the importance of dietary adequacy. For example, iron is an essential nutrient that your body loses daily; it must be replaced continually by iron-rich foods. If your diet does not provide adequate iron—that is, if it lacks food sources of the mineral—you can develop a condition known as *iron-deficiency anemia*. If you add iron-rich foods such as meat, fish, poultry, and legumes to your diet, the condition is likely to disappear soon. (More information about iron appears in Chapter 8.)

Balance   To appreciate the importance of balance, consider a second essential nutrient. Calcium plays a vital role in building a strong frame that can withstand the gradual bone loss that occurs with age. Thus, adults are advised to consume three cups of milk or milk products (the best sources of this bone-building mineral) daily to meet their calcium needs. Foods that are rich in calcium typically lack iron, however, and vice versa; so you have to balance the two in your diet.

Balancing the whole diet is a juggling act that, if successful, provides enough, but not too much, of each of the 40-odd nutrients the body needs for good health. As you will see later in the chapter, you can design a diet that is both adequate and balanced by using food group plans that help you choose from various groups the specific amounts of foods that should be eaten each day.

Calorie Control   To maintain a healthy weight, energy intakes should not exceed energy needs. Calorie control helps ensure a balance between energy we take in from food and energy we expend in activity. A cup and a half of ice cream, for example, has about the same amount of calcium as a cup of milk, but the ice cream may contain more than 500 calories, whereas the milk may supply only 90. When it comes to iron, a 3-ounce serving of beef pot roast provides about twice the amount of the mineral as a 3-ounce serving of canned tuna. But whereas the beef contains 280 calories, the tuna adds only about 100 calories to the diet. The choice of which one to eat depends on personal preferences as well as the nutrient and calorie content of the other foods in the total diet.

Diet-planning principles:

- Adequacy
- Balance
- Calorie control
- Nutrient density
- Moderation
- Variety

adequacy characterizes a diet that provides all of the essential nutrients, fiber, and energy (calories) in amounts sufficient to maintain health.

balance a feature of a diet that provides a number of types of foods in harmony with one another, such that foods rich in one nutrient do not crowd out of the diet foods that are rich in another nutrient.

calorie control control of consumption of energy (calories); a feature of a sound diet plan.

moderation the attribute of a diet that provides no unwanted constituent in excess.

variety a feature of a diet in which different foods are used for the same purposes on different occasions; the opposite of *monotony*.

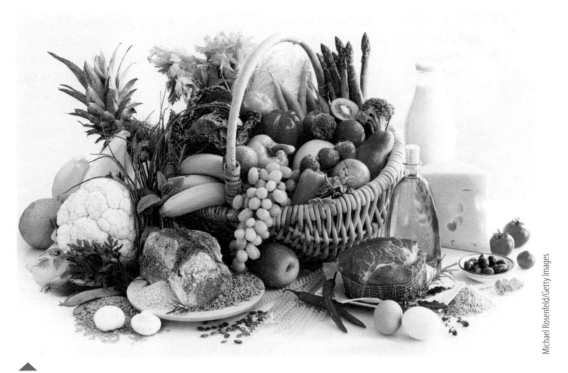

Variety fosters good nutrition.

Those who are trying to ensure optimal intakes of nutrients without excess calories should be sure to include foods that are rich in nutrients (protein, vitamins, and minerals) but relatively low in calories and fat. Such foods are referred to as **nutrient dense**. A baked potato, for example, contains more iron and vitamin C for its calories than French fries. Hence, it is more nutrient dense. Figure 3-2 compares the nutrient density of selected beverages.

nutrient dense refers to a food that supplies large amounts of nutrients relative to the number of calories it contains. The higher the level of nutrients and the fewer the number of calories, the more nutrient dense the food is.

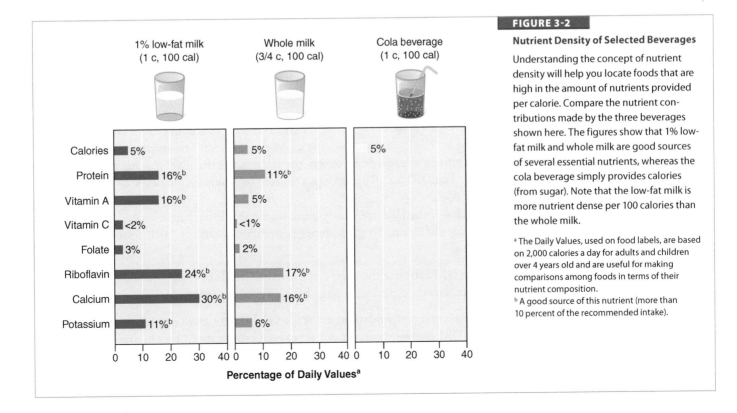

FIGURE 3-2

Nutrient Density of Selected Beverages

Understanding the concept of nutrient density will help you locate foods that are high in the amount of nutrients provided per calorie. Compare the nutrient contributions made by the three beverages shown here. The figures show that 1% low-fat milk and whole milk are good sources of several essential nutrients, whereas the cola beverage simply provides calories (from sugar). Note that the low-fat milk is more nutrient dense per 100 calories than the whole milk.

[a] The Daily Values, used on food labels, are based on 2,000 calories a day for adults and children over 4 years old and are useful for making comparisons among foods in terms of their nutrient composition.
[b] A good source of this nutrient (more than 10 percent of the recommended intake).

Moderation Another characteristic of a healthy diet is moderation. In other words, try to eat meals that do not contain excessive amounts of any one nutrient, such as solid fats, which are major sources of saturated and *trans* fatty acids (discussed in Chapter 5), the culprits linked to a number of chronic diseases. That's not to say that you should choose only foods that supply little or no fat. Such an approach is unrealistic and will only lead to frustration. Practice moderation by choosing such foods only on occasion (milkshake versus fat-free milk) and regularly choosing the most nutrient-dense foods from all food groups without exceeding overall calorie needs.

Variety Aside from avoiding the monotony of eating the same foods day after day, we need variety in our diet for several reasons. First, some foods are better sources of nutrients needed in such small amounts that we don't consciously plan diets around them. Second, variety improves nutrient adequacy, as foods within a specific food group may contain different amounts of nutrients. For example, when selecting fruits, oranges are an excellent source of vitamin C, but a slice of cantaloupe would be a better choice for vitamin A. Finally, a limited diet can supply excess amounts of undesirable substances such as chemical contaminants. Eating many different foods, in contrast, greatly reduces the likelihood that large amounts of a potential toxin will be consumed.

Research underscores that variety is one of the hallmarks of a healthful diet.[1] If your diet lacks variety, chances are good that you're missing out on many nutrients necessary for optimal health. The Japanese, incidentally, recognize variety as such an important part of healthful eating that their dietary guidelines recommend consuming 30 or more different kinds of food *every* day to achieve a balance of essential nutrients.[2]

Nutrient Recommendations

At this point, knowing that foods are made of so many different combinations of nutrients, you may be wondering how to determine whether you are eating the right balance of nutrients. Obviously, if your diet lacks any of the essential nutrients, you may develop deficiencies. Even if you don't develop a full-blown deficiency disease, when you are less than optimally nourished you may get sick more easily and suffer other health problems. To help prevent such problems and provide a benchmark for people's nutrient needs, experts in Canada and the United States devised the **Dietary Reference Intakes (DRI)** for planning and assessing diets of healthy people in both countries.[3]

The Dietary Reference Intakes (DRI) A committee of nutrition experts selected by the National Academy of Sciences (NAS) sets forth the DRI—a set of daily nutrient standards based on the latest scientific evidence regarding diet and health. The DRI for all age groups are listed on Study Cards pages 27–29 at the back of this book.

Although the DRI are widely used, many people have misconceptions about their meaning and intent. To get a proper perspective about the DRI, consider the following facts:

- The DRI estimate the energy and nutrient needs of *healthy* people. People with certain medical problems often have different nutritional needs.

- Separate recommendations are made for different groups of people. For instance, the DRI committee issues one set of recommendations for children ages 4 through 8, another set for adult men, another for pregnant women, and so on. The DRI may evolve over time because of new scientific evidence indicating a need for reevaluation of current concepts and recommended intakes.[4]

Most fats with a high percentage of saturated and/or *trans* fatty acids are solid at room temperature and are referred to as solid fats (see Chapter 5). Common solid fats include butter, beef fat, chicken fat, pork fat (lard), stick margarine, and shortening. The fat in whole milk is also considered to be solid fat since it is solid at room temperature but suspended in milk by the process of homogenization.

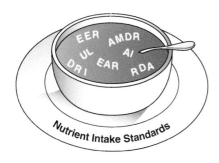

Dietary Reference Intakes (DRI) a set of reference values for energy and nutrients that can be used for planning and assessing diets for healthy people.

FIGURE 3-3

The Correct View of the DRI

This figure shows that people with intakes below the EAR are likely to have dietary adequacy of 50 percent or less. People with intakes between the EAR and RDA are likely to have adequacy between 50 and 97–98 percent. Intakes between the RDA or AI and the UL are likely to be adequate. At intakes above the UL, the risk of harm increases.

People often think that more is better when it comes to nutrients. Too much of a good thing can be dangerous, however, so the RDA, AI, and AMDR fall within an optimal margin of safety, and the UL help people avoid harmful excesses of nutrients.

SOURCE: Adapted from Institute of Medicine, *Dietary Intakes for Energy, Carbohydrate, Fiber, Fat, Fatty Acids, Cholesterol, Protein, and Amino Acids* (Washington, DC: National Academy Press, 2002).

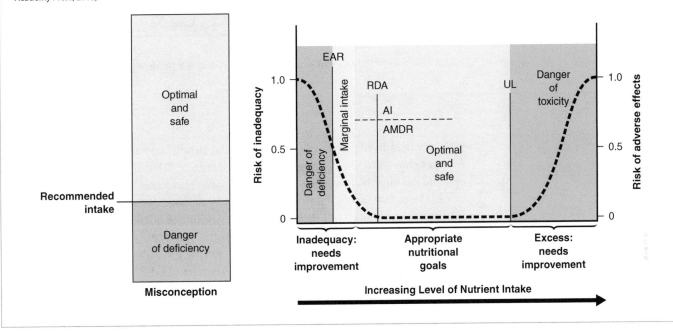

- The DRI take into account differences among individuals and establish a range within which the nutritional needs of virtually all healthy people in a particular age and gender group will be covered (see Figure 3-3).

- The DRI are illustrated in Figure 3-3 and include:
  - Estimated Average Requirement (EAR)
  - Recommended Dietary Allowances (RDA)
  - Adequate Intakes (AI)
  - Tolerable Upper Intake Levels (UL)
  - Estimated Energy Requirement (EER)
  - Acceptable Macronutrient Distribution Ranges (AMDR)

The DRI for Nutrients The DRI aim to prevent nutrient deficiencies in a population as well as reduce risk for chronic diseases such as heart disease, cancer, and osteoporosis. To understand the process of developing the new DRI, consider the following discussion. Suppose we were the committee members, and we were called upon to set the DRI for nutrient X. First, we would determine the **requirement**—how much of that nutrient the average healthy person needs to prevent a deficiency. To do so, we would review scientific research and explore how the body stores the nutrient, what the consequence of a deficiency might be, what causes depletion of the nutrient, and what other factors affect a person's need for nutrient X. We would also consider current concepts regarding the amount of the nutrient needed for reducing risk of chronic disease (for example, optimal calcium intake and reduced risk of bone

requirement the minimum amount of a nutrient that will prevent the development of deficiency symptoms. Requirements differ from the RDA and AI, which include a substantial margin of safety to cover the requirements of different individuals.

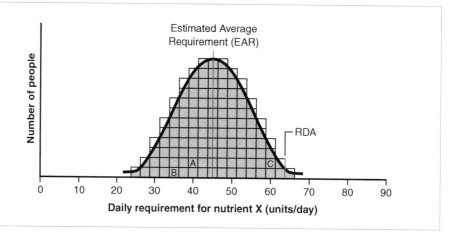

fractures later in life). However, we know that people vary in the amount of a given nutrient they need. Mr. A might need an average of 40 units of nutrient X daily for optimal health; Ms. B might need 35; Mr. C, 60; and so on.

Our next task would be to determine what amount of nutrient X to recommend for the general public. In other words, what amount of nutrient X would we consider optimal for covering most people's needs without posing a hazard? One option would be to set it at the average requirement for nutrient X (shown in Figure 3-4 at 45 units). This is the **Estimated Average Requirement (EAR)**: the amount of a nutrient that is estimated to meet the requirement for the nutrient in half of the people of a specific age and gender. But if we did so and people took us literally, half the population—Mr. C and everyone else whose requirement is greater than 45—would eventually develop deficiencies.

Instead, we use the EAR to set the **Recommended Dietary Allowance (RDA)**. To benefit the most people, the RDA is set at a point high enough to cover most healthy people without creating an excess in people who do not require as much nutrient X. In this case, a reasonable choice might be 63 units, which would add a generous safety margin to ensure that just about all healthy people are covered (see Figure 3-4).

If sufficient scientific evidence is not available for us to set an EAR—the requirement for nutrient X—that is needed to establish an RDA, an **Adequate Intake (AI)** is provided instead of an RDA.* Because sufficient scientific evidence is lacking, the AI is based on our best estimate of the need for nutrient X in practically all apparently healthy individuals of a specific age and gender. Individuals may use both the RDA and the AI as goals for nutrient intake.

For healthy individuals, no established benefits result from consuming amounts of a nutrient that exceed the recommended intake (the RDA or AI). However, the DRI include a **Tolerable Upper Intake Level (UL)**, which is the maximum daily intake of a nutrient that is unlikely to pose risk of *adverse* effects in healthy people. The UL exceeds the RDA and is not intended to be a recommended level of intake (refer to Figure 3-3). The need to set ULs is the result of more and more people using large doses of nutrient supplements and the increasing availability of **fortified foods**. Individuals can use the UL to determine whether their levels of nutrient intakes may pose risk of adverse effects over time.

fortified foods foods to which nutrients have been added, either because they were not already present or because they were present in insignificant amounts; foods to which manufacturers have added 10 percent or more of the Daily Value for a particular nutrient. Examples: margarine with added vitamin A, milk with added vitamin D, certain brands of orange juice with added calcium, and breakfast cereals with added nutrients and nonnutrients.

---

*This text refers to the nutrient recommendations (for example, RDA and AI) as DRI recommended intakes.

Miniglossary of DRI Terms

EAR, Estimated Average Requirement the amount of a nutrient that is estimated to meet the requirement for the nutrient in half of the people of a specific age and gender. The EAR is used in setting the RDA.

RDA, Recommended Dietary Allowance the average daily amount of a nutrient that is sufficient to meet the nutrient needs of nearly all (97–98 percent) healthy individuals of a specific age and gender.

AI, Adequate Intake the average amount of a nutrient that appears to be adequate for individuals when there is not sufficient scientific research to calculate an RDA. The AI exceeds the EAR and possibly the RDA.

UL, Tolerable Upper Intake Level the maximum amount of a nutrient that is unlikely to pose any risk of adverse health effects to most healthy people. The UL is not intended to be a recommended level of intake.

EER, Estimated Energy Requirement the average calorie intake that is predicted to maintain energy balance in a healthy adult of a defined age, gender, weight, height, and level of physical activity, consistent with good health.

AMDR, Acceptable Macronutrient Distribution Range a range of intakes for a particular energy source (carbohydrates, fat, protein) that is associated with a reduced risk of chronic disease while providing adequate intakes of essential nutrients.

Dietary Reference Intakes (DRIs)

DRI for Nutrients:
- EAR
- RDA
- AI
- UL

DRI for Energy & Energy Nutrients:
- EER
- AMDR

The DRI represent a major shift in thinking about nutrient requirements for humans, from prevention of nutrient deficiencies to prevention of chronic disease. They also herald a new way of thinking about the role of dietary supplements in achieving good health—such that, for some individuals at higher risk, use of nutrient supplements may be desirable so as to meet recommended intakes. For example, older women who are at risk of osteoporosis may benefit from dietary calcium supplements to help maintain bone mineral mass. In addition, the development of the UL signals the widespread recognition that high intakes of nutrients can create a degree of risk.

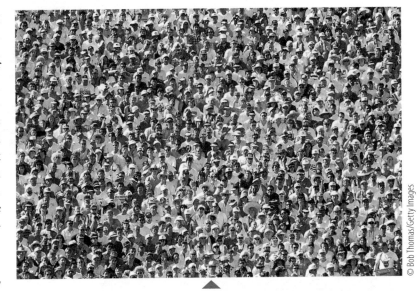

People vary in the amount of a given nutrient they need. The challenge of the DRI is to determine the best amount to recommend for everybody.

The DRI for Energy and the Energy Nutrients

The DRI report on energy and the energy nutrients provides guidelines for the United States and Canada regarding the consumption of energy, carbohydrates, fiber, fat, fatty acids, cholesterol, and protein; it includes guidelines for physical activity as well. To meet the body's daily energy and nutritional needs while minimizing risk for chronic disease, consumption of the energy nutrients should resemble the pattern shown in Figure 3-5.

To reduce the risk of chronic disease, the DRI report stresses the need to balance caloric intake with physical activity, recommending total calories to be consumed by individuals of given heights, weights, and genders for each of four different levels of physical activity (from sedentary to very active). For more about weight management and specific physical activity guidelines, see Chapters 10 and 11 as well as Study Card page 55 at the back of this book.

The Challenge of Dietary Guidelines

As Chapter 1 pointed out, health authorities are as concerned today about widespread nutrient excesses among Americans as they used to be about nutrient deficiencies. This is where dietary guidelines come into play. Among the most widely used of the guidelines are the *Dietary Guidelines for Americans*. The Eating Well with Canada's Food Guide recommendations presented in Appendix B are also commonly used.[5]

FIGURE 3-5

Recommended Dietary Intake Ranges for Energy Nutrients

A balanced diet is composed of approximately 10–35 percent protein, 45–65 percent carbohydrates (with no more than 10 percent of this amount from added sugars or caloric sweeteners), and 20–35 percent from fat, but derived mostly from oils rather than solid fats. Currently, most Americans consume about 15 percent of their calories from protein, 49 percent from carbohydrates (with 16 percent of this amount coming from simple sugars), and 34 percent of their total calories from fat.

Dietary Reference Intakes (DRI) for Carbohydrates, Fats, and Protein

Carbohydrates	45 to 65 percent of total calories
Fats	20 to 35 percent of total calories
Protein	10 to 35 percent of total calories

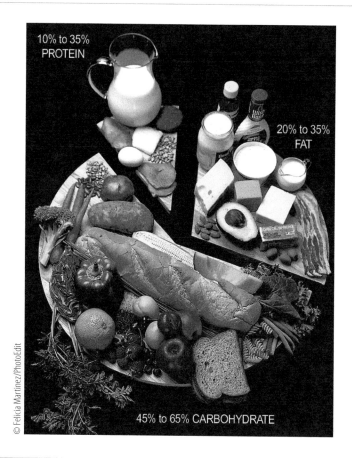

10% to 35% PROTEIN

20% to 35% FAT

45% to 65% CARBOHYDRATE

© Felicia Martinez/PhotoEdit

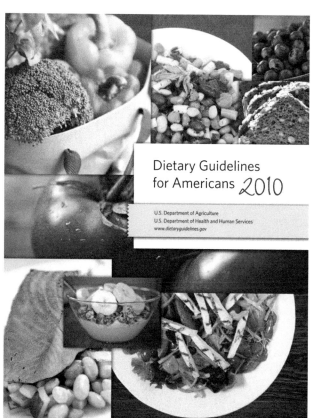

Dietary Guidelines for Americans 2010

U.S. Department of Agriculture
U.S. Department of Health and Human Services
www.dietaryguidelines.gov

USDA

The *Dietary Guidelines for Americans* provide science-based advice to promote health and to reduce risk for chronic diseases through diet and physical activity. They emphasize variety, calorie control, moderation, and nutrient density. The guidelines also emphasize physical activity because it increases energy expenditure and helps in maintaining a healthy weight.

Table 3-2 presents the *Dietary Guidelines for Americans, 2010* grouped into four general topics, along with their key recommendations. The new guidelines incorporate two general themes: maintaining calorie balance over time to achieve and maintain a healthy weight, and consuming more nutrient-dense foods and beverages. Americans currently consume too much sodium and too many calories from solid fats, added sugars, and refined grains. These replace nutrient-dense foods and beverages and make it difficult for people to achieve recommended nutrient intakes without exceeding their energy needs. For this reason, the *Dietary Guidelines* emphasize three major goals for building healthy eating patterns:

- Balance calories with physical activity to manage weight.

- Consume more nutrient-dense foods such as fruits, vegetables, whole grains, fat-free and low-fat (1%) milk products, seafood, lean meats and poultry, eggs, beans and peas, and unsalted nuts and seeds.

Balancing Calories to Manage Weight
- Prevent and/or reduce overweight and obesity through improved eating and physical activity behaviors.
- Control total calorie intake to manage body weight. For people who are overweight or obese, this will mean consuming fewer calories from foods and beverages.
- Increase physical activity and reduce time spent in sedentary behaviors.
- Maintain appropriate calorie balance during each stage of life—childhood, adolescence, adulthood, pregnancy and breastfeeding, and older age.

Foods and Food Components to Reduce
- Reduce daily sodium intake to less than 2,300 milligrams (mg) and further reduce sodium intake to 1,500 mg among persons who are 51 and older and those of any age who are African American or have hypertension, diabetes, or chronic kidney disease.
- Consume less than 10 percent of calories from saturated fat by replacing it with monounsaturated and polyunsaturated fats.
- Consume less than 300 mg per day of dietary cholesterol.
- Keep trans fat consumption as low as possible by limiting foods such as partially hydrogenated oils, and by limiting other solid fats.
- Reduce the intake of calories from solid fats and added sugars.
- Limit the consumption of foods that contain refined grains, especially refined grain foods that contain solid fats, added sugars, and sodium.
- If alcohol is consumed, it should be consumed in moderation—up to one drink per day for women and two drinks per day for men.

Foods and Nutrients to Increase
Individuals should meet the following recommendations as part of a healthy eating pattern while staying within their calorie needs.
- Increase vegetable and fruit intake.
- Eat a variety of vegetables, especially dark-green and red and orange vegetables and beans and peas.
- Consume at least half of all grains as whole grains. Increase whole-grain intake by replacing refined grains with whole grains.
- Increase intake of fat-free or low-fat milk and milk products, such as milk, yogurt, cheese, or fortified soy beverages.
- Choose a variety of protein foods, which include seafood, lean meat and poultry, eggs, beans and peas, soy products, and unsalted nuts and seeds.
- Increase the amount and variety of seafood consumed by choosing seafood in place of some meat and poultry.
- Replace protein foods that are higher in solid fats with choices that are lower in solid fats and calories and/or are sources of oils.
- Use oils to replace solid fats where possible.
- Choose foods that provide more potassium, dietary fiber, calcium, and vitamin D, which are nutrients of concern in American diets. These foods include vegetables, fruits, whole grains, and milk and milk products.

Building Healthy Eating Patterns
- Select an eating pattern that meets nutrient needs over time at an appropriate calorie level.
- Account for all foods and beverages consumed and assess how they fit within a total healthy eating pattern.
- Follow food safety recommendations when preparing and eating foods to reduce the risk of foodborne illnesses.

Note: These guidelines are intended for adults and children ages 2 years and older, including those who are at increased risk of chronic disease. The *Dietary Guidelines for Americans, 2010* contains additional recommendations for specific populations. The full document is available at http://www.cnpp.usda.gov/Publications/DietaryGuidelines/2010/PolicyDoc/PolicyDoc.pdf

SOURCE: U.S. Department of Agriculture and U.S. Department of Health and Human Services, *Dietary Guidelines for Americans, 2010.* 7th ed. (Washington, DC: U.S. Government Printing Office, 2010).

- Consume fewer foods with sodium (salt), saturated fats, trans fats, cholesterol, added sugars, and refined grains.

Healthful eating and regular physical activity enable people of all ages to work productively, enjoy life, and feel their best. They also help children grow, develop, and do well in school. The goal of the *Dietary Guidelines* is to help people decrease their risk of some forms of cancer, heart disease, obesity, diabetes, high blood pressure, stroke, osteoporosis, and liver disease—the so-called **lifestyle diseases**. Following such recommendations certainly makes sense, given the considerable potential health benefits they confer.

Introducing the MyPlate Diet-Planning Tool

Although the DRI and the *Dietary Guidelines* provide good frameworks for healthful eating, planning daily menus requires use of other, more specific tools. Dietitians and other nutrition experts often rely on a number of tools that you, too, can use to assess and plan your own diet.

lifestyle diseases conditions that may be aggravated by modern lifestyles that include too little exercise, poor diets, and excessive drinking and smoking. Lifestyle diseases are also referred to as *diseases of affluence*.

It's 3:30 in the afternoon, and that sound you just heard is coming from your stomach. Physiologically speaking, the human digestive system is customized for us to eat about every four hours to maintain our energy level. So, it's not unreasonable to get a little hungry between meals or before we go to bed. In fact, it is now clear that healthy snacking can fit into any eating plan and is important to everyone's health.[6]

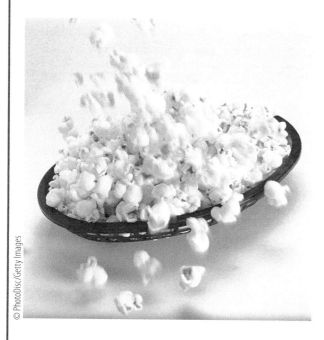

© PhotoDisc/Getty Images

Still, although **grazing** is "in," many people feel a twinge of guilt now and then about between-meal munching. Perhaps parental warnings from childhood that snacks can spoil a meal linger in the back of many minds. Nevertheless, nutritious nibbling can make it easier for many people to eat healthfully.

Snacks can supply essential vitamins, minerals, and calories to diets of young children, who often cannot eat large portions at mealtime because of their small stomachs and appetites. Teenagers typically don't seem to have the time (or inclination) to eat regularly, due to busy school schedules, sports practices, music lessons, or other activities. Snacks account for approximately 25 percent of the calories they eat and are often more energy dense than their meals.[7]

Snacks also contribute to nutritional needs of adults, who may find that fitting meals into a busy schedule is difficult. Even older adults, whose lifestyles tend to be less hectic, can benefit from

grazing eating small amounts of food at intervals throughout the day rather than or in addition to eating regular meals.

grazing. That's because lack of activity, certain medications, and isolation can blunt a formerly hearty appetite, making frequent, small meals more desirable than large breakfasts, lunches, and dinners. And, of course, a college student's busy life makes it difficult, if not impossible, to plan meals and snacks in advance, so snacking is a factor at any age.

The key to healthful snacking for everyone is to choose healthful, high-fiber, nutrient-dense foods instead of snacks that add unhealthful fats and calories to the diet and little else in the way of nutrients. A snack with a balance of carbohydrate, some fat, and some protein will satisfy hunger for a longer period of time than food with only carbohydrate or sugars (such as candy or soft drinks). How do you achieve this balance? Choosing snacks that contain at least two food groups can provide yummy and healthful snack possibilities.

Some snacks that appear nutritious may be deceiving. For example, fruit drinks, mixes, and punches are loaded with sugar (usually in the form of high-fructose corn syrup) and are more similar to soft drinks than to fruit juice. Fruit rolls and bars are nutritionally similar to jams and jelly, not fresh fruit. For these snacks, sugar is added and most of the nutrients are lost when the fruit is processed with heat. Energy and protein bars can also be deceiving because, like candy bars, many are loaded with sugar and fat. Even some varieties of microwave popcorn don't rate well as snacks, because they contain so much oil and salt. (You can easily make your own popcorn in the microwave oven without adding excessive extras.) When you feel like snacking, try some of the alternatives offered in Table 3-3. These snacks provide at least two food groups and 100–250 calories per serving.[8] Use Table 3-4 as a guide for choosing healthful snacks instead of calorie-dense snacks with little nutritional value. In addition, consider the following tips next time you're in the mood to grab a snack:

- Stock your refrigerator and kitchen cupboards with healthful foods like fruit juices, low-fat yogurt, fresh fruits and vegetables, plain popcorn, whole-grain crackers, and low-fat cheeses so that they are close at hand. Nibblers often reach for a snack

TABLE 3-3	Smart Snacking

- Low-fat yogurt with ½ cup cereal
- Fruit and yogurt smoothies
- 1-ounce serving trail mix (nuts, seeds, dried fruits)
- 1 cup cereal with low-fat milk or soy milk
- A *small* handful of tortilla chips with salsa or low-fat bean dip
- Fruit and cheese: apples or grapes with 1 ounce low-fat mozzarella string cheese
- 1–2 tablespoons peanut butter on an apple, celery, or carrots

just to have something to munch on rather than because of a desire for the food itself. If nutritious choices are easy to get to, chances are that's what you'll eat.

- Carry fresh fruit and crackers and cheese in your backpack or book bag so you won't have to resort to buying candy from a vending machine when you get the urge to munch.
- Create your own snacks. Mix together one cup each whole-grain cereal, almonds, raisins, and sunflower seeds to take with you on your next bicycle trip or hike.
- Make new versions of old favorites, such as *Chili Popcorn* and *Mexican Snack Pizzas*.[9]
- Snack with a friend. If you're craving a candy bar or chips and nothing else will do, try splitting a bar or a bag with a friend. That way, you'll satisfy your craving without going too far overboard on calories, fat, or salt.
- Try to brush your teeth—or at least rinse your mouth thoroughly—after snacking to prevent tooth decay. (See pp. 119–120 in Chapter 4 for a detailed explanation of the role of diet in dental health.)

Chili Popcorn

Mix 1 quart popped popcorn with 1 tablespoon melted margarine. In a separate bowl, mix 1¼ teaspoons chili powder, ¼ teaspoon cumin, and a dash of garlic powder. Sprinkle seasonings over popcorn and mix well. Makes about four 1-cup servings, each of which contains approximately 50 calories, 3 grams of fat, and 42 milligrams of sodium.

Mexican Snack Pizzas

Split two whole-grain English muffins and toast lightly. Mix ¼ cup tomato paste; ¼ cup canned, drained, chopped kidney beans; 1 tablespoon each chopped onion and chopped green pepper; and ½ teaspoon oregano. Spread mixture on muffin halves. Top with ¼ cup shredded part-skim mozzarella cheese and broil until cheese is bubbly (about 2 minutes). Garnish with ¼ cup shredded lettuce. Makes four servings, each of which contains 95 calories, 2 grams of fat, and 300 milligrams of sodium.

TABLE 3-4 What's in a Muncher's Healthy Snacking Menu?

100 Calories of Grains				
1½ slices whole wheat bread	or	⅔ Lender's Original® wheat bagel	or	2/7 Dunkin' Donuts® plain bagel
1 c Kellogg's Corn Flakes®	or	scant ½ c Kellogg's Just Right® with fruit and nuts	or	¼ c Kellogg's Healthy Choice Low Fat Granola® (without raisins)
100 Calories of Fruit				
1¼ fresh apple	or	1 c unsweetened applesauce	or	½ c sweetened applesauce
2 heaping cups fresh strawberries	or	½ c frozen, sweetened strawberries	or	2 tbsp strawberry jam
100 Calories of Dairy				
⅗ c 1% cottage cheese	or	4⅓ tbsp grated Parmesan cheese	or	2 tbsp cream cheese
100 Calories of Potato				
½ plain baked potato with skin	or	½ c mashed potato	or	10 French fries
100 Calories of Protein Foods (meats, poultry, fish, beans, nuts)				
2 oz roasted tip round beef	or	1.4 oz extra lean broiled ground beef	or	1.2 oz regular broiled ground beef
2.1 oz roasted chicken breast without skin	or	1.4 oz KFC Original Recipe® chicken breast with skin	or	6 macadamia nuts
3 oz baked/broiled haddock	or	⅛ oz Mrs. Paul's Select Cut® frozen haddock fillets (breaded)		
⅜ c chickpeas	or	¼ c hummus (made with chickpeas)		
29 pistachios	or	15 almonds		
100 Calories of "Eat Sparingly" Foods				
Scant ½ cup soft-serve vanilla frozen yogurt	or	⅜ c regular vanilla ice cream	or	3/16 c Haagen-Dazs® vanilla ice cream
			or	10/11 fudge-covered Oreo®
2⅓ reduced-fat Oreos®	or	1⅖ regular Oreos®	or	5/14 Snickers® bar
⅘ Reese's Peanut Butter Cup®	or	½ Chunky® bar		

SOURCE: Adapted from "For 100 Calories, You Can Have . . . ," *Tufts University Health & Nutrition Letter* (July 2000): 8.

One of the most helpful, easy-to-use diet-planning tools is the **food group plan**, which separates foods into specific groups and then specifies the number of **servings** from each group to eat each day. The MyPlate food guide is presented in detail in Figure 3-6. This tool includes five food groups and presents tips for choosing foods from within each group.

The MyPlate Food Guidance System provides food-based guidance to help implement the recommendations of the *Dietary Guidelines for Americans* and provides a visual aid to assist in improving diet and lifestyle. MyPlate is designed to help you:

- Make smart choices from every food group;

- Find your balance between food and physical activity; and

- Get the most nutrition out of your calories by focusing on nutrient-dense foods in sensible portion sizes.

Using MyPlate to Achieve a Healthy Lifestyle

MyPlate is designed to help consumers choose foods that supply a good balance of nutrients, and it aims to moderate or limit dietary components often consumed in excess, such as saturated fat, *trans* fat, sugar, sodium, and alcohol, in keeping with the U.S. government's *Dietary Guidelines for Americans*. MyPlate includes six key components that can help you achieve a healthy lifestyle, including:

1. **Activity.** The MyPlate website promotes regular physical activity and reduced sedentary activities. As part of an overall healthful diet, balancing caloric intake with energy needs can help reduce the risk of chronic disease, help prevent weight gain, and help sustain weight loss. Adults should do at least 2 hours and 30 minutes each week of aerobic physical activity at a moderate level or 1 hour and 15 minutes each week of aerobic physical activity at a vigorous level.
2. **Variety.** MyPlate creates a foundation for good nutrition and health by guiding us to make food selections from all food groups and subgroups. Different foods contain different nutrients and other substances known to be protective against chronic diseases. No one food or no single food group provides all essential nutrients in amounts necessary for good health.
3. **Proportionality.** MyPlate shows the proportions of foods that should make up a healthful diet. MyPlate illustrates the five food groups using a familiar mealtime visual, a place setting. The plate is split into four sections: red for fruits, green for vegetables, purple for protein, and orange for grains (refer to Figure 3-6). A separate blue section, shaped like a drinking glass, represents dairy foods. MyPlate provides a visual reminder of a key nutrition principle: Fruits and

---

In June 2011, MyPlate replaced MyPyramid (released in April 2005), which replaced the Food Guide Pyramid (1992). The older food guide materials are archived at www.ChooseMyPlate.gov.

Some examples of moderate physical activity are walking briskly, mowing the lawn, dancing, swimming, and bicycling on level terrain. Some examples of vigorous physical activity are jogging, high-impact aerobic dancing, swimming continuous laps, and bicycling uphill.

food group plan a diet-planning tool, such as MyPlate, that groups foods according to similar origin and nutrient content and then specifies the amount of food a person should eat from each group.

serving the standard amount of food used as a reference to give advice regarding how much to eat (such as a 1-cup serving of milk).

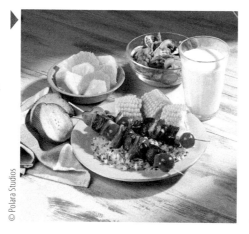

The MyPlate Food Guidance System calls for eating a variety of foods to get the nutrients you need and at the same time the right amount of calories to maintain a healthy weight. Remember to balance the energy consumed with the energy expended in play.

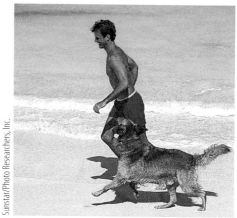

© Polara Studios

Sunstar/Photo Researchers, Inc.

Take Action: Ten Tips to a Great Plate

Use the ideas in this list to balance your calories, to choose foods to eat more often, and to cut back on foods to eat less often.

1. **Balance your calories.** Find out how many calories you need for a day as a first step in managing your weight. Go to www.ChooseMyPlate.gov to find your calorie level. Being physically active also helps you balance calories.

2. **Enjoy your food, but eat less.** Take the time to fully enjoy your food as you eat it. Pay attention to hunger and fullness cues before, during, and after meals. Use them to recognize when to eat and when you've had enough.

3. **Avoid oversized portions.** Use a smaller plate, bowl, and glass. Portion out foods before you eat. When eating out, choose a smaller size option, share a dish, or take home part of your meal.

4. **Eat some foods more often.** Eat more vegetables, fruits, whole grains, and fat-free or 1% dairy products. Make them the basis for meals and snacks.

5. **Make half your plate fruits and vegetables.** Choose red, orange, and dark-green vegetables like tomatoes, sweet potatoes, and broccoli, along with other vegetables for your meals. Add fruit to meals as part of main or side dishes or as dessert.

6. **Switch to fat-free or low-fat (1%) milk.** They have the same amount of calcium and other essential nutrients as whole milk, but fewer calories and less saturated fat.

7. **Make half your grains whole grains.** To eat more whole grains, substitute a whole-grain product for a refined product—such as eating whole-wheat bread instead of white bread or brown rice instead of white rice.

8. **Eat certain foods less often.** Cut back on foods high in solid fats, added sugars, and salt. They include cakes, cookies, ice cream, candies, sweetened drinks, pizza, and fatty meats like ribs, sausages, bacon, and hot dogs. Use these foods as occasional treats, not everyday foods.

9. **Compare sodium in foods.** Use the Nutrition Facts label to choose lower sodium versions of foods like soup, bread, and frozen meals. Select canned foods labeled "low sodium," "reduced sodium," or "no salt added."

10. **Drink water instead of sugary drinks.** Cut calories by drinking water or unsweetened beverages. Soda, energy drinks, and sports drinks are a major source of added sugar and calories in many diets.

Source: Adapted from Center for Nutrition Policy and Promotion, Tip Sheet No. 1. June 2011. Go to www.ChooseMyPlate.gov

GRAINS Make half your grains whole	**VEGETABLES** Vary your veggies	**FRUITS** Focus on fruits	**DAIRY** Get your calcium-rich foods	**PROTEIN FOODS** Go lean with protein
Eat at least 3 oz of whole grain cereals, breads, crackers, rice, or pasta every day.	Eat more dark-green veggies like broccoli, spinach, and other dark leafy greens.	Eat a variety of fruit. Choose fresh, frozen, canned, or dried fruit. Go easy on fruit juices.	Go low-fat or fat-free when you choose milk, yogurt, and other milk products.	Choose low-fat or lean meats and poultry. Bake it, broil it, or grill it.
1 oz is about 1 slice of bread, about 1 cup of breakfast cereal or $1/2$ cup of cooked rice, cereal, or pasta.	Eat more orange vegetables like carrots and sweet potatoes. Eat more dry beans and peas like pinto beans, kidney beans, and lentils.		If you don't or can't consume milk, choose lactose-free products or other calcium sources such as fortified foods and beverages. 1 cup = $1^1/2$ oz natural cheese, or 2 oz processed cheese.	Vary your protein routine—choose more fish, beans, peas, nuts, and seeds. 1 oz = 1 oz meat, poultry, or fish; $1/4$ cup cooked dry beans; 1 egg; 1 tbsp peanut butter; $1/2$ oz nuts/seeds.

For a 2,000-calorie diet, you need the amounts below from each food group. To find the amounts that are right for you, go to www.ChooseMyPlate.gov.

Eat 6 oz every day.	Eat $2^1/2$ cups every day.	Eat 2 cups every day.	Get 3 cups every day; for kids aged 2 to 8, It's 2.	Eat $5^1/2$ oz every day.

*Make most of your fat choices from fish, nuts, and vegetable oils. Find your allowance for oils at www.ChooseMyPlate.gov.

vegetables form the foundation of a healthy diet and should fill at least half of a plate at every meal. The MyPlate food guide advises you to eat more of some foods (fruits, vegetables, whole grains, and fat-free or low-fat milk products), and eat less of others (such as foods high in refined grains and added sugars).

4. **Moderation.** Currently, many of the foods and beverages Americans eat and drink contain *empty calories*—calories from **solid fats** and/or **added sugars**. Solid fats and added sugars add calories to the food but few or no nutrients and are thus called *empty calories*. A small amount of empty calories is fine, but most

solid fats fats that are solid at room temperature, such as butter, lard, and shortening. These fats may be visible or may be a constituent of foods such as milk, cheese, meats, or baked products.

added sugars sugars and other caloric sweeteners that are added to foods during processing or preparation. Added sugars do not include naturally occurring sugars such as those found in milk and fruits.

people eat far more than is healthy. It is important to emphasize nutrient-rich foods in the diet and limit empty calories to the amount that fits your calorie and nutrient needs. Making better choices, like unsweetened applesauce or extra-lean ground beef, can help keep your intake of added sugars and solid fats low. To find your personal total calorie needs and empty calories limit, enter your information into the Daily Food Plan section of www.ChooseMyPlate.gov.

5. **Personalization.** One size doesn't fit all. MyPlate can help you choose the foods and amounts of food that are right for you. For a quick estimate of what and how much you need to eat, enter your age, gender, and physical activity level in the Daily Food Plan box at www.ChooseMyPlate.gov. You can also print out a worksheet based on your personal food plan to help you track your progress.

6. **Gradual improvement.** Individuals can benefit from taking small steps to improve their diet and lifestyle every day (for example, taking the stairs instead of the elevator or escalator, or ordering a green salad instead of fries).

Use the Simplicity of MyPlate to Build a Healthful Diet
You can determine the right amount of foods to eat to meet your personal energy needs and promote a healthy weight in three easy steps.

Step 1: **Estimate Your Daily Energy Needs.** Use Table 3-5 to find your estimated daily energy needs, or go to www.ChooseMyPlate.gov and enter your age, gender, and usual activity level. If you are moderately physically active, you need fewer calories than those who are more active. The calorie levels for the food intake patterns in MyPlate were matched to age and gender groups using the **Estimated Energy Requirement (EER)** for a person of average height, healthy weight, and sedentary activity level in each age and gender group. The sedentary level was selected as a way to help people avoid overestimating their calorie needs.

Step 2: **Build Your Daily Eating Plan.** Use your estimated number of calories to build a daily eating plan that incorporates all five food groups. How much food do you need to eat each day? MyPlate provides guidance by indicating an appropriate amount of food to eat from each food group that will supply not only necessary nutrients but also the adequate amounts of calories. Table 3-6 specifies the amounts of foods from each group that are needed daily to create a healthful diet at several calorie levels.

Step 3: **Let MyPlate Guide Your Food Choices.** Eating is one of life's great pleasures. Different people like different foods and like to prepare the same foods in different ways. Because you can build a healthful menu using many foods in many ways, you have lots of room for choice. MyPlate can provide a starting point to develop healthful eating patterns while still allowing for personal preferences in food choices. Make choices from each major food group and combine them however you like.

The important thing to remember is that you can enjoy all foods as part of a healthy diet as long as you don't overdo it on solid fats (especially saturated fat and *trans* fat), refined carbohydrates, added sugars, sodium, and alcohol. Read labels to identify (and avoid) foods that are higher in saturated fats, *trans* fats, added sugars, and sodium. Certain items in each food group may be difficult to fit into a healthful eating plan on a regular basis.

Using MyPlate to assess and plan your own diet requires an understanding of how much food to consume from the various food groups and how much of a food counts as a serving. For instance, one slice of bread, half a bagel, and ½ cup of pasta each count as 1 ounce from the Grains group. When it comes to vegetables, ½ cup of raw or cooked vegetables or 1 cup of leafy raw vegetables chalks up one serving. Table 3-7 shows the portions that count as a serving from each of the various food groups.

For a hundred more tips, visit www.smallstep.gov.

MyPlate isn't the only food group plan. Canada has one of its own—Canada's Food Guide (shown in Appendix B).

Some popular foods don't fit neatly into one MyPlate food group. For example, a slice of cheese pizza includes servings from several groups: the crust from the grains group, the tomato sauce from the vegetable group, and the cheese from the dairy group. See "Tips and Resources" at www.ChooseMyPlate.gov for a chart showing how to count mixed dishes in a healthy diet.

The Spotlight feature at the end of this chapter shows you how to sort ethnic foods into the MyPlate food groups.

For more information on menu planning with the MyPlate tool, go to www.ChooseMyPlate .gov and click on "Interactive Tools"; also click on "Food Groups" and scroll down to see the Food Gallery photos for each food group for examples of sensible-size portions of the foods you eat.

TABLE 3-5	Estimated Daily Calorie Needs for Adults[a]

Find your gender and age. Then select the activity level that best describes your lifestyle (sedentary, moderately active, or active).

Activity Level:	Sedentary[b]	Moderate[c]	Active[d]
Females			
19–30	1,800–2,000	2,000–2,200	2,400
31–50	1,800	2,000	2,200
51+	1,600	1,800	2,000–2,200
Males			
19–30	2,400–2,600	2,600–2,800	3,000
31–50	2,200–2,400	2,400–2,600	2,800–3,000
51+	2,000–2,200	2,200–2,400	2,400–2,800

[a] The calorie levels in each gender and age group are based on persons of average height and at a healthy weight. If you are overweight, your calorie needs may be higher to maintain your weight. To lose weight, you can follow the calorie level in the chart, depending on your body weight. A range of calories is given to meet needs of different ages within the group. For adults, fewer calories are needed at older ages.

[b] **Sedentary:** less than 30 minutes a day of moderate physical activity in addition to daily activities.

[c] **Moderately active:** at least 30 minutes and up to 60 minutes a day of moderate physical activity in addition to daily activities. Examples of moderate physical activity include walking briskly (about 3-1/2 mph), mowing the lawn, dancing, swimming, or bicycling on level terrain. A person should feel some exertion but should be able to carry on a conversation comfortably during the activity.

[d] **Active:** 60 or more minutes a day of moderate physical activity in addition to daily activities.

NOTE: For more information, visit www.ChooseMyPlate.gov.

SOURCE: U.S. Department of Agriculture, 2005

TABLE 3-6	Build Your Eating Plan with Recommended Daily Amounts from Each Food Group

Find your calorie level at the top of the chart. Follow the column below your estimated calorie level to see how much food to eat from each of the food groups. (Estimated daily energy needs are shown in Table 3-5) Recommended amounts for fruits, vegetables, and dairy are measured in cups and those for grains and meats, in ounces.

Calorie Level:	1,600	1,800	2,000	2,200	2,400	2,600	2,800	3,000
Grains	5 oz	6 oz	6 oz	7 oz	8 oz	9 oz	10 oz	10 oz
Vegetables	2 cups	2½ cups	2½ cups	3 cups	3 cups	3½ cups	3½ cups	4 cups
Fruits	1½ cups	1½ cups	2 cups	2 cups	2 cups	2 cups	2½ cups	2½ cups
Dairy	3 cups	3 cups	3 cups	3 cups	3 cups	3 cups	3 cups	3 cups
Protein Foods	5 oz	5 oz	5½ oz	6 oz	6½ oz	6½ oz	7 oz	7 oz
Oils	5 tsp	5 tsp	6 tsp	6 tsp	7 tsp	8 tsp	8 tsp	10 tsp
Daily Limit for Empty Calories*	120 cal	160 cal	260 cal	265 cal	330 cal	360 cal	400 cal	460 cal

*The *Daily Limit for Empty Calories* (extra fats and added sugars) includes the balance of calories remaining in a person's estimated energy allowance after accounting for the number of calories needed to meet recommended nutrient intakes through consumption of foods in low-fat or no-added-sugar forms. The calories assigned to empty calories may be used to increase intake from the basic food groups; to select foods from these groups that are higher in fat or with added sugars; to add oils, solid fats, or sugars to foods or beverages; or to consume alcohol.

Besides showing what foods are the equivalent of one serving from each food group, Table 3-7 also lists the nutrients supplied by each of the five food groups. To get an idea of how your current diet compares with the recommendations of the interactive MyPlate website, try the Rate Your Plate Scorecard on page 75.

Using MyPlate to Meet Nutrient Needs

MyPlate can help you get the nutrients your body needs each day. The grains, fruits, vegetables, and dairy groups serve as the foundation of a healthful diet because they supply the vitamins, minerals, and fiber lacking in many people's diets. When it comes to the dairy group, low-fat (1%) and fat-free dairy products make the best nutrient-dense choices. Although foods from the Protein foods group provide protein, iron, zinc, and other nutrients, some items can contain large amounts of saturated fat and *trans* fat. Thus, choosing wisely from this group goes a long way in limiting the more unhealthy fat content

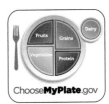

Making Use of MyPlate
- Determine calorie needs.
- Note amount of food to eat from each food group.
- Plan meals and snacks.
- Balance food intake with physical activity.

Food Group	Goal[b]	Nutrients Supplied	Equivalent Amounts
Grain Group Whole grains Other grains	6 oz 3 oz 3 oz	Protein, complex carbohydrate and fiber, folate, niacin, riboflavin, thiamin, magnesium, and iron	**1 ounce is equivalent to:** 1 slice bread, 1 mini bagel, 6" tortilla, ½ English muffin 1 cup dry cereal ½ cup cooked rice, pasta, cereal 1 packet instant oatmeal 3 cups popcorn
Vegetable Group Dark-green vegetables Orange vegetables Legumes (dry beans) Starchy vegetables Other vegetables	2½ cups 3 cups/week 2 cups/week 3 cups/week 3 cups/week 6½ cups/week	Vitamin C, beta-carotene, fiber, potassium, folate, calcium, magnesium	**½ cup is equivalent to:** ½ cup cut-up raw or cooked vegetables 1 cup raw leafy vegetable ½ cup vegetable juice
Fruit Group	2 cups	Vitamin C, beta-carotene, fiber, potassium, folate, magnesium	**½ cup is equivalent to:** ½ cup fresh, frozen, or canned fruit 1 medium fruit ¼ cup dried fruit ½ cup fruit juice
Dairy Group	3 cups	Protein, calcium, riboflavin, vitamin B_{12}, vitamins A and D	**1 cup is equivalent to:** 1 cup low-fat/fat-free milk, yogurt 1½ oz low-fat or fat-free natural cheese 2 oz low-fat or fat-free processed cheese ⅓ cup shredded cheese
Protein Foods Group	5½ oz	Protein, zinc, iron, niacin, thiamin, phosphorus, vitamin B_6, vitamin B_{12}, vitamin E, fiber (legumes)	**1 ounce is equivalent to:** 1 oz cooked lean meats, poultry, fish 1 egg ¼ cup cooked dry beans or tofu 1 tbsp peanut butter ½ oz nuts or seeds ½ cup split-pea soup
Oils[c]	6 tsp (27 grams)	Vitamin E, essential fatty acids (see Chapter 5)	**1 tsp equivalent is:** 1 tsp soft margarine 1 tbsp low-fat mayonnaise 2 tbsp light salad dressing 1 tsp vegetable oil 1 oz peanuts, nuts, or sunflower seeds has 3 teaspoons of oil
Daily limit for empty calories[d]	260 calories		

[a] All servings are per day unless otherwise noted. Vegetable subgroup amounts are per week. To follow this eating pattern, food choices over time should provide these amounts of food from each group on average.

[b] Recommended amounts to eat are based on a 2,000-calorie diet. See Table 3-5 for information about gender/age/activity levels and appropriate calorie intakes. See Table 3-6 for more information on the food groups, amounts, and food intake patterns at other calorie levels, or go to www.ChooseMyPlate.gov.

[c] The oils listed in this table are not considered to be empty calories because they are a major source of the vitamin E and polyunsaturated fatty acids, including the essential fatty acids, in the food pattern. In contrast, solid fats (i.e., saturated and *trans* fats) are included as sources of empty calories.

[d] The empty calorie allowance is the remaining amount of calories in each calorie level after nutrient-dense forms of foods in each food group are selected.

SOURCE: U.S. Department of Agriculture, 2005

of your diet. Because lean cuts of meat, skinless poultry, and fish rank lower in saturated fat than ground beef and chicken with skin, the leaner items should be chosen more often than the high-fat selections. Dry beans, which contain only a trace of fat, are good choices to add to the diet even more often.

In addition to the five food groups, we need a small amount of oil in our diet because oils provide vitamin E and essential fats. The Oils category includes vegetable oils and soft margarines containing no *trans* fat. Heart-healthy oils like olive, canola, and peanut oil are also good choices. (For more about fats, see Chapter 5.)

Using MyPlate to Moderate Energy Intakes   You can follow the MyPlate guidelines to get enough nutrients without overdoing calories. The way to balance your energy needs is to make your food choices count. By incorporating the tips and strategies for healthful eating found in Table 3-8 into your eating plan, you will get the nutrients you need for good health. Choose the most nutrient-dense foods from each of the food groups. This means choosing more whole foods that are naturally high in nutrients, such as whole grains; fruits and vegetables, including legumes; and fat-free and low-fat milk and milk products. This can help you maintain a healthy weight and may lower your risk for developing chronic health problems such as diabetes, heart disease, or cancer. Be flexible and adventurous! Try new food choices in place of some of the less nutritious or higher-calorie foods you usually eat. A sample eating pattern is given in Table 3-9, and Table 3-10 translates that eating pattern into a nutritious menu. The Eat Well Be Well feature on page 78 provides additional tips for including a variety of fruits and vegetables in your diet for maximum health benefits.

Gaining Calorie Control: The Daily Limit for Empty Calories   If you consistently build your diet by choosing mostly nutrient-dense foods that are low in solid fat and added sugars, you may be able to meet your nutrient needs without using your full calorie allowance. If so, you may have what is called a **daily limit for empty calories** for use in meeting the rest of your calorie needs (as illustrated in the margin).

Most empty calorie allowances are very small, between 100 and 300 calories, especially for those who are not physically active. How do we track these extra calories? One example is a regular 12-ounce soda that contains 155 calories—but all 155 of these calories are from added sugars and, thus, are considered "empty" calories. Keep in mind that, for many people, the empty calorie limit is totally used up by the foods they choose with solid fats and added sugars in each food group, such as higher-fat meats, higher-fat cheeses, whole milk, and sweetened bakery products.

Your empty calorie limit can be used to:

- Eat additional nutrient-dense foods from each of the food groups, such as an extra container of fat-free yogurt or an extra piece of fruit

- Select limited amounts of foods that are not in their most nutrient-dense form and/or contain solid fats or added sugars, such as whole milk, full-fat cheese, biscuits, and sweetened cereal

- Add fats or sweeteners to foods, such as sauces, gravies, sugar, syrup, butter, and jelly

- Eat or drink items that contain only fats, caloric sweeteners, and/or alcohol, such as candy, soda, wine, and beer

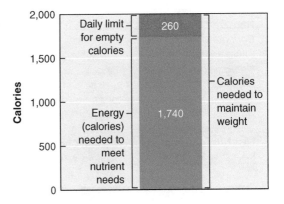

daily limit for empty calories the balance of calories remaining in a person's energy allowance, after accounting for the number of calories needed to meet recommended nutrient intakes through consumption of nutrient-dense foods in low-fat or no-added-sugar forms. These calories may be used to increase intake from the basic food groups; to select foods from these groups that are higher in fat or with added sugars; to add oils, solid fats, or sugars to foods or beverages; or to consume alcohol.

TABLE 3-8 Making the Most of Your Own Personal Food Plan

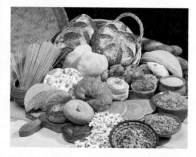

GRAIN GROUP

Tip: Make at least half of your grain selections whole grains.

Strategies:
- Buy products that list a whole grain or whole wheat or other whole-grain flour first on the label's ingredient list.
- Check the Nutrition Facts label for the fiber content of food products. Fiber content is a good clue to the amount of whole grain in the product.
- Choose 100% whole-grain breads, preferably, or mixed flour breads such as multi-grain or cracked wheat.
- To eat more whole grains, substitute a whole-grain product for a refined product—such as eating brown rice instead of white rice.
- Add whole grains to mixed dishes such as soups, stews, and casseroles.

Nutrient-Dense Choices (Choose Most Often)

Whole grains: Barley, brown and wild rice, bulgur, millet, oats, popcorn, quinoa, rye, wheat; whole-grain low-fat breads, cereals, crackers, and pastas

Enriched grain products: breads, bagels, cereals, grits, pastas, rice, rolls, and tortillas

Less Nutrient-Dense Choices (Limit Choices)

Biscuits, cakes, cookies, crackers, cornbread, croissants, Danish, doughnuts, fried rice, French toast, granola, muffins, pancakes, pies, presweetened cereals, taco shells, waffles

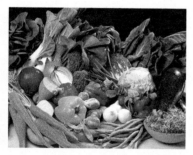

VEGETABLE GROUP

Tip: Choose from all five vegetable subgroups several times a week. Eat more dark-green vegetables, orange vegetables, and dry beans and peas.

Strategies:
- Buy fresh vegetables in season. They cost less and are likely to be at their peak flavor.
- Stock up on frozen vegetables for quick and easy cooking.
- Prepare main dishes, side dishes, and salads that include vegetables.
- Keep a bowl of cut-up vegetables in a see-through container in the refrigerator. Carrot and celery sticks are traditional, but consider broccoli, cucumber slices, or red or green pepper strips.
- Add dark-green or orange vegetables to soups, stews, casseroles, and stir-fries.
- Use romaine, spinach, or other dark leafy greens as salad greens, and eat green salads often.
- Choose main dishes, side dishes, and salads that include cooked dry beans or peas.

Nutrient-Dense Choices (Choose Most Often)

Dark-green vegetables: Broccoli and leafy greens such as arugula, kale, green-leaf and romaine lettuce; spinach, beet, collard, mustard, and turnip greens

Orange vegetables: Carrots, pumpkin, sweet potatoes, winter squash

Legumes: Black beans, black-eyed peas, chickpeas (garbanzo beans), kidney beans, pinto beans, soybeans, split peas, and lentils

Starchy vegetables: Cassava, corn, green peas, and white potatoes

Other vegetables: Artichokes, asparagus, bamboo shoots, beets, bok choy, Brussels sprouts, cabbage, cauliflower, celery, cucumbers, eggplant, green beans, iceberg lettuce, mushrooms, okra, onions, peppers, snow peas, tomatoes, vegetable juices, zucchini

Less Nutrient-Dense Choices (Limit Choices)

Baked beans, candied sweet potatoes, coleslaw, French fries, potato salad, refried beans, scalloped potatoes

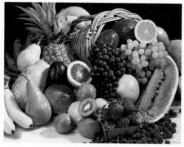

FRUIT GROUP

Tip: Choose a variety of whole or cut-up fruits more often as snacks or with meals, instead of juice.

Strategies:
- Use fruit in salads, toppings, desserts, and/or snacks regularly.
- Use fruit as a topping on cereal, pancakes, and other foods rather than sugars, syrups, or other sweet toppings.
- Buy fresh fruits in season when they may be less expensive and at their peak flavor.
- Buy fruits that are dried, frozen, and canned (in water or juice) as well as fresh, so that you always have a supply on hand.

Nutrient-Dense Choices (Choose Most Often)

Apples, apricots, avocados, bananas, blueberries, cantaloupe, grapefruit, grapes, guava, kiwi, mango, oranges, papaya, peaches, pears, pineapple, plums, raspberries, strawberries, watermelon, dried fruit, unsweetened fruit juices

Less Nutrient-Dense Choices (Limit Choices)

Canned or frozen fruit in syrup; juices, punches, and fruit drinks with added sugars

TABLE 3-8

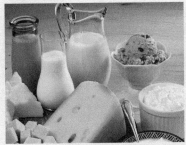

DAIRY GROUP

Tip: Make most milk group choices fat-free or low-fat (1%). Consume other calcium-rich foods or fortified cereals or beverages if milk products are not consumed.

Strategies:
- Drink fat-free or low-fat (1%) milk as a beverage.
- Use fat-free or low-fat milk or yogurt on cereal or as a snack.
- If you drink cappuccinos or lattes, ask for them with fat-free milk.
- Add fat-free or low-fat milk instead of water to oatmeal and hot cereals.
- Choose low-fat cheeses.

Nutrient-Dense Choices (Choose Most Often)

Fat-free milk and fat-free milk products, buttermilk, cheeses, cottage cheese, yogurt, fat-free fortified soy milk

Less Nutrient-Dense Choices (Limit Choices)

Reduced-fat milk, whole milk, reduced-fat milk and whole milk products such as cheeses, cottage cheese, yogurt, chocolate milk, fortified soy milk, custards and puddings, ice cream, ice milk, and frozen yogurt

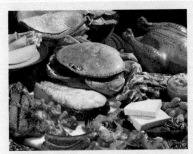

PROTEIN FOODS GROUP

Tip: Make most choices lean or low-fat. Include fish, dry beans and peas, nuts, and seeds as well as meats, poultry, and eggs.

Strategies:
- Select meat cuts that are low in fat and ground beef that is extra lean (at least 90% lean).
- Trim fat from meat and remove poultry skin before cooking or eating.
- Drain fat from ground meats after cooking.
- Use preparation methods that do not add fat, such as grilling, broiling, poaching, or roasting.
- Choose lean turkey, roast beef, ham, or low-fat luncheon meats for sandwiches instead of fatty luncheon meats such as regular bologna or salami.
- Select fish as a choice from this group more often, especially fish rich in omega-3 fatty acids, such as salmon, trout, and herring.
- Choose dry beans or peas as a main dish often.
- Choose unsalted nuts as a snack, on salads, or in main dishes, to replace meat or poultry.

Nutrient-Dense Choices (Choose Most Often)

Lean meat, fish, shellfish, poultry (no skin), eggs, legumes, tofu, tempeh, peanut butter, nuts, and seeds

Less Nutrient-Dense Choices (Limit Choices)

Luncheon meats, ground beef, hot dogs, fried meats, fried fish, fried poultry, or fried eggs, poultry with skin, refried beans, sausages

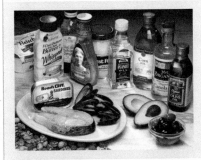

OILS

Tip: Choose most fats from sources of monounsaturated and polyunsaturated fatty acids, such as fish, nuts, seeds, and vegetable oils.

Strategies:
- Substitute vegetable oils for solid fats like butter, stick margarine, shortening, or lard.
- Substitute nuts for meat or cheese as a snack or as part of a meal.

Nutrient-Dense Choices (Choose Most Often)

Liquid vegetable oils, such as canola, corn, flaxseed, olive, peanut, safflower, sesame, soybean oil, and sunflower oils; mayonnaise, oil-based salad dressings, and soft margarine with no *trans* fats; foods naturally high in oils, such as avocados, nuts, seeds, olives, fatty fish, and shellfish

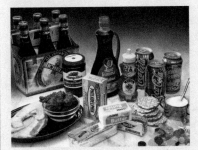

SOLID FATS & ADDED SUGARS

Tip: Limit intakes of foods and beverages with solid fats or added sugars. Choose and prepare foods and beverages with little added sugars or caloric sweeteners.

Strategies:
- Limit products containing saturated fats, such as ground and processed meats, full-fat cheese, cream, ice cream, and fried foods.
- Limit foods containing partially hydrogenated vegetable oils, which contain *trans* fats, such as some commercially fried foods and some bakery goods.
- Select baked, steamed, or broiled rather than fried foods most often.
- Choose water, fat-free milk, or unsweetened tea or coffee as a beverage most often.
- Limit sweet snacks and desserts. Choose canned fruits in 100% fruit juice.
- Select unsweetened cereals.

TABLE 3-9 — A Sample Eating Pattern for 2,000 Calories

Food Group	Recommended Amounts	Breakfast	Lunch	Snack	Dinner	Snack
Grains	6 oz	1½ oz	2 oz		2 oz	½ oz
Vegetables	2½ c		1 c		1½ c	
Fruits	2 c	½ c		1 c	½ c	
Dairy	3 c	1 c			1 c	1 c
Protein Foods	5½ oz		2 oz	1 oz	2½ oz	
Oils	6 tsp		2 tsp		4 tsp	
Empty Calories	260 cal					

TABLE 3-10 — A Sample Menu for 2,000 Calories

The menu below provides about 1,830 calories, leaving about 170 extra calories to spend on additional nutrient-dense foods, or on foods with added sugars or fats.

Amounts	Menu Item	Calories
Breakfast		
1½ oz whole grains	1½ c whole-grain flakes cereal	162
1 c dairy	1 c fat-free milk	90
1 c fruit	1 c sliced banana	105
Lunch		
2 oz whole grains	2 slices rye bread	160
2 oz protein foods	1½ oz tuna, packed in water, drained	55
1 c vegetables	2 tbsp kidney beans	25
	6 baby carrots, shredded	25
	¼ c shredded Romaine lettuce	2
	2 slices tomato	10
2 tsp oils	1 tbsp low-fat mayonnaise	35
	1 tsp Dijon mustard	5
8 oz unsweetened beverage	1 c iced tea, unsweetened	0
Snack		
½ c fruit	¼ c dried apricots	80
1 oz protein foods	½ oz almonds (12 almonds)	80
Dinner		
	Spinach salad:	
½ c vegetables	1 c raw baby spinach leaves	8
½ oz protein foods	2 tbsp chickpeas	34
½ c fruit	½ c tangerine slices	30
2 tsp oils	2 tsp oil and vinegar dressing	60
	Pasta with meat sauce:	
2 oz enriched grains	1 c rigatoni pasta	197
1 c vegetables	½ c tomato sauce with	25
	½ c mixed frozen vegetables	25
2 oz protein foods	2 oz cooked ground turkey breast,	130
2 tsp oils	sautéed in 2 tsp oil	90
1 c dairy	1½ oz Parmesan cheese	190
Snack		
1 c dairy	1 c fat-free fruited yogurt	120
½ oz grains	3 graham crackers	90

How Well Do We Eat?

How are consumers doing in following the nutrition recommendations presented in this chapter? The answer to this question is, "Needs improvement." Undoubtedly, trends such as eating away from home and increased portion sizes in restaurant and carry-out items negatively affect American eating habits.

Figure 3-7 provides insights into how the typical American diet compares to recommended intakes or limits.[10] In general, we eat too many calories and too much solid fat, added sugars, refined grains, and sodium. Solid fats and added sugars should make up only a small proportion of total calories in the diet. However, as illustrated in the margin, Americans consume about 35 percent of total calories from foods high in solid fats and added sugars—soft drinks, desserts, fatty meats, French fries, pizza, and whole milk products, in contrast to a recommended limit of no more than 5 to 15 percent of total calories for most individuals.

We also consume too few vegetables, fruits, whole grains, and fat-free or low-fat milk and milk products. As shown in Figure 3-7, consumers eat only 15 percent of

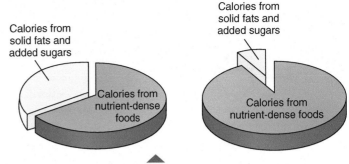

What We Eat versus Recommended Limits

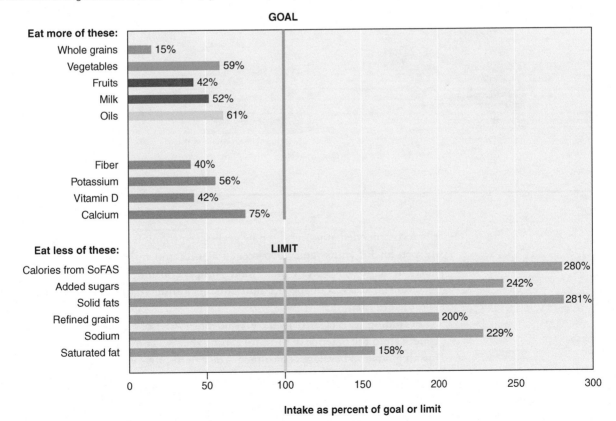

FIGURE 3-7

How the U.S. Diet Measures Up to Recommended Dietary Guidelines

The bars show average intakes for all individuals (2 years or older) as a percent of the recommended intake level or recommended limit.[a]

Eat more of these:
- Whole grains: 15%
- Vegetables: 59%
- Fruits: 42%
- Milk: 52%
- Oils: 61%
- Fiber: 40%
- Potassium: 56%
- Vitamin D: 42%
- Calcium: 75%

Eat less of these:
- Calories from SoFAS: 280%
- Added sugars: 242%
- Solid fats: 281%
- Refined grains: 200%
- Sodium: 229%
- Saturated fat: 158%

Intake as percent of goal or limit

[a] Recommended intakes for food groups and limits for refined grains, SoFAS (solid fats and added sugars) are based on a 2,000-calorie diet.

[*] Recommended intakes for fiber, potassium, vitamin D, and calcium are based on the highest Adequate Intakes (AI) for ages 14 to 70 years. Limits for sodium are based on the AI and for saturated fat on 7 percent of calories.

SOURCE: U.S. Department of Agriculture and U.S. Department of Health and Human Services, *Dietary Guidelines for Americans, 2010*. 7th ed. (Washington, DC: U.S. Government Printing Office, 2010). Data source: What We Eat in America, National Health and Nutrition Examination Survey (WWEIA, NHANES) 2001–2004 or 2005–2006.

In the "more must be better" viewpoint of eating in America today, it can be difficult to balance the energy we take in through the food we eat with the energy we expend on a daily basis. This is evidenced by the larger and larger portion sizes we find in restaurants, on the grocery shelves, and in almost every aspect of eating in the United States today.

What's the difference between a serving and a portion? A *serving* is a standard amount of food used as a reference to give advice regarding how much food to eat (such as 1 cup of milk or its equivalent). The amount of a food that is considered a serving usually stays the same. A *portion,* in contrast, is the amount of food *you* choose to eat, and it may vary from one meal or snack to the next based on your appetite or hunger. How do you determine how much food is in your portion? You can use the following images as a visual reference to "right-size" your portions and avoid consuming extra calories.

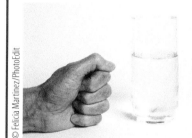
One fist, clenched = 8 fl oz

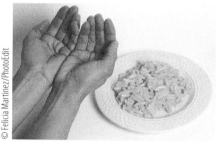
Two hands, cupped = 1 cup

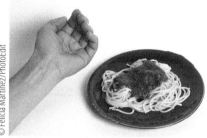
One hand, cupped = 1/2 cup

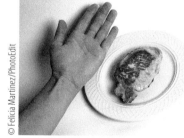
Palm of hand = 3 oz

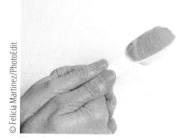
Two thumbs together = 1 tbsp

SOURCE: Adapted from USDA, *Dietary Guidelines for Americans,* 5th ed., 2000.

the recommended amount of whole grains, less than 60 percent for vegetables, about 42 percent for fruits, and 50 percent for milk and milk products. By eating fewer nutrient-dense foods from these food groups, consumers are at risk for lower than recommended levels of specific nutrients, including vitamin D, calcium, potassium, and dietary fiber.

According to the 2010 Dietary Guidelines Advisory Committee, Americans can benefit from the practice of mindful eating, that is, "consciously" and carefully choosing all foods and beverages consumed. You can improve your health with a diet that is:

- Energy balanced, limited in total calories, and portion controlled
- Nutrient-dense and includes:
  - Vegetables, fruits, high-fiber whole grains
  - Fat-free or low-fat dairy products
  - Seafood, lean meat and poultry, eggs, soy products, nuts, seeds, and oils
- Very low in solid fats and added sugars and low in sodium

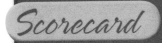

Rate Your Plate Using the MyPlate Food Guide

To see how your diet measures up to the recommendations in the MyPlate food plan, follow these steps.

Step 1: Write down everything you ate yesterday, including meals *and* snacks. Make note of portion sizes as well. (Refer to Table 3-7 for help with conversions.)

Step 2: Identify the food group for each item you ate. (Refer to Figure 3-6 for help.)

Step 3: Using the five food groups, determine the amounts that are right for you. Go to "Interactive Tools" at www .ChooseMyPlate.gov and type in your age, sex, and activity level under the "Daily Food Plan" and click on "submit." This will give you a plan with a good estimate of the amount of -servings you need from each food group. In addition, it will give you the approximate number of calories you require.

Step 4: Circle the estimated amounts you should eat from the middle column. In the right column, write down the amounts you ate yesterday. (Refer to Table 3-7 and the Savvy Diner feature in this chapter for help with conversions.) Compare the two columns to see how your diet rates.

	Amount You Should Eat	Amount You Ate
Grain group servings (ounces)	5 6 7 8 9 10	_____
Vegetable group servings (cups)	2 2½ 3 4	_____
Fruit group servings (cups)	2 2½ 3	_____
Dairy group servings (cups)	3	_____
Protein Foods group (ounces)	5 5½ 6 7	_____
Solid Fats and Added Sugars	Use Empty Calorie Limit	_____

Step 5: Decide what changes in your eating habits will make your diet more healthful. If your diet is "un-proportional," with too many foods coming from one food group, make gradual changes to develop a diet with more variety. The chapters that follow offer tips on how to do so.

More Tools for Diet Planning

In 1990, Congress passed one of the most important pieces of legislation of the 20th century. Known as the Nutrition Labeling and Education Act, the law called for sweeping changes in the way foods are labeled in the United States.[11] For consumers, the law ensures that food companies provide the kind of nutrition information that best allows people to select foods that fit into a healthful eating plan.

Food Labels   Considering the great variety of packaged foods available, using the food label to understand the nutrients a food supplies or lacks is essential (see Figure 3-8). The label is one of the most important tools you can use to eat healthfully.

By law, all labels must contain the following five components:

- The name of the food, also known as the statement of identity.

- The name of the manufacturer, packer, or distributor, as well as the firm's city, state, and ZIP code.

- The net contents of the package, which tells you the quantity of the food product that is in the container and helps you compare prices.

- The **ingredients list**, with items listed in descending order by weight. The first ingredient listed makes up the largest proportion of all the ingredients in the food; the second, the second largest amount; and so on. If the first ingredient

ingredients list a listing of the ingredients in a food, with items listed in descending order of predominance by weight. All food labels are required to bear an ingredients list.

FIGURE 3-8

How to Read a Food Label

You can use food labels to help you make informed food choices for healthy eating practices. The food label allows you to compare similar products, determine the nutritional value of the foods you choose, and can increase your awareness of the links between good nutrition and reduced risk of chronic, diet-related diseases.

SOURCE: Food and Drug Administration

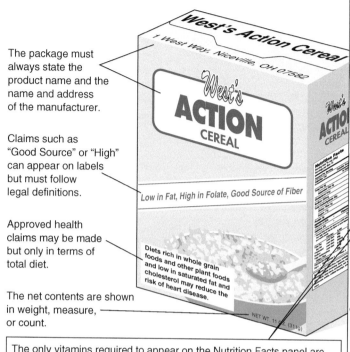

The package must always state the product name and the name and address of the manufacturer.

Claims such as "Good Source" or "High" can appear on labels but must follow legal definitions.

Approved health claims may be made but only in terms of total diet.

The net contents are shown in weight, measure, or count.

The only vitamins required to appear on the Nutrition Facts panel are vitamins A and C. If a manufacturer makes a nutrition claim about another vitamin, however, the amount of that nutrient in a serving of the product must also be stated on the panel. For instance, the cereal shown is touted as "High in Folate," so the percentage of the recommended intake for folate in a serving of the cereal (25%) is stated on the label. The manufacturer has the option of listing any other nutrients as well.

Start here

Serving size, number of servings per container, and calorie information

Limit these nutrients.

Information on sodium is required on food labels.

Get enough of these nutrients.

Guide to the % Daily Value: Quantities of nutrients as a percentage of Daily Value for nutrients based on a 2,000-calorie energy intake.
5% or less is low.
10% or more is good.
20% or more is high.

Calcium and iron are required on the label. Look for foods that provide 10% or more of these minerals.

Reference values

This allows comparison of some values for nutrients in a serving of the food with the needs of a person requiring 2,000 or 2,500 calories per day.

Calorie/gram reminder

Ingredients in descending order of predominance by weight

Nutrition Facts
Serving size ¾ cup (55g)
Servings per Box 5

Amount Per Serving		
Calories 167	Calories from Fat 27	

	% Daily Value*
Total Fat 3g	5%
Saturated Fat 1g	5%
Trans Fat 0g	
Cholesterol 0mg	0%
Sodium 250mg	10%
Total Carbohydrate 32g	11%
Dietary Fiber 4g	16%
Sugars 11g	
Protein 3g	

Vitamin A	0%
Vitamin C	15%
Calcium	10%
Iron	25%
Vitamin D	0%
Thiamin	25%
Riboflavin	25%
Niacin	25%
Folate	25%
Phosphorus	15%
Magnesium	10%
Zinc	6%
Copper	8%

*Percent Daily values are based on a 2,000 calorie diet. Your daily values may be higher or lower depending on your calorie needs:

		Calories:	2,000	2,500
Total Fat	Less than		65g	80g
Sat Fat	Less than		20g	25g
Cholesterol	Less than		300mg	300mg
Sodium	Less than		2,400mg	2,400mg
Total Carbohydrate			300g	375g
Dietary Fiber			25g	30g

Calories per gram
Fat 9 • Carbohydrate 4 • Protein 4

Ingredients: Whole oats, milled corn, enriched wheat flour (contains niacin, reduced iron, thiamin mononitrate, riboflavin, folic acid), dextrose, maltose, high fructose corn syrup, brown sugar, partially hydrogenated cottonseed oil, coconut oil, walnuts, vitamin C (sodium ascorbate), vitamin A (palmitate), iron.

---

in the list is sugar, for example, you know the food contains more sugar than anything else. The list is especially useful in helping people identify ingredients they avoid for health, religious, or other reasons (see Figure 3-9).

- The **Nutrition Facts panel**, unless the package is small—no larger than 12 square inches of surface area (about the size of a small candy bar or a roll of breath mints).* Small packages must carry a telephone number or address that consumers can use to obtain nutrition information.

Nutrition Facts panel a detailed breakdown of the nutritional content of a serving of a food that must appear on virtually all packaged foods sold in the United States.

*A container with less than 40 square inches of surface area for nutrition labeling (e.g., a can of tuna) is allowed to present fewer facts.

Oats 'N' More

Ingredients: whole grain oats, (includes the oat bran), modified corn starch, wheat starch, (sugar) salt, oat fiber, trisodium phosphate, calcium carbonate, vitamin E (mixed tocopherols) added to preserve freshness. **Vitamins and Minerals:** iron and zinc (mineral nutrients), vitamin C (sodium ascorbate), vitamin B_6 (pyridoxine hydrochloride), riboflavin, thiamin mononitrate, niacinamide, folic acid, vitamin A (palmitate), vitamin B_{12}, vitamin D.

Morning Krisps

Ingredients: (Sugar) wheat, (corn syrup) (honey) hydrogenated soybean oil, salt, caramel color, soy lecithin. **Vitamins and Iron:** sodium ascorbate (vitamin C), ferric phosphate (iron), niacinamide, pyridoxine hydrochloride (vitamin B_6), riboflavin, vitamin A palmitate, thiamin hydrochloride, BHT (preservative), folic acid, vitamin B_{12}, and vitamin D.

The cereals shown contain sugars. Learn to read the ingredients list. Labels list ingredients in order of amount by weight with the greatest amount of an ingredient present in the food listed first. Check labels for sugar terms, in addition to sugar, such as: brown sugar, corn syrup, dextrose, fructose, glucose, high-fructose corn syrup, honey, invert sugar, levulose, mannitol, molasses, sorbitol, and sucrose.

Using the Nutrition Facts Panel   The Nutrition Facts panel must indicate the amount of certain mandatory nutrients that one serving of the food contains. You can use the Nutrition Facts panel to help you follow a healthful diet by considering the nutrition information that it provides.

1. Keep serving sizes in mind. Based on the amount of food most people eat at one time, the Food and Drug Administration (FDA) has set forth a list of serving sizes for more than 100 food categories. Manufacturers must use these recommended serving sizes on food labels. For instance, the FDA might say that the serving size for product X must always be 8 ounces. This procedure ensures that consumers can easily compare one brand of a product to another without having to make difficult calculations to compare nutrient quantities for different serving sizes.

2. Notice the total calories and calories from fat per serving.

3. Check out the nutrient information that must appear on the Nutrition Facts panel, including total fat, saturated fat, *trans* fat, cholesterol, sodium, total carbohydrate, dietary fiber, sugars, protein, vitamin A, vitamin C, calcium, and iron (in that order). These nutrients were chosen to appear on the Nutrition Facts panel because they address today's health concerns.

   The FDA spelled out the ranking of the required nutrients to ensure that the label reflects the government's dietary priorities for the public. For example, fat falls near the top of the list because most consumers need to pay closer attention to the amount and type of fat in their diet. Most Americans eat too much saturated fat and trans fat, which raises the risk of developing heart disease. Protein, in contrast, appears near the bottom of the label because the amount of protein most Americans eat does not rate as a major health concern. Note that only vitamins A and C, iron, calcium, and sodium appear on the nutrition panel. Those are the only vitamins and minerals required to be on food labels, unless a manufacturer chooses to make a nutrition claim about another one. For instance, if a manufacturer says that a cereal is *high* in folate or fortified with niacin, the amount of folate or niacin in the product must appear on the label (see Figure 3-8).

4. Look for the percent Daily Values. The **Daily Values** for fats, protein, carbohydrates, and fiber are calculated according to what experts deem a healthful diet for adults (as noted in the Calculation Practice box on page 80). For instance, since the Daily Value for fat recommends that no more than

Daily Value the amount of fat, sodium, fiber, and other nutrients health experts say should make up a healthful diet. The "% Daily Values" that appear on food labels tell you the percentage of a nutrient that a serving of the food contributes to a healthful diet.

The message is simple: *Eat plenty of fruits and vegetables every day for better health.*[12] Most Americans, however, find this simple bit of nutritional advice challenging to put into practice. Overwhelming evidence points to the health benefits available from diets rich in fruits and vegetables because of the vitamins, minerals, and **phytochemicals** (*phyto* is the Greek word for plant) found in plant foods.

In the classic sense, the naturally occurring phytochemicals—for example, lycopene, a pigment that makes tomatoes red and watermelon pink—are not vitamins, minerals, or nutrients because they do not provide energy or building materials. However, scientists who study them say that phytochemicals may have the potential to slow the aging process; boost immune function; decrease blood pressure and cholesterol; prevent cataracts; prevent, slow, or even reverse certain cancers; and strengthen our hearts and circulatory systems. (More about the food sources and beneficial effects of phytochemicals appears in Chapter 7.)

How can you incorporate fruits and vegetables into your diet to achieve the maximum health benefits? Aim for the amounts of fruits and vegetables recommended in MyPlate (about 2 cups of fruits and 2½ cups of vegetables on a 2,000-calorie diet).* Go to www.ChooseMyPlate.gov to determine your own recommended intake of fruits and vegetables. Also consider the following three steps in your daily food planning.

1   Color Your Plate with Health-Protective Foods.

Consume many differently colored fruits and vegetables. Select at least three differently colored fruits and vegetables a day. The red pigment in tomatoes has different bioactive properties than the orange pigments in carrots, sweet potatoes, melon, or winter squash. Add dark-green leafy vegetables such as kale, mustard greens, collards, and spinach, along with broccoli and Brussels sprouts. Fruits are a vital powerhouse of the **antioxidant nutrients** that act to squelch cell-damaging molecules in the body. Blueberries top the list for being one of the highest in antioxidants. Be sure to include citrus fruits such as oranges and grapefruit regularly, as they contain many compounds that have antioxidant and other vital health benefits.

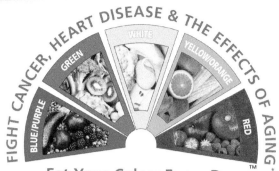

Eat Your Colors Every Day To Stay Healthy & Fit

*Low-fat diets rich in fruits and vegetables and low in saturated fat and cholesterol may reduce the risk of heart disease and some types of cancer—diseases associated with many factors.

SOURCE: © Produce for Better Health Foundation.

2   Be Adventurous: Select from As Wide a Variety of Fruits and Vegetables As Possible.

Foods within each group of the MyPlate Food Guidance System have similar nutrient content. Choosing foods from each group offers a variety of the nutrients necessary for health, but variety within food groups is valuable, too. Even fruits that may seem like comparable foods often provide a number of different nutrients; no food has them all. For example, oranges are an excellent source of vitamin C and folate but do not supply beta-carotene (a precursor of vitamin A); cantaloupe is high in beta-carotene.

3   Make It Easy on Yourself!

Keep fruit and sliced vegetables in easy-to-reach places, such as sliced vegetables in the refrigerator and fresh fruit on the table. For convenience, keep a variety of fresh, frozen, and canned fruits and vegetables on hand to add to soups, salads, rice dishes, and other menu items. Frozen fruits and vegetables are processed right after harvesting and contain nutrient profiles similar to fresh produce. If using canned items, choose fruits packed in fruit juice (not in syrup) and remove excess salt from vegetables by rinsing before using them.

*In general, 1 cup of fruit or 100% fruit juice, or ½ cup of dried fruit is considered 1 cup from the fruit group; 1 cup of raw or cooked vegetables or vegetable juice, or 2 cups of raw leafy vegetables are considered as 1 cup from the vegetable group.

phytochemicals nonnutritive substances in plants that possess health-protective benefits.

antioxidant nutrients vitamins and minerals that protect other compounds from damaging reactions involving oxygen by themselves reacting with oxygen. The antioxidant nutrients are vitamin C, vitamin E, and beta-carotene. The mineral selenium also has a role in antioxidant reactions in the body.

30 percent of total calories should come from fat, the % Daily Value tells you the percentage of fat that a serving of the food contributes to a 2,000-calorie eater's fat "allowance." A 2,000-calorie diet was chosen as a good point of reference because that's about the amount recommended for most moderately active women, teenage girls, and sedentary men. Of course, more calories may be appropriate for many men, teenage boys, and active women. This is why the nutrition panel also shows Daily Values for a 2,500-calorie diet (refer to the bottom of the Nutrition Facts panel in Figure 3-8).

Using the Percent Daily Values (% DV)

To understand how the Daily Values for fats, sodium, carbohydrates, and fiber are calculated, let's go through an example. First, look for the grams of total fat and the % Daily Value for the cereal shown in Figure 3-8. The label shows that a serving supplies 3 grams of fat, with a Daily Value of 5 percent. This means that a serving of the cereal contributes 5 percent of the total fat that a person eating 2,000 calories a day should consume.

Now look at the bottom of the Nutrition Facts panel, which indicates that someone eating 2,000 calories a day should take in no more than 65 grams of fat a day. Divide 3 (the number of fat grams in a serving of the cereal) by 65. Multiply that number by 100 to obtain a percentage. The answer is 5—that is, 5 percent of the total fat.

You can use the % Daily Values to get a good idea of how various foods fit into a healthful diet, regardless of the number of calories you eat. Consider a student who eats only 1,800 calories a day. If she snacks on two servings of potato chips with a Daily Value of 15 percent fat per serving, she has already taken in 30 percent of the fat that someone eating 2,000 calories should have in an entire day. Because she eats less than 2,000 calories, the potato chips contribute slightly more than 30 percent. Thus, the 30 percent Daily Value shows that potato chips add up to a lot of fat for one snack. In short, the % Daily Value column can give you a good idea of how different foods fit into your overall diet.

Some people find it easiest to bypass the % Daily Values and simply check the grams of total fat a serving of food supplies to see how much it adds to a daily fat tally. Let's say a man eats 2,000 calories a day and therefore should consume no more than 65 grams of fat a day. If he eats a muffin (15 grams of fat) and coffee with cream (10 grams) in the morning, he's already up to 25 grams of fat. That means he can have about 40 more grams during the rest of the day to stay within his fat "budget." Once you determine the maximum number of fat grams you should have in a day, you can use the food label to get a good idea of how many grams of total fat the items you buy add to your daily tally. To figure out your fat allowance, check Table 5-4 in Chapter 5.

You can also use the Daily Values to comparison-shop. For example, if you're looking for a high-fiber cereal to increase the amount of fiber in your diet, you can check the % Daily Value for fiber on the labels of several brands of cereal. If a serving of Brand X's cereal has a Daily Value of 20 percent for fiber and Brand Y supplies only 5 percent, you know that Brand X is a better source of fiber, whereas Brand Y is low in fiber.

The % Daily Values for vitamins and minerals are calculated using standard values designed specifically for use on food labels. These values are listed on Study Card page 54 at the back of this book. These standard values for nutrients were created to help manufacturers avoid a stumbling block they face as they label foods. Because manufacturers don't know whether you're an 18-year-old woman or a 30-year-old man, they don't know exactly what your nutritional needs are. You may recall that the DRI include a different set of vitamin and mineral recommendations for each gender and age group.

To help get around this problem, the nutrient recommendations used for vitamins and minerals on labels represent the highest of all the values to ensure that virtually everyone in the population is covered. For most nutrients, the highest recommendation is for an adult man. When it comes to iron, however, the DRI for women is the highest (women require more iron than men), so the women's DRI is used as the standard value on labels.

Nutrient Content Claims

By law, foods carrying terms called **nutrient content claims**—low-fat, low-calorie, light, and so forth—must adhere to specific definitions spelled out by the Food and Drug Administration. For instance, a serving of

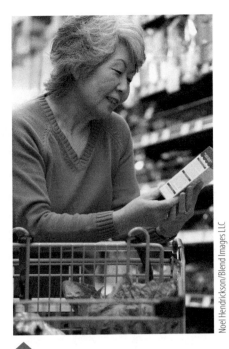

Learn to read food labels to help you achieve a healthful diet.

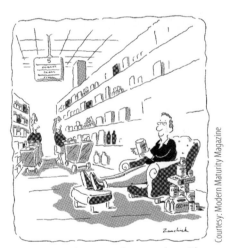

"Henry likes nothing more than to curl up with a good label."

nutrient content claims claims such as "low-fat" and "low-calorie" used on food labels to help consumers who don't want to scrutinize the Nutrition Facts panel get an idea of a food's nutritional profile. These claims must adhere to specific definitions set forth by the Food and Drug Administration.

Calculation Practice: Determining Personal Daily Values (DVs)

The Daily Values (DVs) and % Daily Values (% DVs) can help you choose foods and comparison-shop. As noted earlier, the DVs are designed for persons requiring 2,000 or 2,500 calories to meet their energy needs. The Daily Values for carbohydrates, protein, and fat are calculated using "calculation factors" set forth by the FDA for food labeling purposes as follows:*

Calculation factors:

- Fat: 30% of calories

- Saturated Fat: 10% of calories

- Protein: 10% of calories

- Carbohydrate: 60% of calories

- Fiber: 11.5 grams of fiber per 1,000 calories

To understand how the Daily Values for the macronutrients are calculated if your energy needs differ from 2,000 or 2,500 calories, let's go through an example using the calculation factors. If a person's energy requirement (EER) is 1,800 calories, determine this person's DVs for carbohydrate, protein, and fat.

Carbohydrate:
60% of 1,800 calories = 0.60 × 1,800 = 1,080 calories
1,080 calories of carbohydrate = 270 grams of carbohydrate (1,080 calories ÷ 4 calories/gram)
DV for carbohydrate = 270 grams

Protein:
10% of 1,800 calories = 0.10 × 1,800 = 180 calories
180 calories of protein = 45 grams of protein (180 calories ÷ 4 calories/gram)
DV for protein = 45 grams

Fat:
30% of 1,800 calories = 0.30 × 1,800 = 540 calories
540 calories of fat = 60 grams of fat (540 calories ÷ 9 calories/gram)
DV for fat = 60 grams

*THE FDA may update the DV calculation values soon to reflect the current DRI and AMDR values.

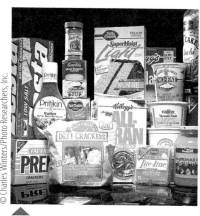

Nutrient content claims are strictly defined by the FDA.

a food dubbed low-fat must contain no more than 3 grams of fat. An item touted as low-calorie may provide no more than 40 calories per serving. Table 3-11 lists the claims commonly used on food labels and their legal definitions.

Health Claims   A statement linking the nutritional profile of a food to a reduced risk of a particular disease is known as a **health claim**. The FDA has set forth very strict rules governing the use of such health claims (see Table 3-11).[13] For example, if a food label bears health claims regarding calcium, a serving of the product must contain at least 20 percent of the Daily Value for calcium, among other restrictions. What's more, the manufacturers are allowed to imply only that the food "may" or "might" reduce risk of disease. They must also note the other factors, such as exercise, that play a role in prevention of the disease. Finally, they must phrase the claim so that the consumer can understand the relationship between the nutrient and the disease. For example, a health claim on a food low in fat, saturated fat, and cholesterol might read, "Whereas many factors affect heart disease, diets low in saturated fat and cholesterol may reduce the risk of this disease." The nutrient–disease relationships about which health claims can be made are listed in Table 3-12.[14]

Exchange Lists   Although food group plans provide sufficient detail to help most healthy people plan a good diet, exchange lists take meal planning a step further. As their name implies, **exchange lists** are simply lists of categories of foods, such as fruit, with portions specified in a way that allows the foods to be mixed and

health claim a statement on the food label linking the nutritional profile of a food to a reduced risk of a particular disease, such as osteoporosis or cancer. Manufacturers must adhere to strict government guidelines when making such claims.

exchange lists lists of foods with portion sizes specified. The foods on a single list are similar with respect to nutrient and calorie content and thus can be mixed and matched in the diet.

TABLE 3-11	Definitions of Nutrient Content Claims

General Terms
- Fresh, Raw: Unprocessed, or minimally processed with no added preservatives.
- Good Source of: A serving of the food supplies 10 to 19% of the Daily Value for a particular nutrient.
- Healthy: A food is low in fat, saturated fat, *trans* fat, cholesterol, and sodium, and provides at least 10% of the Daily Value for vitamin A, vitamin C, protein, calcium, iron, or fiber.
- High, Rich in, Excellent Source of: Contains 20% or more of the Daily Value for a particular nutrient.
- Less, Fewer, Reduced: A serving provides at least 25% less of a nutrient or calories than the comparison food.
- Light or Lite: A serving provides one-third fewer calories than or half the fat of the regular product. If fat supplies 50% or more of the calories to begin with, it must be reduced by half to be called "light." The sodium content of a serving of a low-calorie, low-fat food has been reduced by 50%.
- More, Extra: A serving of the food contains at least 10% more of the Daily Value of a particular nutrient than the regular food.
- Organic: At least 95% of the product's ingredients have been grown and processed according to USDA regulations regarding the use of fertilizers, herbicides, fungicides, insecticides, preservatives, and other substances (see Chapter 13).

Energy Terms
- Calorie-Free: Less than 5 calories per serving.
- Low-Calorie: No more than 40 calories per serving.
- Reduced Calories: Contains at least 25% fewer calories than the regular, unaltered product.

Carboydrates: Sugar and Fiber
- Sugar-Free: Less than 0.5 g of sugar per serving.
- High Fiber: 5 g or more fiber per serving.
- Good Source of Fiber: 2.5 g to 4.9 g per serving.

Fat and Cholesterol Terms
- Fat-Free: Less than 0.5 g of fat per serving.
- Low-Fat: 3 grams of fat or less per serving.
- Saturated Fat-Free: Less than 0.5 g of saturated fat and less than 0.5 g *trans* fat per serving.
- Low Saturated Fat: 1 gram or less saturated fat per serving and less than 0.5 g *trans* fat per serving.
- Less Saturated Fat: at least 25 percent less saturated fat and trans fat combined than the comparison food.
- *Trans* Fat-Free: Less than 0.5 g of *trans* fat *and* less than 0.5 g of saturated fat per serving.
- Cholesterol-Free: Less than 2 mg cholesterol and 2 g or less saturated fat and *trans* fat combined per serving.
- Low in Cholesterol: 20 mg or less of cholesterol and 2 g or less of saturated fat and *trans* fat combined per serving.
- Reduced or Less Cholesterol: at least 25 percent less cholesterol than the comparison food and 2 g or less saturated fat and trans fat combined per serving.
- Percent Fat-Free: An indication of the amount of a food's weight that is fat-free; can be used only on foods that are low-fat or fat-free to begin with, and must reflect the amount of fat in 100 g. For instance, a food that weighs 100 g with 3 g from fat can be labeled "97 percent fat-free." Note that this term refers to the amount of the food that is fat-free by weight, not calories. If that same food supplies 100 calories, the 3 g of fat contribute 27 of them (1 g of fat contains 9 calories). This means that 27 of the 100 calories, or 27% of the total calories, come from fat.
- "Lean" and "Extra Lean" describe the fat content of meat and poultry products:
  Lean:
  Less than 10 g of fat and
  Less than 4.5 g of saturated fat and *trans* fat combined, and
  Less than 95 mg of cholesterol per serving.
  Extra Lean:
  Less than 5 g of fat and
  Less than 2 g of saturated fat and *trans* fat combined, and
  Less than 95 mg of cholesterol per serving.

Sodium Terms
- Sodium-Free: Less than 5 mg of sodium per serving.
- Very Low Sodium: 35 mg or less sodium per serving.
- Low in Sodium: 140 mg sodium or less per serving.
- Reduced Sodium: At least 25% lower in sodium than the regular product.

SOURCE: Food and Drug Administration

matched or exchanged with one another in the diet. For instance, you might strive to eat four servings of fruit each day, and the exchange list shows you that ½ cup of orange juice, a small banana, or a small apple each counts as a fruit.

Portion sizes within groups are determined by considering the calorie, protein, carbohydrate, and fat content of the food. For example, one fruit contains about 60

Appendix A provides more details regarding Choose Your Foods: Exchange Lists for Diabetes (formerly U.S. Food Exchange System).

TABLE 3-12	Health Claims on Food Labels

Approved health claims with significant scientific agreement:[a]

- Diets adequate in calcium and vitamin D, as part of a well-balanced diet, may reduce the risk of osteoporosis.
- Eating a healthful diet low in total fat may help reduce the risk of some types of cancers.
- Low-fat diets rich in fiber-containing grain products, fruits, and vegetables may reduce the risk of some types of cancer.
- Low-fat diets rich in fruits and vegetables may reduce the risk of some types of cancer.
- Diets low in sodium may reduce the risk of high blood pressure.
- Diets low in saturated fat and cholesterol, and as low as possible in trans fat, may reduce the risk of heart disease.
- Diets low in saturated fat and cholesterol and high in fruits, vegetables, and grain products that contain fiber may lower blood cholesterol levels and reduce your risk of heart disease.
- Diets low in saturated fat and cholesterol and rich in fruits, vegetables, and grain products that contain dietary fiber, particularly soluble fiber, may reduce the risk of heart disease.
- Diets that are low in saturated fat and cholesterol and that include soluble fiber in foods such as whole oats may reduce the risk of heart disease.
- Adequate folate in healthful diets may reduce a woman's risk of having a child with a brain or spinal cord birth defect.
- Sugar alcohols may reduce the risk of tooth decay.
- Drinking fluoridated water may reduce the risk of tooth decay.
- Diets low in saturated fat and cholesterol that include 25 grams of soy protein a day may reduce the risk of heart disease.
- Diets rich in whole-grain foods and other plant foods and low in total fat, saturated fat, and cholesterol may reduce the risk of heart disease and certain cancers.
- Diets low in saturated fat and cholesterol that include 2 grams per day of phytosterols [plant sterols, plant stanols, or plant sterols and stanols] eaten with meals or snacks may reduce the risk of heart disease.
- Diets containing foods that are good sources of potassium and low in sodium may reduce the risk of high blood pressure and stroke.

A sampling of qualified health claims:[b]

- Omega-3 fatty acids and reduced risk of heart disease
- Nuts such as walnuts and reduced risk of heart disease
- Calcium and reduced risk of high blood pressure
- Calcium and reduced risk of colorectal cancer
- Monounsaturated fat from olive oil and reduced risk of heart disease
- B vitamins and reduced risk of heart disease

[a] The FDA does not require these claims to carry disclaimers.
[b] FDA requires label disclaimers when these claims are used; for example, "Health claim: Although there is scientific evidence supporting the claim, the evidence is not conclusive."

SOURCE: Food and Drug Administration

calories and 15 grams of carbohydrate. One starch, in contrast, provides about 80 calories, 15 grams of carbohydrate, 3 grams of protein, and a trace of fat. This breakdown makes exchange lists especially useful tools for people who follow carefully planned diets as a result of a health problem such as diabetes.

Exchange lists are also useful for people who are following calorie-controlled diets to lose weight. Dietitians sometimes give clients tailor-made diets centered on the exchange lists—say, a 1,500-calorie daily diet that might include six starches, five vegetables, two fruits, and so forth. A person can take such a framework and use the exchange lists to choose a wide variety of foods that fit into the basic eating plan.

Nutrition on the Web

www.cengage.com/nutrition/boyle/personalnutrition8e
Go to the *Personal Nutrition* section to check for the latest updates to chapter topics or to access links to related websites.

www.nap.edu
The National Academy Press site contains the latest Dietary Reference Intakes (DRI) reports.

www.nal.usda.gov/fnic
The Food and Nutrition Information Center (FNIC) provides credible, accurate, and practical information about nutrition and health. Browse by Subject to access links:

- Click on Dietary Guidance and then select Dietary Guidelines.
- Click on Dietary Guidance and then select MyPlate. Scroll down to access Ethnic/Cultural and Special Audience Food Guides.
- Click on Dietary Guidance and then select Dietary Reference Intakes.
- Click on Food Composition to access Food Composition resources.
- Click on Food Labeling for links to Food Labeling resources.

www.ChooseMyPlate.gov
This interactive website provides tips and resources for planning a healthy diet using MyPlate. Browse Interactive Tools to access links to the following:

- MyPlate Food Planner—an online menu-planning tool.
- MyPlate Tracker—an online dietary and physical activity assessment tool.

www.ars.usda.gov/ba/bhnrc/ndl
Click on Search for free food analyses. Just type in the food you want to analyze, and get a breakdown of its calories, fat, fiber, protein, vitamins, and minerals.

www.fao.org/ag/AGN/nutrition/education_guidelines_country_en.stm
Dietary guidelines and food guides from around the world.

www.cdc.gov/nutrition/index.html
The Centers for Disease Control and Prevention (CDC) maintains a nutrition home page that includes many links.

www.health.gov
This website sponsored by the U.S. Department of Health and Human Services (HHS) is a portal to websites of a number of multi-agency government health initiatives pertaining to health and nutrition.

http://nat.illinois.edu/
A free diet analysis program developed at the University of Illinois–Urbana/Champaign. This site allows anyone to analyze the various nutrients in the foods they eat.

www.fda.gov/Food/LabelingNutrition/default.htm
Useful facts about food labels; updates on label health claims.

Menu of Online Study Tools

A variety of study tools for this chapter are available at our website to deepen your understanding of chapter concepts. Go to

www.cengage.com/sso

to find

- Practice tests
- Flashcards
- Glossary
- Web links
- Animations
- Chapter summaries, learning objectives, and crossword puzzles.

Diet Analysis+ in Action

Go to the Profile report in Diet Analysis+ and record the daily recommended intakes for the following nutrients:

- calories
- protein
- fat
- fiber
- water
- sodium
- vitamin C

Using the three-day diet tracking you created in Chapter 1's assignment, go again to the food guide report and record which food groups were in the preferred range, which food groups were in the less-than-preferred-range, and which food groups exceeded the range.

Make a copy of your Profile (the foods you have recorded will also be copied). Now add one fruit to each meal for all three days. Once you have done that, look again at the food guide report. Have any of the ranges improved?

Try other changes—for example, substitute at least one whole-grain food in each meal for a less-nutritious choice (whole-grain toast instead of a bagel at breakfast; brown rice instead of French fries at lunch, etc.). What difference does that change make in the ranges? Based on this assignment, are there any changes you want to make in your diet?

UNIT 4

Useful Facts about Sugars, Starches, and Fiber

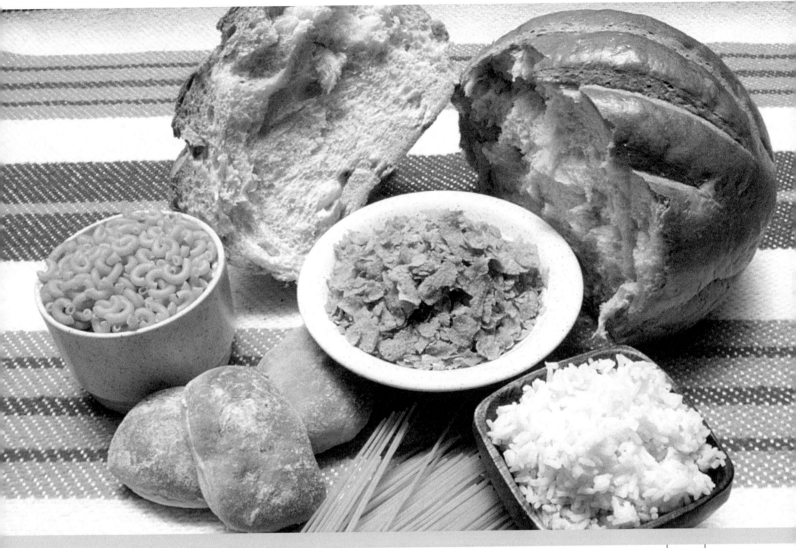

NUTRITION SCOREBOARD

		TRUE	FALSE
1	Pasta, bread, and potatoes are good sources of complex carbohydrates.		
2	Ounce for ounce, presweetened breakfast cereals and unsweetened cereals provide about the same number of calories.		
3	A 12-ounce can of soft drink contains about 3 tablespoons (9 teaspoons) of sugar.		
4	Lettuce, onions, and celery are high in dietary fiber.		
5	Cooking vegetables destroys their fiber content.		
6	Sugar consumption is the leading cause of tooth decay.		

Key Concepts and Facts

- Simple sugars, the "starchy" complex carbohydrates, and dietary fiber are members of the carbohydrate family.

- Ounce for ounce, sugars and the starchy complex carbohydrates supply fewer than half the calories of fat.

- Tooth decay and poor-quality diets are related to high sugar intake.

- Fiber benefits health in a number of ways.

Answers to
NUTRITION SCOREBOARD

	TRUE	FALSE
1 If you get this right, you may be in the minority. In one study of college students, only 38% could identify good sources of complex carbohydrates. Rice, crackers, grits, dried beans, corn, peas, tortillas, biscuits, and oatmeal are also good sources of complex carbohydrates.	✔	
2 That's true! Both sweetened and unsweetened cereals consist primarily of carbohydrate. A gram of carbohydrate provides 4 calories whether the source is sugar or flakes of corn.	✔	
3 That's a lot of sugar!	✔	
4 Although these are healthy food choices, they do not contain very much dietary fiber. (Not all that goes "crunch" is a good source of fiber.)		✔
5 Cooking doesn't destroy dietary fiber.		✔
6 Rates of tooth decay increase in populations as sugar intake increases.[1]	✔	

The Carbohydrates

carbohydrates
Chemical substances in foods that consist of a simple sugar molecule or multiples of them in various forms.

Carbohydrates are the major source of energy for people throughout the world. They are the primary ingredient of staple foods such as pasta, rice, cassava, beans, and bread. On average, Americans consume less carbohydrate than people in much of the world: approximately 50% of total calories.[2] This level of intake is on the low end of the recommended range of carbohydrate intake of 45 to 65% of total calories.[3]

The carbohydrate family consists of three types of chemical substances:

1. Simple sugars

2. Complex carbohydrates ("starch")

3. Total fiber

Some food sources of these different types of carbohydrate are shown in Illustration 4.1. Carbohydrates consist of carbon, hydrogen, and oxygen. They perform a number of functions in the body, but their primary function is to serve as an energy source. Simple sugars and complex carbohydrates supply the body with four calories per gram. Dietary fiber, on average, supplies two calories per gram.[4] Although humans cannot digest any of them, bacteria in the colon can digest some types of dietary fiber. These bacteria excrete fatty acids as a waste product from fiber digestion. The fatty acids are absorbed and used as a source of energy.[4] The total contribution of fiber to our energy intake is modest (around 50 calories) and supplying energy is not a major function of fiber. Certain

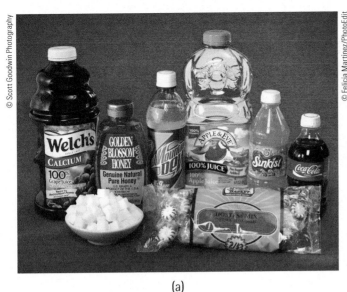

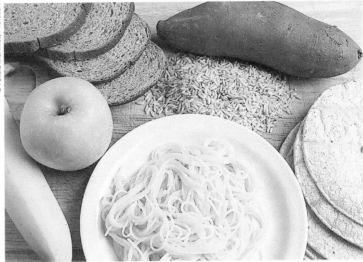

(a)

(b)

carbohydrates perform roles in the functioning of the immune system, reproductive system, and blood clotting. One simple sugar (ribose) is a key a component of the genetic material DNA.

Alcohol sugars and alcohol (ethanol) are similar in chemical structure to carbohydrates (Illustration 4.2) and are presented in this text. The alcohol sugars are presented in this Unit and alcohol in Unit 14. Increasingly, carbohydrates and carbohydrate-containing foods are being classified by their "glycemic index," or the extent to which they increase blood glucose levels. This topic is introduced in this unit and explored further in Unit 13 on diabetes.

Simple Sugar Facts

Simple sugars are considered "simple" because they are small molecules that require little or no digestion before they can be used by the body. They come in two types: **monosaccharides** and **disaccharides**. The monosaccharides consist of one molecule and include glucose ("blood sugar" or "dextrose"), fructose ("fruit sugar"), and galactose. Disaccharides consist of two monosaccharide molecules (see Table 4.1). The combination of a glucose molecule and a fructose molecule makes sucrose (or "table sugar"); maltose ("malt sugar") is made from two glucose molecules; and lactose ("milk sugar") consists of a glucose molecule plus a galactose molecule. Honey, by the way, is a disaccharide. It is composed of glucose and fructose just as sucrose is, but it's a liquid rather than a solid because of the way the two molecules of sugar are chemically linked together. Disaccharides are broken down into their monosaccharide components during digestion; only glucose, fructose, and galactose are absorbed into the bloodstream.

Illustration 4.1 The carbohydrate family. Some food sources of simple sugars (left), and some food sources of starch and dietary fiber (right) are shown.

simple sugars
Carbohydrates that consist of a glucose, fructose, or galactose molecule, or a combination of glucose and either fructose or galactose. High-fructose corn syrup and alcohol sugars are also considered simple sugars. Simple sugars are often referred to as "sugars."

monosaccharides
(*mono* = one, *saccharide* = sugar): Simple sugars consisting of one sugar molecule. Glucose, fructose, and galactose are common examples of monosaccharides.

disaccharides
(*di* = two, *saccharide* = sugar): Simple sugars consisting of two molecules of monosaccharides linked together. Sucrose, maltose, and lactose are disaccharides.

Illustration 4.2 The similar chemical structures of glucose, fructose, xylitol (an alcohol sugar), and ethanol (an alcohol).

Table 4.1

The monosaccharides and the disaccharides they form

Monosaccharides	Disaccharide formed
glucose + glucose	maltose
glucose + fructose	sucrose
glucose + galactose	lactose

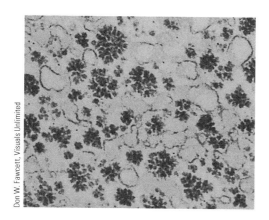

Illustration 4.3 Glycogen in a liver cell. The black "rosettes" are aggregates of glycogen molecules. This cell was photographed under an electron microscope at a magnification of 65,000X.

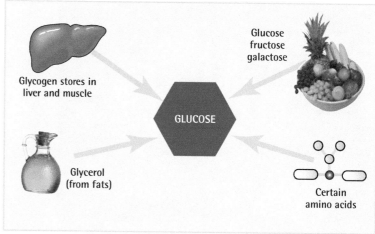

Illustration 4.4 The body's sources of glucose.

glycogen
The body's storage form of glucose. Glycogen is stored in the liver and muscles.

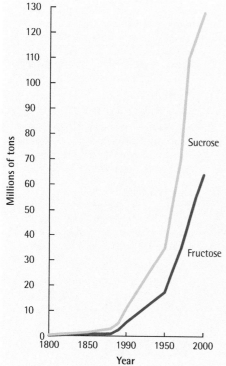

Illustration 4.5 Worldwide trends in sucrose and fructose consumption between 1800 and 2000.[a]

[a] Source: Figure drawn from data presented in Bray GA.[7]

High-fructose corn syrup—a liquid sweetener used in many soft drinks, fruit drinks, breakfast cereals, and other products is also considered a simple sugar. It generally consists of 55% fructose and 45% glucose.[5] Most of the simple sugars have a distinctively sweet taste.

The simple sugars the body uses directly to form energy are glucose and fructose. Galactose is readily converted by the body to glucose. When the body has more glucose than it needs for energy formation, it converts the excess to fat and to **glycogen**, the body's storage form of glucose. Glycogen is a type of complex carbohydrate. It consists of chains of glucose units linked together in long strands. Glycogen is produced only by animals and is stored in the liver (Illustration 4.3) and muscles. When the body needs additional glucose, glycogen is broken down, making glucose available for energy formation. Glucose can also be derived from certain amino acids and the glycerol component of fats. Illustration 4.4 shows the various ways glucose becomes available to the body. A constant supply of glucose is needed because the brain, red blood cells, white blood cells, and specific cells in the kidneys require glucose as an energy source.[2]

Simple Sugar Intake Most of the simple sugar in our diet comes from foods and beverages sweetened with sucrose and high fructose corn syrup. As a matter of fact, simple sugars are the most commonly used food additive.[6] Per person consumption of added sucrose and fructose has increased dramatically across the globe over time (Illustration 4.5). Added sugars now make up 17% of the total calorie intake of Americans.[8] Combined with naturally occurring simple sugars in fruits and some vegetables, total simple sugar consumption in the United States averages 23% of total calories.[2] That's a lot of sugar and far more than is good for health.[7,9]

The largest source of simple sugar in the diet is beverages, particularly soft drinks.[9] One 12-ounce serving of soft drink contains about 9 teaspoons of simple sugar. Sucrose and high fructose corn syrup are commonly added to fruit drinks, breakfast cereals, and candy. Simple sugars are also present in fruits, and small amounts are found in some vegetables (Table 4.2). Milk is the only animal product that contains a simple sugar (lactose).

Nutrition Labeling of Sugars Nutrition labels must list the total amount of mono- and diglycerides per serving of food under the heading "sugars" (Illustration 4.6). In addition, in the ingredient list, all simple sugars contained in the product must be listed in order of weight.[10] Labels contain information on total sugars per serving and do not distinguish between sugars naturally present in foods and added sugars.

Table 4.2

The simple sugar content of some common foods

	Amount	Simple Sugars (grams)[a]	% Total Calories from Simple Sugars
Sweeteners:			
Corn syrup	1 tsp	5	100%
Honey	1 tsp	6	100
Maple syrup	1 tsp	4	100
Table sugar	1 tsp	4	100
Fruits:			
Apple	1 medium	16	91
Peach	1 medium	8	91
Watermelon	1 wedge (4" × 8")	25	87
Orange	1 medium	14	86
Banana	1 medium	21	85
Vegetables:			
Broccoli	1/2 cup	2	40
Corn	1/2 cup	3	30
Potato	1 medium	1	4
Beverages:			
Fruit drinks	1 cup	29	100
Soft drinks	12 oz	38	100
Skim milk	1 cup	12	53
Whole milk	1 cup	11	28
Candy:			
Gumdrops	1 oz	25	100
Hard candy	1 oz	28	100
Caramels	1 oz	21	73
Fudge	1 oz	21	73
Milk chocolate	1 oz	16	44
Breakfast cereals			
Apple Jacks	1 oz	13	52
Raisin Bran	1 oz	19	40
Cheerios	1 oz	14	4

[a] 4 grams sucrose 5 1 teaspoon.

What's So Bad about Sugar? Foods to which simple sugars have been added are often not among the top sources of nutrients. Simple sugars are among the few foods that provide only calories. Many foods high in simple sugars, such as cake, sweet rolls, cookies, pie, candy bars, and ice cream, are also high in fat. The likelihood that diets will provide insufficient amounts of vitamins and minerals increases along with sugar intake.[2] High levels of consumption of sucrose and fructose are related to increased blood levels of triglycerides.[5] Neither sucrose or high fructose corn syrup has been found to cause obesity or type 2 diabetes. However, high intakes of these sweeteners may contribute to the risk of both disorders due to excessive calorie intake.[9,11] Furthermore, it is perfectly clear that the frequent consumption of sticky sweets causes tooth decay.[6]

Advice on Sugar Intake What's the bottom line on eating sugary foods? Enjoy them in limited amounts as part of a healthful diet. The World Health Organization and other health authorities in 26 countries recommend limiting added sugars to 10% of calories or less.[13] If you are concerned about the amount of sugar in your diet and your teeth, don't wait until it's time for a New Year's resolution. Get some suggestions for small changes that will have a positive impact in this Unit's Take Action feature.

Illustration 4.6 Labeling the sugar content of breakfast cereal

	% Daily Value**	
Total Fat 1 g*	2%	2%
Saturated Fat 0 g	0%	0%
Monounsaturated Fat 0 g		
Polyunsaturated Fat 0.5 g		
Trans Fat 0 g		
Cholesterol 0 mg	0%	0%
Sodium 5 mg	0%	3%
Potassium 200 mg	6%	12%
Total Carbohydrate 48 g	16%	18%
Dietary Fiber 6 g	24%	24%
Sugars 12 g		
Other Carbohydrate 30 g		
Protein 6 g		
Vitamin A	0%	4%
Vitamin C	0%	0%
Calcium	0%	15%
Iron	90%	90%
Thiamin	25%	30%
Riboflavin	25%	35%
Niacin	25%	25%
Vitamin B$_6$	25%	25%
Folic Acid	25%	25%
Vitamin B$_{12}$	25%	35%
Phosphorus	15%	25%
Magnesium	15%	20%
Zinc	10%	15%
Copper	10%	10%

	Calories	2,000	2,500
Total Fat	Less than	65 g	80 g
Saturated Fat	Less than	20 g	25 g
Cholesterol	Less than	300 mg	300 mg
Sodium	Less than	2,400 mg	2,400 mg
Potassium		3,500 mg	3,500 mg
Total Carbohydrate		300 g	375 g
Dietary Fiber		25 g	30 g

Calories Per gram: Fat 9 • Carbohydrate 4 • Protein 4

INGREDIENTS: WHOLE GRAIN WHEAT, SUGAR, HIGH FRUCTOSE CORN SYRUP, GELATIN, **VITAMINS AND MINERALS:** REDUCED IRON, NIACINAMIDE, ZINC OXIDE, PYRIDOXINE HYDRO-CHLORIDE (VITAMIN B$_6$), RIBOFLAVIN (VITAMIN B$_2$), THIAMIN HYDROCHLORIDE (VITAMIN B$_1$), FOLIC ACID AND VITAMIN B$_{12}$, TO MAINTAIN QUALITY, BHT HAS BEEN ADDED TO THE PACKAGING.

The Alcohol Sugars—What Are They?

alcohol sugars
Simple sugars containing an alcohol group in their molecular structure. The most common are xylitol, mannitol, and sorbitol. They are a subgroup of chemical substances called "polyols."

Nonalcoholic in the beverage sense, the **alcohol sugars** (or "polyols") are like simple sugars except that they include a chemical component of alcohol. Like simple sugars, the alcohol sugars have a sweet taste. Xylitol is by far the sweetest alcohol sugar—it's much sweeter than the other two common alcohol sugars, mannitol and sorbitol.

Alcohol sugars are found naturally in very small amounts in some fruits. They are mostly used as sweetening agents in gums and candy (Illustration 4.7). Unlike the simple sugars, xylitol, mannitol, and sorbitol do not promote tooth

Take Action Lower Your Sugar Intake

Concerned about your sugar intake? Want to consider some ways to lower it and to protect your teeth?

Consider these actions and check the options you'd be willing to try.

_____ 1. When you want something sweet to eat, try:

_____ raisins
_____ sweet cherries
_____ melon
_____ a banana
_____ other fruit: _____
_____ a mango
_____ unsweetened applesauce

_____ 2. Replace a serving of soft drink or fruit drink with a no-added sugar, 100% juice serving such as:

_____ tomato juice
_____ vegetable juice
_____ dark grape juice
_____ apple cider/juice
_____ other juice: _____
_____ pineapple juice
_____ cranberry juice
_____ grapefruit-tangerine juice

_____ 3. Taste-test beverages or gum sweetened with alcohol sugars or artificial sweeteners for acceptability. Try:

_____ ice tea sweetened with aspartame or sucrolose
_____ soft drinks sweetened with Reb A or aspartame
_____ gum sweetened with xylitol or other alcohol sugar

_____ 4. Keep sugar off your teeth. After you eat a food with added sugar:

_____ rinse your mouth with water
_____ brush your teeth
_____ floss in between your teeth

decay because bacteria in the mouth that cause tooth decay cannot digest them.[6] Foods sweetened with alcohol sugars can use the health claim "Does not promote tooth decay" on labels.

Like dietary fiber, the alcohol sugars are slowly and incompletely broken down in the gastrointestinal tract, and provide fewer calories per gram than other carbohydrates. On average, alcohol sugars provide two calories per gram, so foods labeled "sugar free" will not be calorie-free. High intake of alcohol sugars can, like fiber, cause diarrhea. This characteristic limits their use in foods. The "diarrhea dose" for alcohol sugars defined by the FDA equals 50 grams of sorbitol, and 20 grams of mannitol. A food product's content of alcohol sugars per serving must be listed on the nutrition label as "Sugar Alcohols" or by the name of the sugar alcohol.[10]

Artificial Sweetener Facts

Unwanted calories in simple sugars, the connection of sucrose with tooth decay, the need for a sugar substitute for people with diabetes, and sugar shortages such as occurred during the two world wars have all provided incentives for developing sugar substitutes. Six artificial sweeteners are currently on the market in the United States, (Table 4.3) more are being developed. None of the artificial sweeteners that are currently approved for use exactly mimic the taste and properties of sugar.[14,15]

Artificial sweeteners are also known as non-nutritive sweeteners because they are not a significant source of energy or nutrients.[14] Although they are not carbohydrates, they have chemical properties that invoke an intensively sweet taste on the tongue. Gram for gram, artificial sweeteners are 160 to 13,000 times sweeter than sucrose and only small amounts are needed to sweeten food products. Of the artificial sweeteners, only aspartame provides calories (4 calories/gram).[6]

Table 4.3

Artificial sweeteners currently approved for use in the United States

Trade name	Product name	Calories/gram
Saccharin	Sweet and Low	0
Aspartame	NutraSweet, Equal Sugar Twin	4
Sucralose	Splenda	0
Acesulfame potassium	Acesulfame K, Sunnette, Sweet One	0
Neotame	–	0
Rebiana	Reb-A, Truvia, PureVia	0

Illustration 4.8 Some of the thousands of foods that contain artificial sweeteners.

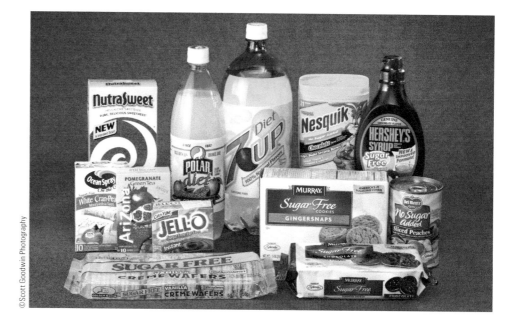

©Scott Goodwin Photography

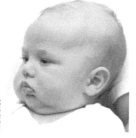

Photo Disc

phenylketonuria (feen-ol-key-tone-u-re-ah), PKU
A rare genetic disorder related to the lack of the enzyme phenylalanine hydroxylase. Lack of this enzyme causes the essential amino acid phenylalanine to build up in blood.

The artificial sweeteners currently on the market do not promote tooth decay because they are not utilized by bacteria in the mouth that cause decay.[6] They do not appear to promote weight loss without calorie restriction.[14] Artificial sweeteners are used to sweeten thousands of products, a few of which are shown in Illustration 4.8.

Saccharin Saccharin was the first artificial sweetener developed. Did you know that it was discovered in a laboratory in the late 1800s? That's right—saccharin is over 100 years old. The availability of this artificial sweetener, which is 300 times as sweet as sucrose, helped relieve the sugar shortages that occurred during World Wars I and II.

In 1977 saccharin was taken off the market after very high doses were found to cause cancer in laboratory animals. At that time, however, saccharin was the only no-calorie, artificial sweetener available, and its removal sparked a public outcry. After many people complained to Congress, saccharin was returned to the market by congressional mandate. Saccharin was deemed safe in 2000 after scientists concluded there was no clear evidence that it causes cancer in humans.[16]

Aspartame Early in the 1980s, the artificial sweetener aspartame was approved for use in the United States and more than 90 other countries. Primarily known as Nutrasweet, this artificial sweetener is about 200 times sweeter than sucrose.

Aspartame is made from two amino acids (phenylalanine and aspartame). Both are found in nature, but it took chemists to arrange their chemical partnership. Because aspartame is made from amino acids (the building blocks of protein), it supplies four calories per gram. Aspartame is so sweet, however, that very little is needed to sweeten products. Illustration 4.9 shows the relative sweetening power of various artificial sweeteners and naturally occurring sugars.

Aspartame is used in more than 6000 products worldwide, including soft drinks, whipped toppings, jellies, cereals, puddings, and some medicines. Products containing aspartame must carry a label warning people with **phenylketonuria** (an inherited disease) and others with certain liver conditions about the presence of phenylalanine. People with these disorders are unable to utilize the amino acid phenylalanine, causing it to build up in the blood. Because high temperatures tend to break down aspartame, it is not used in baked or heated products.[6]

■ Is Aspartame Safe? A safe level of aspartame intake is defined as 50 milligrams per kilogram of body weight per day in the United States and as

40 milligrams per kilogram of body weight in Canada.[18] In food terms, the limit in the United States is equivalent to approximately 20 aspartame-sweetened soft drinks or 55 desserts per day (Illustration 4.10). The average intake of aspartame in the United States, Canada, Germany, and Finland, for example, ranges from 2 to 10 milligrams per day, well below the level of intake considered safe.[21] A small proportion of individuals, however, report that they are sensitive to aspartame and develop headaches, dizziness, or anxiety when they consume small amounts. Studies have failed to confirm these effects.[19] Aspartame has not been found to promote cancer, nerve disorders, or other health problems in humans.[20]

Sucralose   This noncaloric, intense sweetener is made from sucrose, is safe, is very sweet (600 times sweeter than sucrose), and does not leave a bitter aftertaste. Known primarily as "Splenda" on product labels, it is used in both hot and cold food products, including soft drinks, baked goods, frosting, pudding, and chewing gum.

Acesulfame Potassium   Acesulfame potassium, also known as acesulfame K, "Sunette" and "Sweet One," was approved by the FDA in 1988. It is added to at least 4000 foods and is used in food production in about 90 countries. It is 200 times as sweet as sucrose, provides zero calories, and does not break down when heated.

Neotame   Neotame is derived from the same amino acids as aspartame and is extraordinarily sweet. (Its sweetness potency is 7000 to 13,000 times that of sucrose.) Only minute amounts of neotame are absorbed and it is not considered harmful to individuals with PKU. It is marketed as having a clean sweet taste with little bitter or metallic aftertaste.[6]

Rebiana   In December 2008 the FDA approved Rebiana for use as an artificial sweetener. Called Reb-A, Truvia, and Purevia, this sweetener is derived from the herb stevia (Illustration 4.11). Stevia grows in sub-tropical and tropical areas and has been known in these areas as "sugar leaf" for centuries.

Stevia leaves contain the chemical rebaudioside that imparts a sweet taste and it is used in purified form in Reb-A. It is currently used to sweeten beverages (Illustration 4.12) and reportedly tastes best with citrus flavors.[15]

NEOTAME

SUCRALOSE

SACCHARIN

REB-A

ACESULFAME K

ASPARTAME

FRUCTOSE

SUCROSE

XYLITOL

GLUCOSE

SORBITOL

MANNITOL

GALACTOSE

MALTOSE

LACTOSE

Illustration 4.9   A ranking of various types of artificial sweeteners and naturally occurring sugars in order of sweetness.

Illustration 4.10   You would have to consume more than 20 cans of soft drinks sweetened with aspartame (Nutrasweet) a day to exceed the safe limit set for this artificial sweetener.

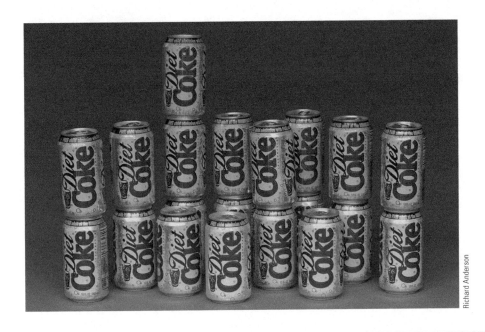

Richard Anderson

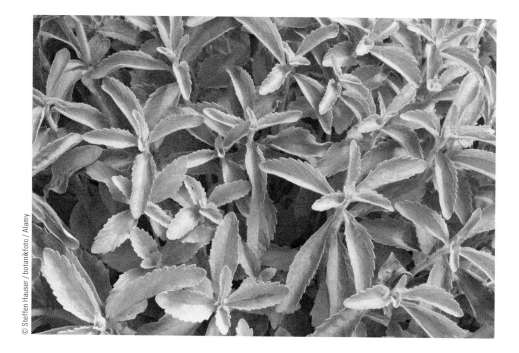

Illustration 4.11 The stevia plant is the source of the artificial sweetener rebiana.

complex carbohydrates
The form of carbohydrate found in starchy vegetables, grains, and dried beans and in many types of dietary fiber. The most common form of starch is made of long chains of interconnected glucose units.

polysaccharides
(*poly* = many, *saccharide* = sugar): Carbohydrates containing many molecules of monosaccharides linked together. Starch, glycogen, and dietary fiber are the three major types of polysaccharides. Polysaccharides consisting of 3 to 10 monosaccharides may be referred to as oligosaccharides.

Illustration 4.12 Example of beverages sweetened with rebiana (Reb-A).

Complex Carbohydrate Facts

Starches, glycogen, and dietary fiber constitute the **complex carbohydrates** known as **polysaccharides.** Only plant foods such as grains, potatoes, dried beans, and corn that contain starch and dietary fiber are considered dietary sources of complex carbohydrates (Table 4.4). Very little glycogen is available from animal products.

Which Foods Have Carbohydrates? Food sources of complex carbohydrates include whole-grain breads, cereals, pastas, and crackers, as well as these same foods produced from refined grains. Whole grain products provide more fiber and beneficial substances naturally present in grains than do refined grain products. Whole grain foods reduce the risk of heart disease and some types of cancer.[21]

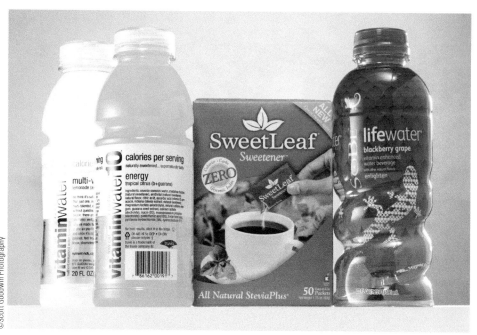

Table 4.4

The complex carbohydrate content of some common foods

	Amount	Complex Carbohydrate (grams)	% Total Calories from Complex Carbohydrates
Grain and grain products:			
Rice (white), cooked	¹/₂ cup	21	83%
Pasta, cooked	¹/₂ cup	15	81
Cornflakes	1 cup	11	76
Oatmeal, cooked	¹/₂ cup	12	74
Cheerios	1 cup	11	68
Whole wheat bread	1 slice	7	60
Dried beans (cooked):			
Lima beans	¹/₂ cup	11	64
White beans	¹/₂ cup	13	63
Kidney beans	¹/₂ cup	12	59
Vegetables:			
Potato	1 medium	30	85
Corn	¹/₂ cup	10	67
Broccoli	¹/₂ cup	2	40

Are They Fattening?   Starchy foods are caloric bargains (Illustration 4.13, next page). A medium baked potato weighs in at only 122 calories, a half-cup of corn at 85 calories, and a slice of bread at 70 calories. You can expand the caloric value of complex carbohydrates quite easily by adding fat, sauces, and cheese. One cup of macaroni (about 200 calories) gains around 180 calories when it comes as macaroni and cheese. Adding a quarter-cup of gravy to potatoes elevates calories by 150.

United States Fiber Facts   What is low in calories, prevents constipation, may lower the risk of heart disease, obesity, and diabetes; and is generally underconsumed by people in the United States? The answer is fiber.

Total fiber intake by U.S. children and adults (15 grams per day) is well below the amount recommended (28 grams for women and 35 grams for men).[41] People who consume the recommended amount of fiber tend to select whole-grain breads, high-fiber cereal, and dried beans most days and eat at least five servings of vegetables and fruits daily.[22] Food sources of fiber are listed in Table 4.5. It doesn't matter whether the fiber foods are mashed, chopped, cooked, or raw. They retain their fiber value through it all.

In the past it was assumed that fiber had no calorie value because it is not broken down by human digestive enzymes. Recent studies suggest that the calorie contribution of dietary fiber be re-considered. Bacteria in the colon are able to break down many types of fiber to some extent. The bacteria excrete fatty acids as a waste product and they are used as an energy source by the colon and the rest of the body. On average, fiber provides two calorie per gram.[4] Although not yet required on U.S. or Canadian nutrition information labels, those in the European Union must include the calorie contribution of fiber in food products.[23]

Types of Fiber   A new classification system for defining edible fibers based on source of fiber and effects on body processes has been developed.[3] Fibers are classified as **functional fiber**, **dietary fiber**, and **total fiber**. All fiber shares the property of not being digested by human digestive enzymes.

Functional fibers perform specific, beneficial functions in the body, including decreasing food intake by providing a feeling of fullness, reducing postmeal rises in blood glucose levels, preventing constipation, and decreasing fat and

functional fiber
Specific types of nondigestible carbohydrates that have beneficial effects on health. Two examples of functional fibers are psyllium and pectin.

dietary fiber
Naturally occurring, intact forms of nondigestible carbohydrates in plants and "woody" plant cell walls. Oat and wheat bran, and raffinose in dried beans, are examples of this type of fiber.

total fiber
The sum of functional and dietary fiber.

Illustration 4.13 Which has more calories?
Check your answers below.[a]

One medium baked potato (four ounces) OR three ounces of lean hamburger?

One slice of bread OR a half-cup of low-fat cottage cheese?

One cup of spaghetti noodles OR 17 french fries (three ounces)?

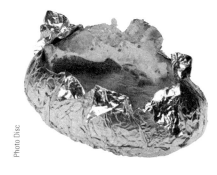

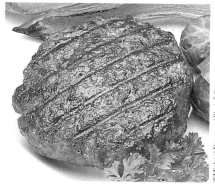

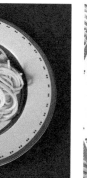

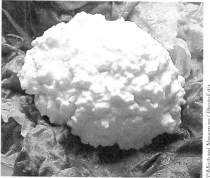

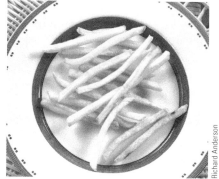

[a]*Answers*
Potato = 122 calories;
Lean hamburger = 239 calories.
Bread = 70 calories;
Cottage cheese = 102 calories.
Spaghetti = 197 calories;
French fries = 265 calories.

Who gets thumbs up?
Answers on page 98

Reality Check

Carbohydrate craving   Have you ever pined or whined for something sweet? Is a meal not complete unless there's a "starch?" Do you think you can get addicted to carbohydrates?

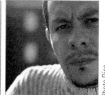

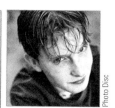

Terry:
Maybe you could really love to eat them, but addicted? I don't think so.

Wolfgang:
The more I don't eat candy, the more I want to eat some. I swear, I'm addicted.

Table 4.5

Examples of good sources of fiber

The recommended intake of total fiber for men is 38 grams per day and 25 grams per day for women.

	Amount	Fiber (grams)
Grain and grain products:		
Bran Buds	$^1/_2$ cup	12.0
All Bran	$^1/_2$ cup	11.0
Raisin Bran	1 cup	7.0
Granola (homemade)	$^1/_2$ cup	6.0
Bran Flakes	$^3/_4$ cup	5.0
Oatmeal	1 cup	4.0
Spaghetti noodles	1 cup	4.0
Shredded Wheat	1 biscuit	2.7
Whole wheat bread	1 slice	2.0
Bran (dry; wheat, oat)	2 tbs	2.0
Fruits:		
Raspberries	1 cup	8.0
Avocado	$^1/_2$ medium	7.0
Mango	1 medium	4.0
Pear (with skin)	1 medium	4.0
Apple (with skin)	1 medium	3.3
Banana	6" long	3.1
Orange (no peel)	1 medium	3.0
Peach (with skin)	1 medium	2.3
Strawberries	10 medium	2.1
Vegetables:		
Lima beans	$^1/_2$ cup	6.6
Green peas	$^1/_2$ cup	4.4
Potato (with skin)	1 medium	3.5
Brussels sprouts	$^1/_2$ cup	3.0
Broccoli	$^1/_2$ cup	2.8
Carrots	$^1/_2$ cup	2.8
Green beans	$^1/_2$ cup	2.7
Collard greens	$^1/_2$ cup	2.7
Cauliflower	$^1/_2$ cup	2.5
Corn	$^1/_2$ cup	2.0
Nuts:		
Almonds	$^1/_4$ cup	4.5
Peanuts	$^1/_4$ cup	3.3
Peanut butter	2 tbs	2.3
Dried beans (cooked):		
Pinto beans	$^1/_2$ cup	10.0
Peas, split	$^1/_2$ cup	8.2
Black beans (turtle beans)	$^1/_2$ cup	8.0
Lentils	$^1/_2$ cup	7.8
Kidney or navy beans	$^1/_2$ cup	6.9
Black-eyed peas	$^1/_2$ cup	5.3
Fast foods:		
Big Mac	1	3
French fries	1 regular serving	3
Whopper	1	3
Cheeseburger	1	2
Taco	1	2
Chicken sandwich	2	1
Egg McMuffin	1	1
Fried chicken, drumstick	1	1

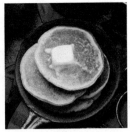

Photo Disc

Have you ever had buckwheat pancakes (three grams of fiber per serving)? Did you know that buckwheat is a member of the rhubarb family—not a grain?

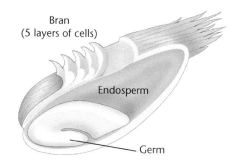

Illustration 4.14 Diagram of a grain of wheat showing the bran that is a rich source of dietary fiber. The germ contains protein, unsaturated fats, thiamin, niacin, riboflavin, iron, and other nutrients. (The bran and germ are removed in the refining process.) The endosperm primarily contains starch, the storage form of glucose in plants.

cholesterol absorption.[3] This type of fiber can be extracted from foods or produced commercially for use in fortifying foods with fiber, as well as in fiber supplements.[4] Psyllium, pectin, gels, and seed and plant gums are classified as functional fibers.

Dietary fiber consists of nondigestible carbohydrates found in plant foods. Because functional fibers are components of plant foods, this type of fiber comes with all of the other beneficial nutrients and other substances found in plants. Dietary fibers are found in the bran component of oats and wheat (Illustration 4.14), in cellulose (a rigid component of plant cell walls), in vegetables and fruits, and in the nondigestible starch components of dried beans. The recommended daily intake of fiber is based on total fiber, which is the sum of functional plus dietary fiber intake.[3]

■ **Soluble and Insoluble Fiber.** Soluble fiber is a functional fiber because it benefits health in several ways. Soluble fiber slows glucose absorption, thereby lowering peak blood levels of glucose, and reduces fat and cholesterol absorption. Soluble fibers are found in oats, barley, fruit pulp, and psyllium. They are called "soluble" because of their ability to combine chemically with water.[41]

Insoluble fibers, such as wheat bran and other brans, and the fiber in legumes, do not combine chemically with water. They offer some of the same health benefits as do soluble fiber and are particularly beneficial in preventing constipation.[41]

Be Cautious When Adding More Fiber to Your Diet Newcomers to adequate fiber diets often experience diarrhea, bloating, and gas for the first week or so of increased fiber intake. These side effects can be avoided. They occur when too much fiber is added to the diet too quickly. Adding sources of dietary fiber to the diet gradually can prevent these side effects. In addition, dietary fiber can be constipating if consumed with too little fluid. Your fluid intake should increase along with your intake of dietary fiber. You know you've got the right amount of fiber in your diet when stools float and are soft and well formed.

The "Health Action" on the next page suggests some food choices that will put fiber into your meals and snacks. Fiber should be added carefully to children's diets, because the large volume of some high-fiber diets can fill the children up before they consume enough calories.[24]

Glycemic Index of Carbohydrates

In the not-too-distant past it was assumed that "a carbohydrate is a carbohydrate is a carbohydrate." It was thought that all types of carbohydrates had the same effect on blood glucose levels and health, so it didn't matter what type was consumed. As is the case with many untested assumptions, this one fell by the wayside. It is now known that some types of simple and complex carbohydrates in

Carbohydrate craving The popular theory about carbohydrate craving and addiction goes like this: Carbohydrates increase blood levels of glucose, then insulin level surges to drop blood glucose levels. Resulting low blood glucose levels send a message to your brain telling you that carbohydrates are needed to bring your blood glucose levels back up. The truth is there are no biological processes that make healthy people crave carbohydrate. (There may be psychological cravings, however.) Any source of calories will relieve hunger.[21]

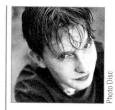

Terry

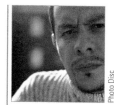

Wolfgang

HIGH-FIBER OPTIONS FOR BREAKFAST

Whole grain toast		2 g per slice
Bran cereal:		
Bran flakes	1 cup	7 g
All Bran	¹/₂ cup	11 g
Raisin bran	1 cup	7 g
Oat bran	¹/₃ cup	5 g
Bran muffin, with fruit:	1 small	3 g
Strawberries	10	2 g
Raspberries	¹/₂ cup	3 g
Bananas	1 medium	2 g

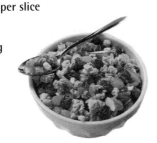

LUNCHES THAT INCLUDE FIBER

Whole grain bread		2 g per slice
Baked beans	¹/₂ cup	10 g
Carrot	1 medium	2 g
Raisins	¹/₄ cup	2 g
Peas	¹/₂ cup	4 g
Peanut butter	2 tablespoons	2 g

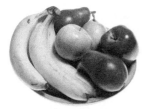

FIBER ON THE MENU FOR SUPPER

Brown rice	¹/₂ cup	2 g
Potato	1 medium	3 g
Dried cooked beans	¹/₂ cup	8 g
Broccoli	¹/₂ cup	3 g
Corn	¹/₂ cup	3 g
Tomato	1 medium	2 g
Green beans	¹/₂ cup	3 g

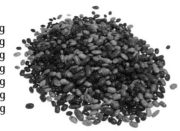

FIBER-FILLED SNACKS

Peanuts	¹/₄ cup	3 g
Apple	1 medium	2 g
Pear	1 medium	4 g
Orange	1 medium	3 g
Prunes	3	2 g[a]
Sunflower seeds	¹/₄ cup	2 g
Popcorn	2 cups	2 g

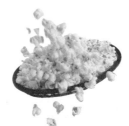

Photo Disc

[a]Prunes contain fiber, but their laxative effect is primarily due to a naturally occurring chemical substance that causes an uptake of fluid into the intestines and the contraction of muscles that line the intestines.

foods elevate blood glucose levels more than do others. Such differences are particularly important to people with disorders such as **insulin resistance** and **type 2 diabetes.**[25]

Carbohydrates and cabohydrate-containing foods are now being classified by the extent to which they increase blood glucose levels. This classification system is called the **glycemic index.** Carbohydrates that are digested and absorbed quickly have a high glycemic index and raise blood glucose levels to a higher extent than do those with lower glycemic index values. Carbohydrates and carbohydrate-containing foods with high glycemic index values include glucose, white bread, baked potatoes, and jelly beans. Fructose, xylitol, hummus, apples, and all-bran cereal are examples of carbohydrates and carbohydrate-containing

insulin resistance
A condition is which cell membranes have a reduced sensitivity to insulin so that more insulin than normal is required to transport a given amount of glucose into cells.

type 2 diabetes
A disease characterized by high blood glucose levels due to the body's inability to use insulin normally or to produce enough insulin.

glycemic index
A measure of the extent to which blood glucose is raised by a 50-gram portion of a carbohydrate-containing food compared to 50 grams of glucose or white bread.

foods with low glycemic indexes. Fructose has a low glycemic index because it does not raise blood glucose levels. It is absorbed as fructose and does not require insulin for passage into cells.[26]

Diets providing low glycemic index carbohydrates have been found to improve blood glucose control in people with diabetes, to reduce elevated levels of blood cholesterol and triglycerides, increase levels of beneficial HDL cholesterol, and decrease the risk of developing type 2 diabetes, some types of cancer, and heart disease.[27]

Carbohydrates and Your Teeth

tooth decay
The disintegration of teeth due to acids produced by bacteria in the mouth that feed on sugar. Also called dental caries or cavities.

The relationship between sugar and **tooth decay** is very close, and the history of tooth decay closely parallels the availability of sugar. The incidence of tooth decay is estimated to have been very low (less than 5%) among hunter-gatherers who had minimal access to sugars.[29] Tooth decay did not become a widespread problem until the late 17th century, when great quantities of sucrose were exported from the New World to Europe and other parts of the world. When sugar shortages occurred in the United States and Europe during World War I and World War II, rates of tooth decay declined; they rebounded when sugar became available again.[29] Rates of tooth decay in children vary substantially among countries, but the highest rates are in countries where sugar is widely available in processed foods and beverages. Tooth decay is spreading rapidly in developing countries where sugar, candy, soft drinks, and fruit drinks are becoming widely available.[30]

Sweets are not the only culprit. Simple sugars that promote tooth decay can also come from starchy foods, especially pretzels, crackers, and breads that stick to your gums and teeth. Some of the starch is broken down to simple sugars by enzymes in the mouth.

To reduce the incidence of tooth decay, a number of countries have developed campaigns to help inform consumers about cavity-promoting foods. Switzerland and other countries label foods that are safe for the teeth with a "happy tooth" symbol (Illustration 4.15) and encourages the use of alcohol sugars (which don't promote tooth decay) in sweets.[23] Other countries recommend that sweets be consumed with meals or that teeth be brushed after sweets are eaten.

There's More to Tooth Decay Than Sugar Per Se How frequently sugary and starchy foods are consumed and how long they stick to gums and teeth make a difference in their tooth-decay-promoting effects. Marshmallows, caramels, and taffy, for example, are much more likely to promote tooth decay than are apples and milk chocolate. Nevertheless, all of the foods listed in Table 4.6 can promote

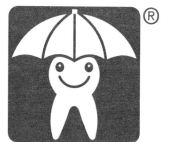

Illustration 4.15 Switzerland's "happy tooth" symbol. It has became an internationally used symbol.

Table 4.6

The "stickiness" value of some foods

The stickier the food, the worse it is for your teeth.

Very Sticky	Sticky	Somewhat Sticky	Barely Sticky
Caramels	Doughnuts	Bagels	Apples
Chewy cookies	Figs	Cake	Bananas
Crackers	Frosting	Cereal	Fruit drinks
Cream-filled cookies	Fudge	Dry cookies	Fruit juices
Granola bars	Hard candy	Milk chocolate	Ice cream
Marshmallows	Honey	Rolls	Oranges
Pretzels	Jelly beans	White bread	Peaches
Taffy	Pastries		Pears
	Raisins		
	Syrup		

Table 4.7

Foods that don't promote tooth decay.[3,39,40]

Artificial sweeteners	Gum and candy sweetened with	Peanut butter
Cheese	alcohol sugars	Tea
Coffee (no sugar)	Meats	Water
Eggs	Milk	Yogurt (plain)
Fats and oils	Nuts	Vegetables
		Fresh fruit

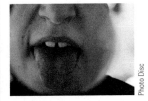
On the Side

Bacteria on the tongue have recently been identified as the primary cause of bad breath. Mouthwash gets rid of bad breath for about an hour; brushing teeth with toothpaste takes care of it in 25% of people, but brushing the tongue eliminates it in 70 to 80%.[33]

tooth decay if allowed to remain in contact with the gums and teeth. Drinking coffee or tea with sugar throughout the day or consuming three or more regular soft drinks between meals hastens tooth decay (more than if these beverages are consumed with meals) Candy, cookies, and crackers eaten between meals are much more likely to promote tooth decay than are the same foods consumed as part of a meal. Chewing as few as two sticks of sugar-containing gum a day also significantly increases tooth decay.[31,32]

Why Does Sugar Promote Tooth Decay? Sugar promotes tooth decay because it is the sole food for certain bacteria that live in the mouth and excrete acid that dissolves teeth. In the presence of sugar, bacteria in the mouth multiply rapidly and form a sticky, white material called **plaque.** Tooth areas covered by plaque are prime locations for tooth decay because they are dense in acid-producing bacteria. Acid production by bacteria increases within 5 minutes of exposure to sugar. It continues for 20 to 30 minutes after the bacteria ingest the sugar.[34] If teeth are frequently exposed to sugar, the acid produced by bacteria may erode the enamel, producing a cavity. If the erosion continues, the cavity can extend into the tooth and allow bacteria to enter the inside of the tooth. That can cause an infection and the loss of the tooth. It can be prevented if the plaque is removed before the acid erodes much of the enamel. Teeth are capable of replacing small amounts of minerals lost from enamel.[35] Table 4.7 lists foods that do not promote tooth decay.

plaque
A soft, sticky, white material on teeth; formed by bacteria.

"Water fluoridation is one of the ten great public health achievements of the twentieth century."

—W. Bailey[36]

Water Fluoridation In the early 1930s, lower rates of tooth decay were observed among children living in areas where water naturally contained fluoride. This provided the initial evidence that led to the fluoridation of many community water supplies. Fluoridated water reduces the incidences of tooth decay by 50% or more and is primarily responsible for declining rates of tooth decay and loss.[36]

Credit for declines in tooth decay and tooth loss in the United States is also shared by fluoride supplements, toothpastes, rinses and gels, protective sealants, and improved dental hygiene and care.[1] Further improvements in rates of dental caries will occur with reduced intake of sugars and sticky carbohydrates. Fluoridation is a safe, effective, and cheap method of controlling dental disease; providing fluoridated community water supplies costs about 50 cents per person per year.[38] Despite the advantages of fluoride, 31% of Americans consume water from a less than optimally fluoridated water supply.[36]

Baby Bottle Caries A startling example of the effect that frequent and prolonged exposure to sugary foods can have is "baby bottle caries" (Illustration 4.16). Infants and young children who routinely fall asleep while sucking a bottle of sugar water, fruit drink, milk, or formula—or while breastfeeding—may develop severe decay. After the child falls asleep, the fluid may continue to drip into the

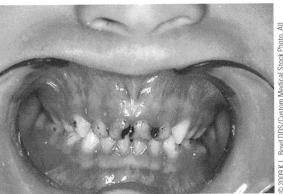

Illustration 4.16 "Baby bottle caries" (also called "nursing bottle syndrome") occurs in infants who habitually receive sweet fluids or milk in bottles when they go to sleep. Cavities occur first in the upper front teeth because that's where fluid pools when babies sleep.

mouth. A pool of the fluid collects between the tongue and the front teeth, bathing the teeth in the sweet fluid for as long as the child sleeps. The upper front teeth become decayed first because the tongue protects the lower teeth. Baby bottle caries occur in 5 to 10% of infants and young children and can lead to the destruction of all baby teeth.[38]

A number of other health problems related to carbohydrates are presented in other Units within this text. Diabetes, insulin resistance, and hypoglycemia are covered in Unit 13, and lactose intolerance in Unit 7.

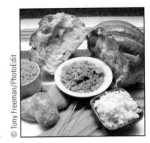

Up Close

Does Your Fiber Intake Measure Up?

Focal Point: Approximate the amount of fiber your diet contains.

Are you meeting your fiber quota, or do you consume the typical low-fiber American diet? To determine if your fiber intake is adequate, award yourself the allotted number of points for each serving of the following foods that you eat in a typical day. For example, if you normally eat one slice of whole grain bread each day, give yourself two points. If you eat two slices daily, give yourself four points. After tallying your score, refer to the Feedback section for the results.

High-fiber food choices

Fruits:

    1 whole fruit (e.g., apple, banana)

    $1/2$ cup cooked fruit

    $1/4$ cup dried fruit

Grains:

    $1/2$ cup cooked brown rice

    1 whole grain slice of bread, roll, muffin, or tortilla

    $1/2$ cup hot whole-grain cereal (e.g., oatmeal)

    $3/4$ cup cold whole-grain cereal (e.g., Cheerios)

    2 cups popcorn

Nuts and seeds:

    $1/4$ cup seeds (e.g., sunflower)

    2 tablespoons peanut butter

Vegetables: **3 points for each serving**

    1 whole vegetable (e.g., potato)

    $1/2$ cup cooked vegetable (e.g., green beans)

Bran cereals: **7 points for each serving**

    $1/2$ cup cooked oat bran cereal

    1 cup cold bran cereal

Legumes: **8 points for each serving**

    $1/2$ cup cooked beans (e.g., baked beans, pinto beans)

                                           Total score

2 points for each serving

_____

_____

_____

_____

_____

_____

_____

_____

_____

_____

_____

_____

_____

_____

_____

_____

Special note: You can also calculate your fiber intake using the Diet Analysis Plus software. Input your food intake for one day. Then go to the Analyses/Reports section to view the total number of grams of fiber in your diet on that day.

FEEDBACK (including scoring) can be found at the end of Unit 4.

[Key Terms

alcohol sugars, page **90**
carbohydrates, page **86**
complex carbohydrates, page **94**
dietary fiber, page **95**
disaccharides, page **87**
functional fiber, page **95**

glycemic index, page **99**
glycogen, page **88**
insulin resistance, page **99**
monosaccharides, page **87**
phenylketonuria (PKU), page **92**
plaque, page **101**

polysaccharides, page **94**
simple sugars, page **87**
tooth decay, page **100**
total fiber, page **95**
type 2 diabetes, page **99**

[Review Questions

TRUE FALSE

1. Excluding fiber, one gram of carbohydrate provides four calories. ☐ ☐

2. Fructose is a monosaccharide, maltose is a diasaccharide, and glycogen is a trisaccharide. ☐ ☐

3. When the body has more glucose than it needs for energy formation, the excess glucose is converted to glycogen and fat. ☐ ☐

4. Sugars are the most commonly used food additive. ☐ ☐

5. Excess sugar intake causes obesity. ☐ ☐

6. Xylitol and sorbitol are examples of alcohol sugars. ☐ ☐

TRUE FALSE

7. Excess intake of aspartame (also called Nutrasweet) causes headaches in a majority of children and adults. ☐ ☐

8. Complex carbohydrates are also known as polysaccharides. ☐ ☐

9. All types of fiber share the characteristic of providing four calories per gram. ☐ ☐

10. Carbohydrates and carbohydrate-containing foods are classified by their glycemic index, or the extent to which they increase blood glucose levels. ☐ ☐

11. Declining rates of dental caries in the United States are primarily related to increased access to fluoridated water supplies. ☐ ☐

[Media Menu

**www.cancer.gov/cancertopics/factsheet/
Risk/artificial-sweeteners**
The National Cancer Institute provides information on artificial sweeteners and cancer from this site.

**www.nlm.nih.gov/medlineplus/dietaryfiber.
html**
This site offers specific suggestions on how to fit more fiber into your diet, fiber and health information, fiber content of foods, and the latest research on fiber.

www.mendosa.com/gilists.htm
This site provides a table of the glycemic index of foods.

www.ada.org
It's not the American Dietetic Association, it's the American Dental Association; they have a column called "The Public" that provides information on oral health, finding a dentist, videos, tooth whitening, and tips for teachers.

**www.nlm.nih.gov/medlineplus/dentalhealth.
html**
The long menu of topics on this site includes answers to FAQs about caring for your teeth and gums; information on diet and dental health, gum chewing and caries prevention, causes of periodontal disease, facts about fluoride, and an atlas of teeth.

www.adha.org
The American Dental Hygienists Association Web site provides dental health education tools and information on dental health and care here.

www.ific.org
This is an industry-sponsored site offering information on carbohydrates and sugars, artificial sweeteners, and oral health.

www.mchoralhealth.org
The Bureau of Maternal and Child Health offers webcasts and information on practices and programs aimed at improving oral health in children.

Notes

1. Touger-Decker R et al. Sugars and dental caries. Am J Clin Nutr 2003;78(suppl):881S–92S.

2. What we eat in America, NHANES, 2005–2006, USDA, 2008, available at www.are.usda.gov/ba/bhnrc/fsrg.

3. Dietary reference intakes: energy, carbohydrate, fiber, fat, fatty acids, cholesterol, protein, and amino acids. Institute of Medicine, National Academies of Sciences. Washington, DC: National Academies Press, chapter 11, 2002.

4. Grabitske HA et al. Low-digestible carbohydrates in practice. J Am Diet Assoc 2008;108:1677–81.

5. Fulgoni III, V. High-fructose corn syrup: everything you wanted to know, but were afraid to ask, Am J Clin Nutr 2008;88(suppl):1715S.

6. Position of the American Dietetic Association: Use of nutritive and nonnutritive sweeteners. J Am Diet Assoc 2004;104:255–58.

7. Bray GA. Fructose—how worried should we be? Medscape J Med 2008;10:159, www.medscape.com/viewarticle/575891, accessed 2/09.

8. Duffey KJ et al. High-fructose corn syrup: is this what's for dinner? Am J Clin Nutr 2008;88(suppl):1722S–32S.

9. Vos MB et al. Dietary fructose consumption among U.S. children and adults: the Third National Health and Nutrition Examination Survey, Medscape J Med 2008, www.medscape.com/viewarticle/575891, accessed 3/09.

10. Food and Drug Administration (Department of Health and Human Services), Nutrition labeling, Federal Register 1991 Nov 27.

11. American Medical Association, AMA finds high fructose corn syrup unlikely to be more harmful to health than other caloric sweeteners, AMA Press Release, 12/08, www.ama.org, accessed 12/08.

12. Dietary reference intakes, NAS, chap. 11; and National Institutes of Health Consensus Development Conference Statement: Diagnosis and management of dental caries throughout life. March 28, 2001; 18:1–24.

13. Dietary reference intakes, NAS, chap. 11; and Joint WHO/FAO Expert Consultation on Diet, Nutrition, and the Prevention of Chronic Diseases, Geneva, Switzerland; 2002.

14. Mattes RD et al. Nonnutritive sweetener consumption in humans: effects on appetite and food intake and their putative mechanisms. Am J Clin Nutr 2009;8:1–14.

15. McKay B. Beverage wars take on new flavor, Wall Street Journal 8/31/08, p. B12.

16. Saccharin deemed safe. Community Nutrition Institute, 2000; June 2:8.

17. Taddio A et al. Sucrose as a pediatric analgesia, Pediatrics 2009;123:e425–e429.

18. Butchko HH et al. Acceptable daily intake vs. actual intake: the aspartame example. J Am Coll Nutr 1991;10:258–66.

19. Spiers PA et al. Aspartame: neuropsychologic and neurophysiologic evaluation and chronic effects. Am J Clin Nutr 1998;68:531–7.

20. Magnuson B et al. Safety of Aspartame, Crit Rev Toxicol 10/07, accessed at www.medscape.com/viewarticle/564923, 3/09.

21. American Association of Cereal Chemists Report: All fibers are essentially functional, Cereal Foods World 2003;48:128.

22. Marlett JA et al. Position of the American Dietetic Association: health implications of dietary fiber. J Am Diet Assoc 1997;97:1157–9.

23. Scott-Thomas C. Prepare for higher calorie count for fibre, say scientists, 19-Dec-2008, www.foodnavigator/europe.com, accessed 12/08.

24. Williams CL. A summary of conference recommendations on dietary fiber in childhood. Pediatrics 1995; 96:1023–8.

25. Rizkella SW et al. Low glycemic index diet and glycemic control in type 2 diabetes. Diabetes Care 2004;27:1866–72.

26. Stanhope KL et al. Endocrine and metabolic effects of consuming beverages sweetened with fructose, glucose, sucrose, or high-fructose corn syrup, Am J Clin Nutr 2008;88(suppl):1733S–7S.

27. Riccardi G et al. Role of glycemic index and glycemic load in the healthy state, in prediabetes, and in diabetes. Am J Clin Nutr 2008;87(Suppl):269S–74S.

28. Jordan M. Colgate brings dental care to Brazilian Indian tribes; ravages of tobacco and rice. Wall Street Journal, 7/23/02, page B1.

29. Cornero S et al. Diet and nutrition of prehistoric populations at the alluvial banks of the Parana River. Medicina 2000;60:109–14.

30. Parajas IL. Sugar content of commonly eaten snack foods of school children in relation to their dental health status. J Phillipine Dent Assoc 1999;51:4–21.

31. Ismail A. Food cariogenicity in Americans aged from 9 to 29 years accessed in a national cross-sectional study, 1971–1974, J Dental Res 1986; 65:1435–40.

32. Edgar WM. Sugar substitutes, chewing gum, and dental caries—a review, British Dental J 1998;184:29–32.

33. Bad breath. Nutr Today 2000;35:6.

34. Schachtele CF et al. Will the diets of the future be less cariogenic? J Canadian Dental Assoc 1984;3:213–9.

35. Palmer CA et al. Position of the American Dietetic Association: the impact of fluoride on dental health. J Am Diet Assoc 2005;105: 1620–28.

36. Bailey W et al. Populations receiving optimally fluoridated public drinking water—United States, 1992–2006. MMWR 2008;57(27):737–41.

37. Position of the American Dietetic Association: oral health and nutrition. J Am Diet Assoc 2003;103:615–25.

38. Trends in children's oral health. National Maternal and Child Oral Health Resource Center, www.ncemch.org, 1999.

39. Moynihan P et al. Diet, nutrition and the prevention of dental diseases, Public Health Nutr 2004;7:201–26.

40. Sheihan A. Dietary effects on dental diseases, Public Health Nutr 2001;4:569–91.

41. Position of the American Dietetic Association: health implications of dietary fiber, J Am Diet Assoc 2008;108:1716–31.

NUTRITION | Up Close

Does Your Fiber Intake Measure Up?

Feedback for Unit 4

The total number of points you scored approximates the **grams** of total fiber you typically consume daily.[a] Use this scale to find out if your fiber intake meets the recommended goal:

- **0–10 grams:** You consume less than the average American. Increase your fiber intake by including more fruits, vegetables, whole grains, and legumes in your diet overall.
- **11–15 grams:** Like other Americans, you consume too little fiber. Increase the number of servings of high-fiber foods you already enjoy, while substituting more high-fiber foods for refined food products. A quick way to add fiber to your diet is to consume more of the two fiber powerhouses: legumes and bran cereal.
- **15–20 grams:** You currently consume more fiber than the average American. Make sure you're including 5 or more servings of fruits and vegetables. Eat 6 to 11 servings of bread, cereal, rice, and pasta daily; choose whole-grain versions of these foods often.
- **20–40 grams:** Congratulations! Your dietary fiber intake is in the vicinity of that recommended. Keep up the good work.

[a]Because different foods within a food group contribute varying amounts of dietary fiber, the point values have been average. Make sure to check the Nutrition Facts panel on bran cereals because these cereals vary in the amount of dietary fiber they contain.

UNIT 5

Fats and Cholesterol in Health

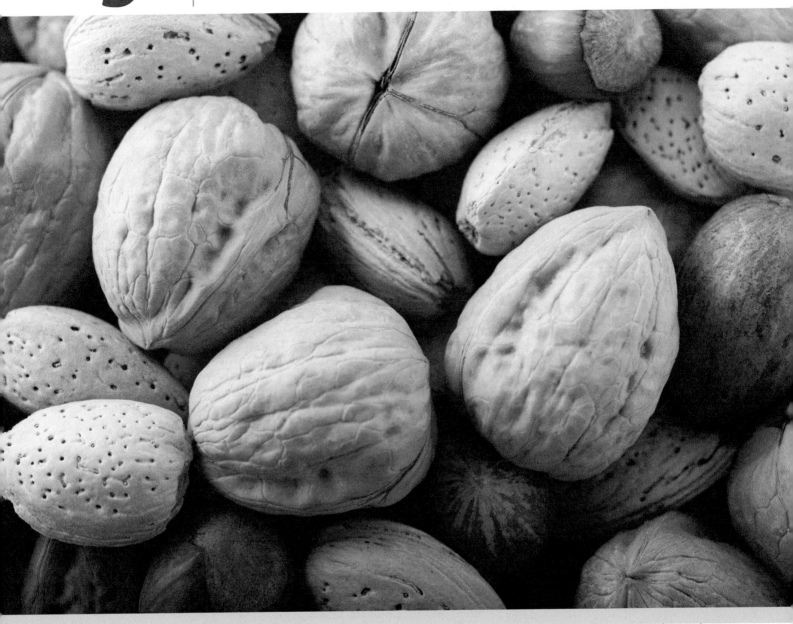

NUTRITION SCOREBOARD

		TRUE	FALSE

1 It is currently recommended that adults consume diets providing less than 30% of calories from fat.

2 The types of fat consumed are more important to health than is total fat intake.

3 Most all of the cholesterol in our diets comes from animal products.

4 Saturated fat intake has a much stronger influence on blood cholesterol levels than does cholesterol intake.

107

Key Concepts and Facts

- Fats are our most concentrated source of food energy. They supply nine calories per gram.

- Dietary fats "carry" the essential fatty acids, fat-soluble vitamins, and healthful phytochemicals along with them in foods.

- Fats are not created equal. Some types of fat have positive effects, and some have negative effects on health.

- Saturated fats and trans fats raise blood cholesterol levels more than does dietary cholesterol or any other type of fat.

Changing Views about Fat Intake and Health

Scientific evidence and opinions related to the effects of fat on health have changed substantially in recent years—and so have recommendations about fat intake. In the past, it was recommended that Americans aim for diets providing less than 30% of total calories from fat. However, recent evidence indicates that the type of fat consumed is more important to health than total fat intake. The watchwords for thinking about fat have become "Not all fats are created equal: Some are better for you than others." American adults are being urged to select food sources of "healthy" fats while keeping fat intake within the range of 20 to 35% of total caloric intake. Concerns that high-fat diets encourage the development of obesity have been eased by studies demonstrating that excessive caloric intakes—and not just diets high in fat—are related to weight gain.[2]

New recommendations regarding fat intake do not encourage increased fat consumption. Rather, they emphasize that healthy diets include certain types of fat and that total caloric intake and physical activity are the most important components of weight management. Diets providing as low as 20% of calories from fat, and those providing 30 to 35%, can be healthy—depending on the types of fat consumed and the quality of the rest of the diet.[1] This unit provides facts about fats, explains the reasons behind recent changes in recommendations for fat intake, and addresses the practical meaning of it all.

Facts about Fats

Fats are a group of substances found in food. They have one major property in common: They are not soluble (or, in other words, will not dissolve) in water. If you have ever tried to mix vinegar and oil when making salad dressing, you have observed the principle of water and fat solubility firsthand.

Fats are actually a subcategory of the fat-soluble substances known as **lipids**. Lipids include fats, oils, and cholesterol. Dietary fats such as butter, margarine, and shortening are often distinguished from oils by their property of being solid at room temperature. This physical difference between fats and oils is due to their chemical structures.

lipids
Compounds that are insoluble in water and soluble in fat. Triglycerides, saturated and unsaturated fats, and essential fatty acids are examples of lipids, or "fats."

Functions of Dietary Fats

Fats in Foods Supply Energy and Fat-Soluble Nutrients Dietary fats are a concentrated source of energy. Each gram of fat consumed supplies the body with 9 calories worth of energy. That's enough energy for a 160-pound person to walk casually for a little over two minutes or to jog at a slow pace for about a minute. Fats in food supply the **essential fatty acids** (linoleic acid and alpha-linolenic acid) and provide the fat-soluble vitamins D, E, K, and A (the "deka" vitamins). So, part of the reason we need fats in our diet is to get a supply of the essential nutrients they contain (Table 5.1). Diets containing little fat (less than 20% of total calories) often fall short on delivering adequate amounts of essential fatty acids and fat-soluble vitamins.[1]

Fat Contributes to the Body's Energy Stores Fat consumed as part of a dietary intake that exceeds calorie need is converted to triglycerides and stored in fat cells (Illustration 5.1). A pound of body fat can provide approximately 3,500 calories of energy to the body when needed.

Body fat is not just skin deep. Fat is also located around organs such as the kidneys and heart. It's there to cushion and protect the organs and keep them insulated. Cold-water swimmers can attest to the effectiveness of fat as an insulation material. They purposefully build up body fat stores because they need the extra layer of insulation (Illustration 5.2).

Fats Increase the Flavor and Palatability of Foods Although "pure" fats by themselves tend to be tasteless, they absorb and retain the flavor of substances that surround them. Thus, fats in meats and other foods pick up flavors from their environment and give those flavors to the food. This characteristic of fat is why butter, if placed next to the garlic in the refrigerator, tastes like garlic.

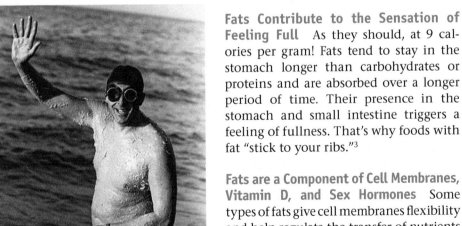

AP Images

Illustration 5.2 Although their body fat stores don't fit the image of the superathlete, cold-water swimmers need the fat to help stay warm.
Pictured here is the English swimmer Mike Read, who had swum the English Channel 20 times by age 39. The narrowest width of the English Channel is 22 miles, or 35 km.

Fats Contribute to the Sensation of Feeling Full As they should, at 9 calories per gram! Fats tend to stay in the stomach longer than carbohydrates or proteins and are absorbed over a longer period of time. Their presence in the stomach and small intestine triggers a feeling of fullness. That's why foods with fat "stick to your ribs."[3]

Fats are a Component of Cell Membranes, Vitamin D, and Sex Hormones Some types of fats give cell membranes flexibility and help regulate the transfer of nutrients into and out of cells.[4] Others serve as precursors to vitamin D and sex hormones, such as estrogen and testosterone.

essential fatty acids
Components of fats (linoleic acid, pronounced *lynn-oh-lay-ick,* and alpha-linolenic acid, pronounced *lynn-oh-len-ick*) required in the diet.

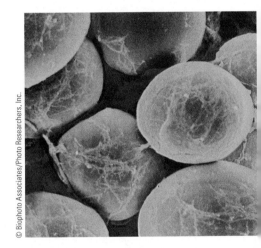

© Biophoto Associates/Photo Researchers, Inc.

Illustration 5.1 A close look at fat cells (color-enhanced microphotograph).

Fats Come in Many Varieties

There are many types of fat in food and our bodies (Table 5.2). Of primary importance are *triglycerides* (or "triacylglycerols"), *saturated and unsaturated fats,*

Table 5.2

Basic facts about the types of fat

Fats can be:
- Monoglycerides
- Diglycerides
- Triglycerides

Fats can be:
- Saturated
- Monounsaturated
- Polyunsaturated

Unsaturated fats come in:
- "Cis" forms
- "Trans" forms

Table 5.3

A glossary of fats

Triglycerides: Fats in which the glycerol molecule has three fatty acids attached to it; also called triacylglycerol. Triglycerides are the most common type of fat in foods and in body fat stores.

Saturated fats: Molecules of fat in which adjacent carbons within fatty acids are linked only by single bonds. The carbons are "saturated" with hydrogens; that is, they are attached to the maximum possible number of hydrogens. Saturated fats tend to be solid at room temperature. Animal products and palm and coconut oil are sources of saturated fats.

Unsaturated fats: Molecules of fat in which adjacent carbons are linked by one or more double bonds. The carbons are not saturated with hydrogens; that is, they are attached to fewer than the maximum possible number of hydrogens. Unsaturated fats tend to be liquid at room temperature and are found in plants, vegetable oils, meats, and dairy products.

Glycerol: A syrupy, colorless liquid component of fats that is soluble in water. It is similar to glucose in chemical structure.

Cholesterol: A fat soluble, calories liquid primarily found in animals. Cholesterol is used by the body to form hormones such as testosterone and estrogen and is a component of cell membranes. Cholesterol is present in plant cell membranes but the quantity is small and plants are not considered to be a significant dietary source of cholesterol.

Diglyceride: A fat in which the glycerol molecule has two fatty acids attached to it; also called diacylglycerol.

Monoglyceride: A fat in which the glycerol molecule has one fatty acid attached to it; also called monoacylglycerol.

Monounsaturated fats: Fats that contain a fatty acid in which one carbon-carbon bond is not saturated with hydrogen.

Polyunsaturated fats: Fats that contain a fatty acid in which two or more carbon–carbon bonds are not saturated with hydrogen.

Trans **fats:** Fats containing fatty acids in the trans form. Also called trans fatty acids.

Glycerol + 3 fatty acids = Triglyceride

Illustration 5.3 A triglyceride.

cholesterol, and *trans* fats (for definitions, see Table 5.3). The different types of fats have different effects on health.

Triglycerides, which consist of one *glycerol* unit (a glucose-like substance) and three fatty acids (Illustration 5.3), make up 98% of our dietary fat intake and the vast majority of our body's fat stores. Triglycerides are transported in blood attached to protein carriers and are used by cells for energy formation and tissue maintenance. A minority of fats take the form of *diglycerides* (glycerol plus two fatty acids) and *monoglycerides* (glycerol and one fatty acid). Diglycerides are present in some oils and small amounts are used in food products as emulsifiers—or to increase the blending of fat- and water-soluble substances. Monoglycerides are present in small amounts in some oils; we don't consume very much of them in foods.

As far as health is concerned, the glycerol component of fat is relatively unimportant. It's the fatty acids that influence what the body does with the fat we eat; and they are responsible, in part, for how fat affects health. Many different types of fatty acids are found in triglycerides. You've heard of the major ones: those that make fat "saturated" or "unsaturated."

Saturated and Unsaturated Fats Fatty acids found in fats consist primarily of hydrogen atoms attached to carbon atoms (Illustration 5.4). When the carbons are attached to as many hydrogens as possible, the fatty acid is "saturated"—that is, saturated with hydrogen. Saturated fats tend to be solid at room temperature. Except for palm and coconut oil, only animal products are rich in saturated fats (Illustration 5.5, p. 112). Fatty acids that contain fewer hydrogens than the maximum are "unsaturated." They tend to be liquid at room temperature. By and large, plant foods are the best sources of unsaturated fats.

Unsaturated fats are classified by their degree of unsaturation. If only one carbon–carbon bond in the fatty acid is unsaturated, the fat is called

Illustration 5.4 A look at the difference between a saturated and an unsaturated fatty acid.

Hydrogen
Oxygen
Oxygen Carbon **Saturated fatty acid** CH₃

CH CH
Monounsaturated fatty acid

CH CH   CH CH
Polyunsaturated fatty acid

Two hydrogens are missing from each of these carbon–carbon links, making the fatty acid polyunsaturated. With fewer hydrogens to attach to, these carbons are doubly bonded to each other. Monounsaturated fatty acids have only one carbon–carbon bond that is "unsaturated" with hydrogen atoms.

"monounsaturated." If two or more carbon–carbon bonds are unsaturated with hydrogen, the fat qualifies as "polyunsaturated."

The Omega-6 and Omega-3 Fatty Acids

The essential fatty acids linoleic acid and alpha-linolenic acid are members of the fatty acid families of omega-6 (also called n-6 fatty acids) and omega-3 fatty acids (also known as n-3 fatty acids), respectively. Both are polyunsaturated, can be used as a source of energy, and are stored in fat tissue. Because they are essential, both linoleic and alpha-linolenic acid are required in the diet.

Linoleic acid is required for growth, maintenance of healthy skin, and normal functioning of the reproductive system. It is a component of all cell membranes and is found in particularly high amounts in nerves and the brain. A number of biologically active compounds produced in the body that participate in regulation of blood pressure and blood clotting are derived from linoleic acid. The major food sources of linoleic acid are sunflower, safflower, corn, and soybean oils.

Alpha-linolenic acid is a structural component of all cell membranes and is found in high amounts in the brain and other nervous system tissues. It also forms biologically active compounds used in the regulation of blood pressure and blood clotting; but these compounds have the opposite effects on blood pressure and blood clotting as do some of the derivatives of linoleic acid.[5] Omega-3 fatty acids are found in walnuts, dark, leafy green vegetables; and flaxseed, canola, and soybean oils in the form of alpha-linolenic acid.

Other, biologically important omega-3 fatty acids exist, and the two primary ones are EPA (eicosapentaenoic acid, pronounced *e-co-sah-pent-tah-no-ick*) and DHA (docosahexaenoic acid, pronounced *dough-cos-ah-hex-ah-no-ick*). These omega-3 fatty acids can be produced from alpha-linolenic acid, but the conversion process is slow and results in the availability of relatively small amounts of EPA and DHA.[6]

EPA and DHA   DHA and EPA are primarily ingredients of fish oils and perform a number of important functions in the body. DHA is a structural component of the brain and is found in high amounts in the retina of the eye. During the

On the Side

Fried fish is generally not a good source of EPA and DHA. The fish used is typically low-fat and a poor source of these omega-3 fatty acids.[7]

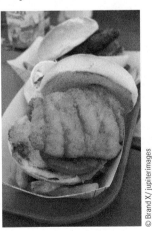

© Brand X/jupiterimages

Omega-3 fatty acids are not just good fats, they affect heart health in positive ways.

—Penny Kris-Etherton, Distinguished Professor of Nutrition

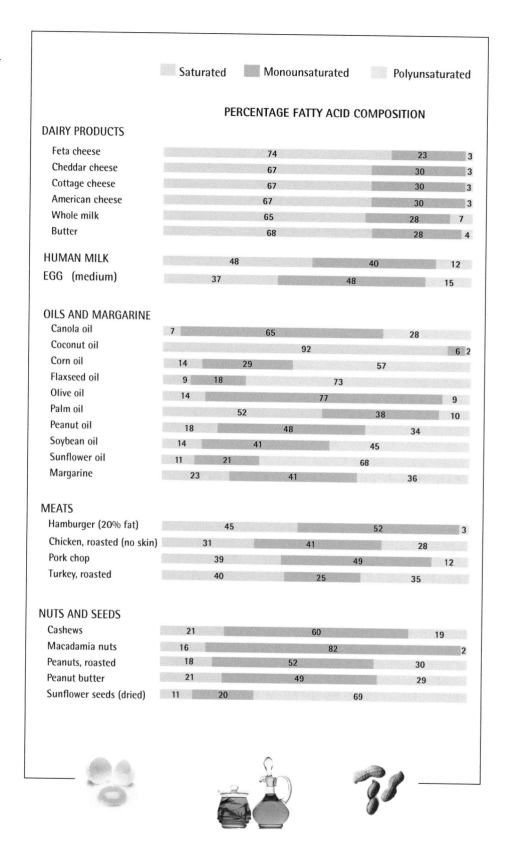

Illustration 5.5 Fat profiles of selected foods.

last three months of pregnancy and during infancy, DHA accumulates in these tissues and promotes optimal intellectual and visual development.[8]

EPA serves as a precursor of a number of biologically active compounds involved in blood pressure regulation, blood clotting, and anti-inflammatory reactions. Inflammation is a central component of many chronic diseases, including heart disease, type 2 diabetes, osteoporosis, cancer, Alzheimer's disease, and rheumatoid arthritis. It is part of the body's response to the presence of infectious agents or irritants. A by-product of the body's inflammatory processes, however, are oxidation reactions that can harm cells and tissues. Derivatives of EPA limit the harmful effects of inflammatory and oxidation reactions.[9]

Adequate intake of EPA and DHA for adults is considered to be 500 mg per day.[8] This level of intake can be achieved by consuming 8 ounces of fatty fish weekly. Fish and shellfish content of EPA and DHA is listed in Table 5.4. The table only includes fish and shellfish that contain relatively low amounts of mercury. Mercury can cause nerve tissue damage and learning problems if consumed in excessive amounts. Pregnant and breast-feeding women are advised to limit their intake to 12 ounces per week of low-mercury fish and shellfish.[10]

Consumption of two fish meals a week reduces the risk of heart disease, heart attack, sudden death, and stoke and improves fetal and infant development.[8] Higher amounts of EPA and DHA (1 to 3 grams), generally provided by fish oils, are being used clinically to lower blood triglyceride levels, reduce the incidence of heart disease in people at risk, and reduce the need for anti-inflammatory drugs in people with rheumatoid arthritis.[12] The Food and Drug Administration recommends that consumers ingest no more than a total of 3 grams of EPA and DHA daily and limit supplementary intakes to 2 grams a day. Fish liver oils should be used with caution because they contain relatively high amounts of vitamins A and D. Fish oils, made from the body of the fish, do not.[4]

Table 5.4

EPA and DHA content of fish and seafoods containing, on average, less than 0.2 ppm mercury in a 3-ounce serving.[11]

	EPA + DHA, mg
Shad	2,046
Salmon, farmed	1,825
Anchovies	1,747
Herring	1,712
Salmon, wild	1,564
Whitefish	1,370
Mackerel	1,023
Sardines	840
Tilefish	796
Whiting	440
Flounder	426
Trout, fresh water	420
Oysters	375
Snapper	273
Shrimp	268
Clams	241
Haddock	202
Catfish, wild	201
Crawfish	187
Sheepshead	162
Tuna, light, canned in oil	109
Lobster	71

Increasing Omega-3 Fatty Acid Intake In the past it was thought that consuming high amounts of omega-6 fatty acids compared to omega-3 fatty acids could interfere with the availability of omega-3 fatty acids, particularly EPA and DHA. Although still somewhat controversial, it appears that rather high intakes of omega-6 fatty acids do not interfere with the availability of EPA and DHA.[5] What interferes most with the availability of EPA and DHA for body functions is inadequate intake. On average, adults in the United States and Canada consume 100 mg EPA plus DHA daily, far short of the recommended intake of 500 mg daily.[8]

■ **EPA and DHA Fortified Foods.** Fatty fish are clearly the richest sources of EPA and DHA. But what if you don't like fish? In that case you can turn to EPA and DHA fortified foods.[13] (For more information on specific EPA and DHA fortified foods see this Unit's Take Action feature.) Purified fish oils with no fishy taste are increasingly being added to products from fruit juice to yogurt, and to animal feeds. The EPA and DHA in feed are incorporated into the animal's tissues. Consequently, beef, pork, eggs, milk and milk products consumed from animals "fortified" with EPA and DHA are fortified, too. Some animal feeds contain DHA from algae and only provide DHA in their food products.

To make sure you're choosing foods with EPA and DHA, or DHA, confirm that the label specifies that these fatty acids are contained in the product. Just because a product announces "Omega-3" on the label doesn't mean it contains EPA and DHA. It may contain flax oil, walnut oil, alpha-linolenic acid, or other sources of omega-3 fatty acids that are not equivalent to EPA or DHA.

Hydrogenated Fats

Unsaturated fats aren't as stable as saturated fats. They are more likely to turn rancid with time and exposure to air and heat than are saturated fats. Additionally, solid fats are preferable to oils for some cooking applications. These problems with unsaturated fats have a solution. It's called hydrogenation.

Take Action

To Consume Enough EPA and DHA from Foods Other than Fish

If you would like to increase your EPA and DHA intake, here are some of your non-fish food choices. Indicate with a check mark foods you would likely consume. At the bottom of the list, answer this question: Based on your choices, about how much EPA and DHA would you be adding to your daily diet by consuming the foods you checked?

	EPA and DHA/DHA content, mg
___ DHA fortified eggs, 1	150
___ Healthy Heart Omega-3 orange juice, 8 oz	50
___ Omega Farm nonfat yogurt, 8 oz	75
___ Egg Creations Liquid, $1/4$ cup	260
___ Smart Balance Omega Buttery Spread, 1 Tbsp	32
___ Italica Omega-3 Olive Oil, 1 Tbsp	120
___ Omega Farms Low-Fat Milk, 1 cup	75
___ Omega Farms Mild Cheddar, 1 oz	75
___ Smart Balance Lactose-Free Milk with Omega-3, 1 cup	32
___ Minute Maid 100% Fruit Juice Blend with Omega 3/DHA, 1 cup	50
___ Shrimp, 3 oz	268
___ Clams, 3 oz	241
___ Crab, 3 oz	375
___ Scallops, 3 oz	161

The approximate amount of EPA and DHA I would be adding to my diet daily based on my food choices is: _____ mg. If not at 500 mg, you would be getting closer.

---

hydrogenation
The addition of hydrogen to unsaturated fatty acids.

trans fats
Unsaturated fatty acids in fats that contain atoms of hydrogen attached to opposite sides of carbons joined by a double bond:

```
      H
—C=C—              H H
      H           —C=C—
Trans fatty        Cis fatty
   acid              acid
```

Fats containing fatty acids in the *trans* form are generally referred to as *trans* fats. *Cis* fatty acids are the most common, naturally occurring form of unsaturated fatty acids. They contain hydrogens located on the same side of doubly bonded carbons.

What's Hydrogenation? **Hydrogenation** is a process that adds hydrogen to liquid unsaturated fats, thereby making them more saturated and solid. The shelf life, cooking properties, and taste of vegetable oils are improved in the process. Hydrogenation has two drawbacks, however. Hydrogenated vegetable oils contain more saturated fat than the original oil. Corn oil, for example, contains only 6% saturated fats; but corn oil margarine has 17%. The other negative is that hydrogenation causes a change in the structure of the unsaturated fatty acids. Specifically, hydrogenation converts some unsaturated fats into **trans fats.**

Trans Fatty Acids The bulk of *trans* fats in our diets comes from hydrogenated vegetable oils. Hydrogenation causes some of the unsaturated fatty acids to be converted from their naturally occurring *cis* to the *trans* form. Ruminant animals like cows, goats, and sheep form a small amount of *trans* fats in their stomachs. Consequently, milk and milk products from these animals will contain *trans* fats.[14]

Repositioned hydrogen molecules in *trans* fats change the way the body uses the fat. *Trans* fats raise blood cholesterol levels more than any other type of fat. They increase the risk of heart disease, stroke, sudden death from heart disease, and type 2 diabetes, and they promote inflammation. Intake of *trans* fats as low as 1% of total calories per day strongly increases the risk of heart disease. An intake of 2.2 grams of *trans* fat daily would place a person consuming 2000 calories a day at increased risk of heart disease.[15]

It is recommended that Americans consume as little *trans* fats as possible,[1] and nutrition information labeling requirements that began in 2006 are making that easier to accomplish. Nutrition Facts panels must include the *trans* fat content of food products (Illustration 5.6). The %DV column (for percent of Daily Value) is not used for *trans* fats because there is no recommended level of intake. Products labeled "*trans* fat-free" (Illustration 5.7) must contain less than 0.5 gram of both *trans* and saturated fats. The requirement to label the *trans* fat content of food products, regulations by various states and cities that ban their use in restaurant foods, and increased consumer awareness of the adverse effects of trans fat have forced food producers to take trans fats out of many prepared and processed foods.[16,17] Prepared foods contain less trans fats than they did just a few years ago. A sampling of some of the remaining food products that contain trans fats is given in Table 5.5.

Checking Out Cholesterol

Cholesterol is a lipid found *primarily* in animal products. It is tasteless and odorless and contained in both the lean and fat parts of animal products. Table 5.6 lists some sources of cholesterol. Cholesterol is present in plant cell membranes, but the quantity is small and plants are not considered to be a significant dietary source of cholesterol.

Sources of Cholesterol

The cholesterol used by the body comes from two sources. Most (about two-thirds) of the cholesterol available to the body is produced by the liver. The rest comes from the diet (Illustration 5.8). Because the liver produces cholesterol from other substances in our diet, it does not qualify as an essential nutrient.

The Contributions of Cholesterol

Would you be surprised to learn that cholesterol:

- is found in every cell in your body?
- serves as the building block for estrogen, testosterone, and the vitamin D that is produced in your skin on exposure to sunlight?
- is a major component of nerves and the brain?
- cannot be used for energy (so it provides no calories)?

The body has many uses for cholesterol (Table 5.7). It doesn't just accumulate in arteries!

Nutrition Facts

Serving Size 1 Entree
Serving Per Container 1

Amount Per Serving

Calories 380 Calories from Fat 170

	%Daily Value
Total Fat 19g	**29%**
Saturated Fat 10g	**50%**
Trans Fat 2g	
Cholesterol 85mg	**28%**
Sodium 810mg	**34%**
Total Carbohydrate 33g	**11%**
Dietary Fiber 3g	**12%**
Sugars 5g	
Protein 20g	

Vitamin A 10%	Vitamin C 0%
Calcium 10%	Iron 15%

Percent Daily Values are based on a 2000 calorie diet. Your daily values may be higher or lower depending on your calorie needs:

		Calories	2000	2500
Total Fat	Less Than		65g	80g
Sat Fat	Less Than		20g	25g
Cholesterol	Less Than		300mg	300mg
Sodium	Less Than		2400mg	2400mg
Total Carbohydrate			300g	375g
Dietary Fiber			25g	30g

Illustration 5.6   *Trans* fat: the newest addition to nutrition facts panels.

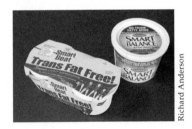
Richard Anderson

Illustration 5.7   Products that feature "no *trans* fats" and "*trans* fat-free" labels.

Table 5.5

Where are the trans fats now?

Values may change as companies lower the trans fat content of foods.

Food	Trans Fatty Acids (Grams)
Frosting, canned, 2 Tbsp	2
Pound cake, 2.5 oz	1
Lemon Bar mix, 1–2″ bar	1
Chocolate syrup Brownie mix, 1–2″ bar	1
Sugar cookies mix, 2 cookies	1

Source: Trans fat content of foods is based on a "trans fat search" conducted by the author in supermarkets, 4/09.

Table 5.6

Food sources of cholesterol

Note that all the leading food sources are animal products. Cholesterol in foods is a clear, oily liquid found in the fat and lean portions of many animal products.

Animal product	Amount	Cholesterol (Milligrams)
Brain	3 oz	1746
Liver	3 oz	470
Egg	1	212
Veal	3 oz	128
Shrimp	3 oz	107
Prime rib	3 oz	80
Chicken (no skin)	3 oz	75
Turkey (no skin)	3 oz	65
Hamburger, regular	3 oz	64
Pork chop, lean	3 oz	60
Fish, baked (haddock, flounder)	3 oz	58
Ice cream	1 cup	56
Sausage	3 oz	55
Hamburger, lean	3 oz	50
Milk, whole	1 cup	34
Crab, boiled	3 oz	33
Lobster	3 oz	29
Cheese (cheddar)	1 oz	26
Milk, 2%	1 cup	22
Yogurt, low-fat	1 cup	17
Milk, 1%	1 cup	14
Butter	1 tsp	10
Milk, skim	1 cup	7

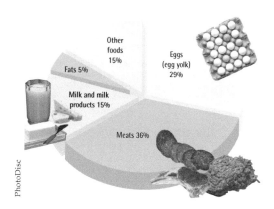

PhotoDisc

Illustration 5.8 Food sources of cholesterol in the U.S. diet.[11] Percentages indicate the proportion of cholesterol each type of food contributes to the diet.

Finding Out about the Fat Content of Food

Not all of the fat in food is visible. To avoid being fooled, it helps to use a reference on the fat composition of foods. Table 5.8 lists the fat content of common food sources of fat, including candy. Vegetables and fruits (except avocado and coconut) and grains are not listed because they contain relatively little fat. Other references can also be used, such as the food composition tables in Appendix A, the Diet Analysis Plus Program software, and the nutrition labels on food products.

Knowledge of the caloric and fat content of a food can be used to calculate the percentage of calories provided by fat. For example, suppose that a slice of cherry pie provides 350 calories and 15 grams of fat. To calculate the percentage of fat calories, multiply 15 grams by 9 (the number of calories in each gram of fat), divide the result by 350 calories, and then multiply this result by 100:

$$15 \text{ grams fat} \times 9 \text{ calories/gram} = 135 \text{ calories}$$
$$135 \text{ calories}/350 = 0.39$$
$$0.39 \times 100 = 39\% \text{ of total calories from fat}$$

Fat Labeling

Nutrition labeling regulations for fat require that food manufacturers adhere to standard definitions of "low fat," "fat-free," and related terms used on food labels. Similarly, claims made about the cholesterol content of food products must comply with standard definitions (Table 5.9, p. 118). If a claim is made about the fat content of a food, the nutrition facts panel must specify the food's fat, saturated fat, *trans* fat, and cholesterol content. If a claim is made about cholesterol content

Table 5.7

How the body uses cholesterol

- Cholesterol is a component of all cell membranes, the brain, and nerves.
- Cholesterol is needed to produce estrogen, testosterone, and vitamin D.

Table 5.8

The fat content of some foods

Food	Amount	Grams	Percentage of Total Calories From Fat
Fats and oils			
Butter	1 tsp	4.0	100%
Margarine	1 tsp	4.0	100
Oil	1 tsp	4.7	100
Mayonnaise	1 tbs	11.0	99
Heavy cream	1 tbs	5.5	93
Salad dressing	1 tbs	6.0	83
Meats and fast foods			
Hot dog	1 (2 oz)	17.0	83
Bologna	1 oz	8.0	80
Sausage	4 links	18.0	77
Bacon	3 pieces	9.0	74
Salami	2 oz	11.0	68
Hamburger, regular (20% fat)	3 oz	16.5	62
Chicken, fried with skin	3 oz	14.0	53
Big Mac	6.6 oz	31.4	52
Quarter Pounder with cheese	6.8 oz	28.6	50
Whopper	8.9 oz	32.0	48
Steak (rib eye)	3 oz	9.9	47
Veggie pita	1	17.0	38
Chicken, baked without skin	3 oz	4.0	25
Flounder, baked	3 oz	1.0	13
Shrimp, boiled	3 oz	1.0	10
Milk and milk products			
Cheddar cheese	1 oz	9.5	74
American cheese	1 oz	6.0	66
Milk, whole	1 cup	8.5	49
Cottage cheese, regular	$1/2$ cup	5.1	39
Milk, 2%	1 cup	5.0	32
Milk, 1%	1 cup	2.7	24
Cottage cheese, 1% fat	$1/2$ cup	1.2	13
Milk, skim	1 cup	0.4	4
Yogurt, frozen	$3/4$ cup	0.0–6.6	0–3
Other			
Olives	4 medium	1.5	90
Avocado	$1/2$	15.0	84
Almonds	1 oz	15.0	80
Sunflower seeds	$1/4$ cup	17.0	77
Peanuts	$1/4$ cup	17.5	75
Cashews	1 oz	13.2	73
Egg	1	6.0	61
Potato chips	1 oz (13 chips)	11.0	61
French fries	20 fries	20.0	49
Taco chips	1 oz (10 chips)	6.2	41
Candy			
Peanut butter cups, 2 regular	1.6 oz	15.0	54
Milk chocolate	1.6 oz	14.0	53
Almond Joy	1.8 oz	14.0	50
Kit Kat	1.5 oz	12.0	47
M & M's, peanut	1.7 oz	13.0	47

(and claims can be made only for products that normally contain a meaningful amount of cholesterol), the nutrition panel must also reveal the product's fat and saturated fat content. To prevent the use of unrealistically small serving sizes as a way to appear to cut down on a product's fat content, standard serving sizes must be used on food labels.

Table 5.9

What claims about the cholesterol content of foods that normally contain cholesterol must mean

- No cholesterol or cholesterol-free: Contains less than three milligrams of cholesterol per serving

- Low cholesterol: Contains 20 milligrams or less of cholesterol per serving

- Reduced cholesterol: Contains at least 75% less cholesterol than normal

- Less cholesterol: Contains at least 25% less cholesterol than normal; the percentage less must be stated on the label

Illustration 5.9   A look at the cuisine of the Mediterranean diet.

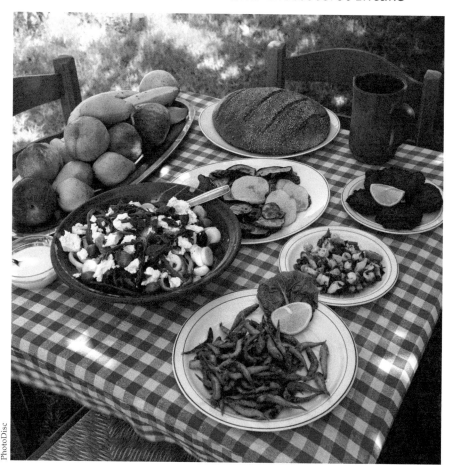

PhotoDisc

Recent Changes in Recommendations for Fat and Cholesterol Intake

Adherence to certain types of diets that are relatively high in total calories from fats, such as the Mediterranean diet highlighted in Illustration 5.9, reduce the risk of heart disease, stroke, obesity, or a number of other diseases.[18] Evidence established on the healthful effects of the Mediterranean diet and other examples of dietary fat intake and health in different populations prompted the development of new recommendations based primarily on the healthfulness of various types of fats.[1]

"Good" Fats, "Bad" Fats   Fats come in many types in foods, and with few exceptions, they serve as a source of energy and provide a number of essential functions in the body. With regard to raising or lowering the risk of heart disease and stroke, however, fats differ. Those that elevate total cholesterol and LDL-cholesterol levels are regarded as "bad" or unhealthy fats. Those that lower total cholesterol and LDL-cholesterol and raise blood levels of HDL-cholesterol (the one that helps the body get rid of cholesterol in the blood) are considered "good" or healthy."[19]

The list of unhealthy fats includes *trans* fats, saturated fats, and cholesterol. Fats labeled "bad" are generally solid at room temperature and are included in foods such as high-fat meats and dairy products, hard margarines, shortening, and crispy snack foods.[19] Monounsaturated fats, polyunsaturated fats, alpha-linolenic acid, DHA, and EPA are considered healthy fats and are present in food in the form of oils (Table 5.10).

Recommendations for Fat and Cholesterol Intake

Current recommendations for adults call for consumption of 20 to 35% of total calories from fat. Average fat consumption in the United States is at the upper end of this range (35% of total calories).[20] The AIs (Adequate Intakes) for the essential

Table 5.10

Healthy and unhealthy fats and examples of food sources

Healthy Fats	Unhealthy Fats
DHA, EPA (omega-3 fatty acids) fish and seafood	**_Trans_ fats** Snack and fried foods, bakery goods
Monounsaturated fats Olive and peanut oil, nuts, avocados	**Saturated fats** Animal fats
Polyunsaturated fats Vegetable oils	**Cholesterol** eggs, seafood, and meat
Alpha-linolenic acid Soybeans, walnuts, flaxseed	

fatty acid linoleic acid is set at 17 grams a day for men and 12 grams for women. AIs for the other essential fatty acid, alpha-linolenic acid, are 1.6 grams per day for men and 1.1 grams for women. It is recommended that intake of _trans_ fats and saturated fats be as low as possible while consuming a nutritionally adequate diet. Only a small proportion of Americans consume too little linoleic acid, but intakes of alpha-linolenic acid tend to be low. Americans are being encouraged to increase consumption of EPA and DHA by eating fish more often. In addition, saturated fat intake averages 11 to 12% of calories, an amount that increases the risk of heart disease.[8, 20]

There is no recommended level of cholesterol intake, because there is no evidence to indicate that cholesterol is required in the diet. The body is able to produce enough cholesterol, and people do not develop a cholesterol deficiency disease if it is not consumed. Because blood cholesterol levels tend to increase somewhat as consumption of cholesterol increases, it is recommended that intake should be minimal. Although cholesterol intake averages 237 mg per day in the United States,[20] a more health-promoting level of intake would be less than 200 mg a day.[21]

Recent recommendations for fat intake represent an unusually large but necessary change in dietary intake guidance. Much remains to be understood about the effects of dietary fats on health, and how other components of diet, lifestyle, and genetic traits modify relationships between fat intake and health.

Reality Check

Good fats, bad fats   What foods provide "healthy" fats?

Who gets thumbs up?
Answers on page 120

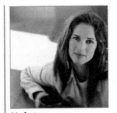

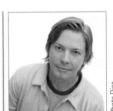

Photo Disc

Kristen:
How can I be wrong? Low-fat food products are best for healthy fat because they contain almost no fat!

Butch:
I'm thinking foods like fish, peanut butter, and _trans_ fat–free margarine contain healthy fats.

"Good" fats, "bad" fats Low-fat foods contain less fat than the regular version of the foods. But that doesn't mean the products contain no fat, or only good fats. Food sources of fish oils, unsaturated fat, and *trans* fat–free products provide the healthy fats. As always, healthy diets aren't based on individual foods, they are based on overall diets. You can emphasize foods providing healthy fats without feeling bad about occasionally eating foods branded with the "bad fat" label.

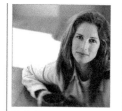

Kristen:

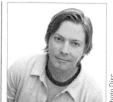

Butch:

NUTRITION

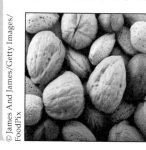

© James And James/Getty Images/FoodPix

Up Close

The Healthy Fats in Your Diet

FOCAL POINT: Identify your healthy fat food choices.

Are the fats in your diet the healthy type? Check it out by answering these questions:

How Often Do You Eat:	Seldom or Never	1–2 Times per Week	3–5 Times per Week	Almost Daily
1. Sausage, hot dogs, ribs, and luncheon meats?	☐	☐	☐	☐
2. Heavily marbled steaks or roasts and chicken with the skin?	☐	☐	☐	☐
3. Soybean products such as tofu or soynuts?	☐	☐	☐	☐
4. Nuts or seeds?	☐	☐	☐	☐
5. Whole milk, cheese, or ice cream?	☐	☐	☐	☐
6. Soft margarine or olive oil?	☐	☐	☐	☐
7. French fries, snack crackers, commercial bakery products?	☐	☐	☐	☐
8. Rich sauces and gravies?	☐	☐	☐	☐
9. Fish or seafood?	☐	☐	☐	☐
10. Peanut butter?	☐	☐	☐	☐

FEEDBACK (including scoring) can be found at the end of Unit 5.

Key Terms

essential fatty acids, page 109
hydrogenation, page 114

lipids, page 108

trans fats, page 114

Review Questions

	TRUE	FALSE
1. Animal products are by far the leading source of saturated fats in the American diet.	☐	☐
2. Flaxseed oil and dark, leafy green vegetables are excellent sources of the essential fatty acid alpha-linolenic acid.	☐	☐
3. The best food sources of EPA and DHA are fish and shellfish.	☐	☐
4. Cholesterol is not a required nutrient because it serves no essential, or life-sustaining, function in the body.	☐	☐
5. Thanks in part to nutrition labeling requirements, there are lower amounts of *trans* fats in food products now than in the recent past.	☐	☐

	TRUE	FALSE
6. *Trans* fats raise blood cholesterol levels more than any other type of fat.	☐	☐
7. If a claim is made on a food package about the product's fat content, the nutrition facts panel must list the food's fat, saturated fat, *trans* fat, and cholesterol content.	☐	☐
8. The type of fat consumed is more important to health than is total fat consumption.	☐	☐
9. Unhealthful, or "bad," fats include *trans* fats and saturated fats.	☐	☐
10. It is recommended that adults consume 20 to 25% of total calories from fat.	☐	☐

Media Menu

www.nlm.nih.gov/medlineplus/dietaryfat.html
This site provides a menu that connects you to other sites such as good and bad fats, interpreting blood lipid profiles, benefits of omega-3 fatty acids, and fat substitutes.

www.nal.usda.gov/fnic
Find out more about fats and fat replacers from the extensive list of topics covered under the search term "fats."

www.healthfinder.gov
Here is a good source of information on fats, *trans* fat, and cholesterol through search terms such as dietary fat and healthy fats.

www.mayoclinic.com
Healthy fats, bad fats, know your fats, fats and heart disease, and other topics are intelligently covered in sites available through the Mayo Clinic's home page.

www.epa.gov/waterscience/fish
The Environmental Protection Agency's site is good for looking up national and local advisories on fish contamination and consumption.

1. Dietary Reference Intakes, Energy, carbohydrate, fiber, fat, fatty acids, cholesterol, protein, and amino acids. Institute of Medicine, National Academy of Sciences, Washington, DC: National Academies Press; 2002

2. Shai I et al. Weight loss with a low-carbohydrate, Mediterranean, or low-fat diet. N Engl J Med. 2008;359:229–241.

3. Schwartz GJ et al. The lipid messenger OEA links dietary fat intake to satiety, Cell Metab, 2008;8:281–8.

4. Oh R. Practical applications of fish oil (omega-3 fatty acids) in primary care. J Am Board Fam Pract 2005;18:28–36.

5. Harris WS et al. Omega-6 fatty acids and risk for cardiovascular disease, Circulation 2009; available at http://circ.ahajournals.org, accessed 1/09.

6. Stark AH et al. Update on alpha-linolenic acid, Nutr Rev 2008;66:326–32.

7. Chung H et al. Frequency and type of seafood consumed influence plasma (n-3) fatty acid concentrations J Nutr 2008;138:2422–7.

8. Position of the American Dietetic Association and Dietitians of Canada: dietary fatty acids, J Am Diet Assoc 2007;107:1599–1611.

9. Kornman KS. Interleukin 1 genetics, inflammatory mechanisms, and nutrigenetic opportunities to modulate diseases of aging. Am J Clin Nutr 2006;83(suppl):475S–83S.

10. FDA affirms position on mercury in fish. www.fda.gov, issued 6/7/06.

11. Nutrient Composition of foods, USDA Nutrient Database, www.ars.usda.gov/nutrientdata and www.ars.usda.gov/ba/bhnrc/ndl, accessed 6/10/06, 9/08.

12. American Heart Association. Guidelines for the secondary prevention of cardiovascular disease. Circulation, posted online May 15, 2006, www.medscape.com/viewarticle/532327.

13. Harris WS. International recommendations for consumption of long-chain omega-3 fatty acids, J Cardiovasc Med 2007;8 Suppl:1:S50–2.

14. Stuppy P. Transitioning away from trans fatty acids, Today's Dietitian 2003;Jan.:12–14; and Dietary Reference Intakes.

15. Mozaffarian D et al. Trans fatty acids and cardiovascular disease. N Engl J Med 2006;345:1602–12.

16. Eckel RH et al. Americans' awareness, knowledge, and behaviors regarding fats 2006–2007, J Am Diet Assoc 2009;109:288–96.

17. Okie S. New York to trans fats: You're out! N Engl J Med 2008;356:2017–12.

18. Trichopoulou A et al. Adherence to a Mediterranean diet and survival in a Greek population. N Engl J Med 2003;348:2599–608.

19. Fats: the good and the bad (www.mayoclinic.com/invoke.cfm?id=NU00262); and Kris-Etherton et al., New guidelines.

20. What we eat in America, NHANES, 2005–2006, USDA, 2008, available at www.are.usda.gov/ba/bhnrc/fsrg.

21. Krauss RM et al., Revision 2000: a statement for healthcare providers from the Nutrition Committee of the American Heart Association, J Nutr 2001;131:132–46.

Answers to Review Questions

1. True, see page 110.
2. True, see page 111.
3. True, see page 113.
4. False, see page 119.
5. True, see page 115.
6. True, see page 114.
7. True, see page 116.
8. True, see pages 108. 118.
9. True, see page 119.
10. False, see page 118.

NUTRITION | # Up Close

The Healthy Fats in Your Diet

Feedback for Unit 5

Give yourself a point for each time you checked the "3–5 Times per Week" or "Almost Daily" columns for numbers 3, 4, 6, 9, and 10. These foods are sources of healthy unsaturated fats or DHA and EPA. Take a point away for each time your answer ended up in the same columns for foods listed in numbers 1, 2, 5, 7, and 8. These foods provide saturated or *trans* fats. If you have any points left, your selection of food sources of fat regularly include healthy fats.

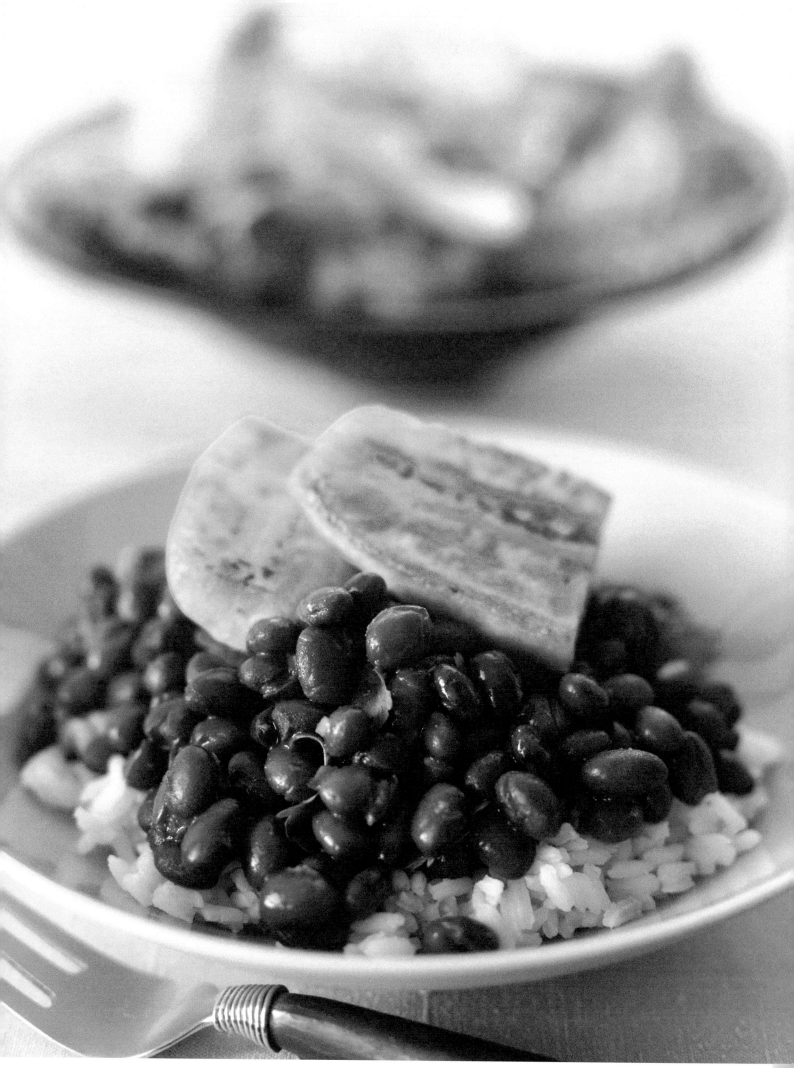

The Proteins and Amino Acids

Chapter 6

Ask Yourself . . .

Which of the following statements about nutrition are true, and which are false? For each false statement, what is true?

1. When more protein is eaten than the body needs, it is stored intact in the body (the way fat is stored) so that it can be used when a person's diet falls short of supplying the day's need for essential proteins.
2. No new living tissue can be built without protein.
3. Whenever cells are lost, protein is lost.
4. All enzymes and hormones are made of protein.
5. When antibodies enter the body, they produce illness.
6. When a person doesn't eat enough food to meet the body's energy needs, the body devours its own protein tissue.
7. Once the body has assembled its proteins into body structures, it never lets go of them.
8. Milk protein is the standard against which the quality of other proteins is usually measured.
9. It is impossible to consume too much protein.
10. People who eat no meat need to eat a lot of special foods to get enough protein.

Answers found on the following page.

The **proteins** are perhaps the most highly respected of the three energy nutrients, and the roles they play in the body are far more varied than those of carbohydrate or fat. First named 150 years ago after the Greek word *proteios* ("of prime importance"), proteins have revealed countless secrets about how living processes take place, and they account for many nutrition concerns. How do we grow? How do our bodies replace the materials they lose? How does blood clot? What makes us able to become immune to diseases we have been exposed to? To a great extent, the answers to these and many other such questions are found in an understanding of the nature of the proteins.

Chapter Objectives

- *Differentiate between essential amino acids and nonessential amino acids.*
- *List the functions of protein in the body.*
- *Describe the impact of animal-based proteins and plant-based proteins on health.*

Contents

The amino acids of proteins are the raw materials of heredity, the keys to life chemistry, handed from generation to generation.

R. M. DEUTSCH (1928–1988, NUTRITION AUTHOR AND EDUCATOR)

proteins compounds composed of atoms of carbon, hydrogen, oxygen, and nitrogen and arranged as strands of amino acids. Some amino acids also contain atoms of sulfur.

An Amino Acid: glycine

Amine group | Acid group

Side group

An Amino Acid: phenylalanine

amino (uh-MEEN-oh) acids building blocks of protein; each is a compound with an amine group at one end, an acid group at the other, and a distinctive side chain.

amine (a-MEEN) group the nitrogen-containing portion of an amino acid.

essential amino acids amino acids that cannot be synthesized by the body or that cannot be synthesized in amounts sufficient to meet physiological need.

protein synthesis the process by which cells assemble amino acids into proteins. All individuals are unique because of minute differences in the ways their body proteins are made. The instructions for making all the proteins in our bodies are transmitted in the genetic information we receive at conception.

peptide bond a bond that connects one amino acid with another.

What Proteins Are Made Of

To appreciate the many vital functions of proteins, we must understand their structure. One key difference from carbohydrate and fat, which contain only carbon, hydrogen, and oxygen atoms, is that proteins contain nitrogen atoms. These nitrogen atoms give the name *amino* ("nitrogen containing") to the **amino acids** of which protein is made. Another key difference is that in contrast to the carbohydrates—whose repeating units, glucose molecules, are identical—the amino acids in a strand of protein are different from one another.

All amino acids have the same, simple chemical backbone, with an **amine group** (the nitrogen-containing part) at one end and an acid group at the other end. The differences among the various amino acids are due to the varying structures of the chemical side chains that are attached to the backbone. Twenty amino acids with 20 different side chains make up most of the proteins of living tissue.

The side chains vary in complexity from a single hydrogen atom, like that on glycine, to a complex ring structure, like that on phenylalanine. Not only do these structures differ in composition, size, and shape, but they also differ in electrical charge. Some are negative, some are positive, and some have no charge. These side chains help to determine the shapes and behaviors of the larger protein molecules that the amino acids make up.

Essential and Nonessential Amino Acids The body can make about half of the amino acids (known as *nonessential amino acids*) for itself, when it has the needed parts: nitrogen to form the amine group and backbone fragments, which are derived from carbohydrate or fat. But even the healthy body cannot make some amino acids. These are known as **essential amino acids**.* If the diet does not supply them, the body cannot make the proteins it needs to do its work. The indispensability of the essential amino acids makes it necessary for people to eat protein food sources every day.

Proteins as the Source of Life's Variety In the first step of **protein synthesis**, each amino acid is hooked to the next. A bond, called a **peptide bond**, is formed between the amino end of one and the acid end of the next. Proteins are made of many amino acid units, from several dozen to many hundred.

A strand of protein is not straight; it is more like a tangled chain. The amino acids at different places along the strand are attracted to one another, and this attraction causes the strand to coil into a shape similar to that of a metal spring. Not only does the strand of amino acids form a long coil, but the coil tangles, forming a globular structure.

The charged amino acids are attracted to water, and in the body fluids they orient themselves on the outside of the globular structure. The neutral amino acids are

ASK YOURSELF ANSWERS: 1. False. When more protein is eaten than the body needs, it is *not* stored in the body (the way fat is stored), so it must be eaten every day to avoid protein depletion. **2.** True. **3.** True. **4.** False. All enzymes, but not all hormones, are made of protein. **5.** False. Antibodies protect the body from illness caused by antigens. **6.** True. **7.** False. Your body loses protein every day. **8.** False. Egg-white protein, not milk protein, is the standard against which the quality of other proteins is usually measured. **9.** False. It is possible to consume too much protein. **10.** False. People who eat no meat can easily get enough protein without eating a lot of special foods.

*The distinction between essential and nonessential amino acids is not quite as clear-cut as the list in the margin makes it appear. For example, cysteine and tyrosine normally are not essential, because the body makes them from methionine and phenylalanine. However, if there are not enough of these precursors from which to make cysteine and tyrosine, they must be supplied by the diet.

repelled by water and are attracted to one another; they tuck themselves into the center, away from the body fluids. All these interactions among the amino acids and the surrounding fluid result in the unique architecture of each type of protein. Additional steps may be needed for the protein to become functional. A mineral or a vitamin may be needed to complete the unit and activate it, or several proteins may gather to form a functioning group.

The differing shapes of proteins enable them to perform different tasks in the body. In proteins that give strength and elasticity to body parts, several springs of amino acids coil together and form rope-like fibers. Other proteins, like those in the blood, do not have such structural strength but are water-soluble, with a globular shape like a ball of steel wool. Some are shaped like hollow balls that can carry and store minerals in their interiors. Still others provide support to tissues. Some—the enzymes—act on other substances to change them chemically.

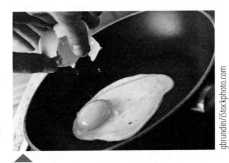
Cooking an egg denatures its proteins.

Denaturation of Proteins
Proteins can undergo **denaturation**, resulting in distortion of shape by heat, alcohol, acids, bases, or the salts of heavy metals. The denaturation of a protein is the first step in breakdown of the protein. Denaturation is useful to the body in digestion. During the digestion of a food protein, an early step is denaturation by the stomach acid, which opens up the protein's structure, permitting digestive enzymes to break the peptide bonds (see Figure 6-1 later in this chapter). Denaturation can also occur during food preparation. For example, cooking an egg denatures the proteins of the egg and makes the egg firmer. Perhaps more important, cooking denatures two raw-egg proteins that bind the B vitamin biotin and the mineral iron, as well as a protein that slows the digestion of other proteins. Thus, cooking eggs liberates biotin and iron and aids in protein digestion.

The Functions of Body Proteins

No new living tissue can be built without protein, for protein is part of every cell. About 20 percent of our total body weight is protein. Proteins come in many forms: enzymes, antibodies, hormones, transport vehicles, oxygen carriers, tendons and ligaments, scars, the cores of bones and teeth, the filaments of hair, the materials of nails, and more (see Table 6-1). A few of the many vital functions of proteins are

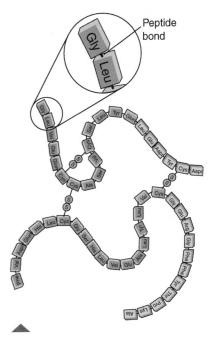

A Molecule of Insulin

Amino acids are linked together with peptide bonds to form strands of protein. The sulfur groups (S) on two cysteine (cys) molecules can bond together, creating a "sulfur bridge" between the two protein strands.

TABLE 6-1	The Functions of Body Proteins

1. Growth and Maintenance
- Proteins provide *building materials*—amino acids—for growth and repair of body tissues.
- *Body structures.* Proteins form vital parts of most body structures, such as skin, nails, hair, membranes, muscles, teeth, bones, organs, ligaments, and tendons.

2. Regulatory Roles
- *Enzymes.* Proteins facilitate numerous chemical reactions in the body; all enzymes are proteins.
- *Hormones.* Some proteins act as chemical messengers, regulating body processes; not all hormones are proteins.
- *Antibodies.* Proteins assist the body in maintaining its resistance to disease by acting against foreign disease-causing substances.
- *Fluid balance.* Proteins help regulate the quantity of fluids in body compartments.
- *Acid–base balance.* Proteins act as buffers to maintain the normal acid and base concentrations in body fluids.
- *Transportation.* Proteins move needed nutrients and other substances into and out of cells and around the body.

3. Energy Production
- *Energy.* Protein can be used to provide calories (4 calories per gram) to help meet the body's energy needs.

denaturation a change in the shape of a protein brought about by heat, alcohol, acids, bases, salts of heavy metals, or other agents.

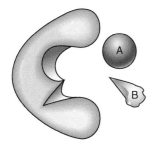

Enzyme plus two compounds, A and B

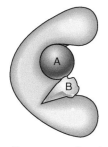

Enzyme complexed with A and B

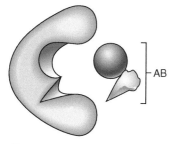

Enzyme plus new compound AB

Enzyme Action

Each enzyme facilitates a specific chemical reaction.

hormones chemical messengers. Hormones are secreted by a variety of glands in the body in response to altered conditions. Each affects one or more target tissues or organs and elicits specific responses to restore normal conditions.

antibodies large proteins of the blood and body fluids that are produced by one type of immune cell in response to invasion of the body by unfamiliar molecules (mostly foreign proteins). Antibodies inactivate the foreign substances and so protect the body. The foreign substances are called *antigens*.

immunity specific disease resistance derived from the immune system's memory of prior exposure to specific disease agents and its ability to mount a swift response against them.

described here to show why they have rightfully earned their position of importance in nutrition.

Growth and Maintenance
One function of dietary protein is to ensure the availability of amino acids for building the proteins of new tissue. New tissue is needed in an embryo; in a growing child; in the blood that replaces that which has been lost in burns, hemorrhage, or surgery; in the scar tissue that heals wounds; and in new hair and nails. Not so obvious, but equally important, is the protein that helps replace worn-out cells. The cells that line the digestive tract live for only about three days, and they are constantly being shed and excreted. You have probably observed that the cells of your skin die, rub off, and are replaced from underneath. For this new growth, amino acids must constantly be resupplied by food.

Enzymes
All enzymes are proteins, and they are among the most important proteins formed in living cells. Enzymes are *catalysts*—biological spark plugs—that help chemical reactions take place. There are thousands of enzymes inside a single cell, each type facilitating a specific chemical reaction. Enzymes are involved in such processes as the digestion of food, the release of energy from the body's stored energy supplies, and the growth and repair of tissue.

The mystery of how an enzyme can be specific for a particular reaction is only partially understood. Scientists believe that the surface of the enzyme is contoured so that it can recognize only the substances it works on, and ignore others. The surface provides a site that attracts one or more specific chemical compounds and promotes a specific chemical reaction. For example, two substances might first become attached to the enzyme and then to each other. The newly formed product is then expelled by the enzyme into the fluid of the cell. Enzymes are the hands-on workers in the production and processing of all substances needed by the body.

Hormones
Hormones are similar to enzymes in creating profound effects. However, hormone molecules differ from enzyme molecules. For one thing, not all of them are made of protein. For another, hormones do not catalyze chemical reactions directly; rather, they act as messengers that elicit the appropriate responses to maintain a normal environment in the body. Hormones regulate overall body conditions, such as the blood glucose level (the hormones insulin and glucagon) and the metabolic rate (thyroid hormone).

Antibodies
Of all the great variety of proteins in living organisms, **antibodies** best demonstrate that proteins are specific to individual organisms. Antibodies form in response to the presence of *antigens* (foreign proteins or other large molecules) that invade the body. The foreign protein may be part of a bacterium, a virus, or a toxin, or it may be something present in food that causes a reaction we call an *allergy*. The body, after recognizing that it has been invaded, manufactures antibodies that deactivate the foreign substance. Without sufficient protein to make antibodies, the body cannot maintain its resistance to disease.

One of the most fascinating aspects of the antibody response to foreign substances is that each antibody is uniquely designed to destroy a specific foreign substance. An antibody that has been manufactured to combat one strain of flu virus is of no help in protecting a person against another strain. Once the body has learned to make a particular antibody, it never forgets, and the next time it encounters that same foreign substance, it will be equipped to destroy it even more rapidly. In other words, the body develops an **immunity**. This is the principle underlying the effectiveness of the vaccines that have nearly eradicated most childhood diseases in the Western world.

Clearly, malnutrition injures the immune system. Without adequate protein in the diet, the immune system will not be able to make its specialized cells and the other tools required to function optimally. Often, protein deficiency and immune incompetence appear together. For this reason, measles can be fatal to a malnourished child.

Many nutrients other than proteins participate in conferring immunity, and many factors other than antibodies are involved.[1] Nevertheless, the immune system is extraordinarily sensitive to nutrition, and almost any nutrient deficit can impair its efficiency and reduce resistance to disease.

Fluid Balance Proteins help regulate the quantity of fluids in the compartments of the body. To remain alive, a cell must contain a constant amount of fluid; this is known as the **fluid balance**. Too much fluid might cause a cell to rupture, and too little would make it unable to function. Although water can diffuse freely into and out of the cell, proteins cannot—and proteins attract water. By maintaining a store of internal proteins, the cell retains the fluid it needs. (It also uses minerals this way.) Similarly, the cells secrete proteins (and minerals) into the spaces between them to keep the fluid volume constant in those spaces. Also, because the proteins secreted into the blood cannot cross the blood vessel walls, they help to maintain the blood volume in the same way.

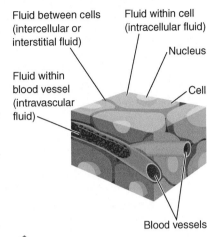

Fluid between cells (intercellular or interstitial fluid)

Fluid within cell (intracellular fluid)

Nucleus

Fluid within blood vessel (intravascular fluid)

Cell

Blood vessels

Shown here are the fluids within and surrounding a cell. Body proteins help hold fluid within cells, tissues, and blood vessels.

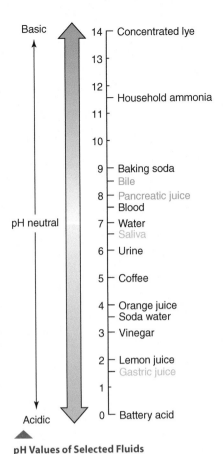

Basic

14 — Concentrated lye
13
12 — Household ammonia
11
10
9 — Baking soda
  — Bile
8 — Pancreatic juice
  — Blood

pH neutral   7 — Water
  — Saliva
6 — Urine
5 — Coffee
4 — Orange juice
  — Soda water
3 — Vinegar
2 — Lemon juice
  — Gastric juice
1
Acidic   0 — Battery acid

pH Values of Selected Fluids

A fluid's acidity or alkalinity is measured in pH units.

Acid–Base Balance Normal processes of the body continually produce **acids** and their opposite, **bases**, which must be carried by the blood to the organs of excretion. The blood must do this without allowing its own **acid–base balance** to be affected. To accomplish this, some proteins act as **buffers** to maintain the blood's normal **pH**. They pick up hydrogen **ions** when there are too many in the blood (the more hydrogen, the more concentrated the acid). Likewise, protein buffers release hydrogens again when there are too few in the blood. The secret is that the negatively charged side chains of the amino acids can accommodate additional hydrogens (which are positively charged) when necessary.

The acid–base balance of the blood is one of the most accurately controlled conditions in the body. If it changes too much, either the dangerous acidic condition called **acidosis** or the opposite basic condition, **alkalosis**, can cause coma or death. The hazards of these conditions are a result of their effect on proteins. When the proteins' buffering capacity is exceeded—for example, when proteins have taken on board or released all the acid hydrogens they can—additional acid or base deranges protein structures by pulling them out of shape; that is, it denatures the proteins—rendering them useless. Knowing how indispensable the structures of proteins are to their functions and how vital protein functions are to life, you can imagine how many body processes would be halted by such a disturbance.

Transport Proteins A specific group of the body's proteins specializes in moving nutrients and other molecules into and out of cells. Some of these **transport proteins** act as pumps, picking up compounds on one side of the membrane and depositing them on the other, and thereby regulating what substances the cell will

fluid balance distribution of fluid among body compartments.

acids compounds that release hydrogens in a watery solution; acids have a low pH.

bases compounds that accept hydrogens from a watery solution; bases have a high pH.

acid–base balance equilibrium between acid and base concentrations in the body fluids.

buffers compounds that help keep the acidity (amount of acid) or alkalinity (amount of base) of a solution constant.

pH the concentration of hydrogen ions. The lower the pH, the stronger the acid: pH 2 is a strong acid, pH 7 is neutral, and a pH above 7 is alkaline (base).

ions (EYE-onz) electrically charged particles, such as sodium (positively charged) and chloride (negatively charged).

acidosis (a-sih-DOSE-is) blood acidity above normal, indicating excess acid.

alkalosis (al-kuh-LOW-sis) blood alkalinity above normal.

transport proteins proteins that carry nutrients and other molecules in body fluids. Some transport proteins reside in cell membranes and act as "pumps" by picking up compounds on one side of the membrane and releasing them on the other side as needed.

take up or release. One such pump is the "sodium–potassium pump," which resides in the cell membrane and acts as a revolving door, picking up potassium from outside the cell and depositing it inside the cell, and picking up sodium from within the cell and depositing it outside the cell as necessary. The protein machinery of cell membranes can be switched on or off in response to the body's needs. Often hormones do the switching with marvelous precision.

Other transport proteins move about in the body fluids, carrying nutrients and other molecules from one organ to another. Those that carry lipids in the lipoproteins are examples. Special proteins also can carry fat-soluble vitamins, water-soluble vitamins, and minerals. As a result, a protein deficiency can cause a vitamin A deficiency or a deficiency of whatever other nutrient needs a transport protein to reach its destination in the body.

This sampling of the major roles proteins play in the body illustrates their versatility, uniqueness, and importance. All the body's tissues and organs—muscles, bones, blood, skin, and nerves—are made largely of proteins. No wonder proteins are said to be the primary material of life.

Protein as Energy   Only protein can perform all the functions previously described, but it will be sacrificed to provide needed energy if insufficient fat and carbohydrate are available from the diet. The body's number one need is for energy. All other needs have a lower priority.

When amino acids are degraded so they can be used for energy, their amine groups are usually incorporated by the liver into **urea** and sent to the kidney for excretion in the urine. The remaining components are carbon, hydrogen, and oxygen, which are available for immediate energy use by the body.

Only when the **protein-sparing** calories from carbohydrate and fat are sufficient to power the cells are the amino acids used for their most important function: making proteins. Thus, energy deficiency (starvation) is always accompanied by the symptoms of protein deficiency.

When amino acids are oversupplied, the body has no place to store them. It removes them, excretes their amine groups, and converts the remaining fragments into glucose and glycogen or into fat for energy storage. Amino acids are not stored in the body except in the sense that they are present in proteins in all the tissues. When there is a great shortage of amino acids, the body must break down such tissues as blood, muscle, and skin so that it can use their amino acids to maintain the heart, lungs, and brain.

How the Body Handles Protein

When a person eats a food protein, whether from cereals, vegetables, meats, or dairy products, the digestive system breaks down the protein and delivers the separated amino acids to the body cells. The cells then put the amino acids together in the order necessary to produce the particular proteins they need. (To review the digestive and absorptive systems relevant to the body's handling of protein, turn to Chapter 3.)

The stomach initiates protein digestion (see Figure 6-1). By the time proteins move into the small intestine, they are already broken into different-sized pieces: some single amino acids and many strands of two amino acids, **dipeptides**; some strands of three amino acids, **tripeptides**; and some longer chains. Digestion continues until almost all pieces of protein are broken into dipeptides, tripeptides, and free amino acids. Absorption of amino acids takes place all along the small intestine. Dipeptides and tripeptides are captured on the surface of the cells that line the small intestine. These cells split the peptides into amino acids, absorb them, and then release them into the bloodstream.

urea (yoo-REE-uh) the principal nitrogen excretion product of metabolism, generated mostly by the removal of amine groups from unneeded amino acids or from those amino acids being sacrificed to a need for energy.

protein-sparing a description of the effect of carbohydrate and fat, which, by being available to yield energy, allow amino acids to be used to build body proteins.

dipeptides (dye-PEP-tides) protein fragments two amino acids long. A *peptide* is a strand of amino acids.

tripeptides (try-PEP-tides) protein fragments three amino acids long.

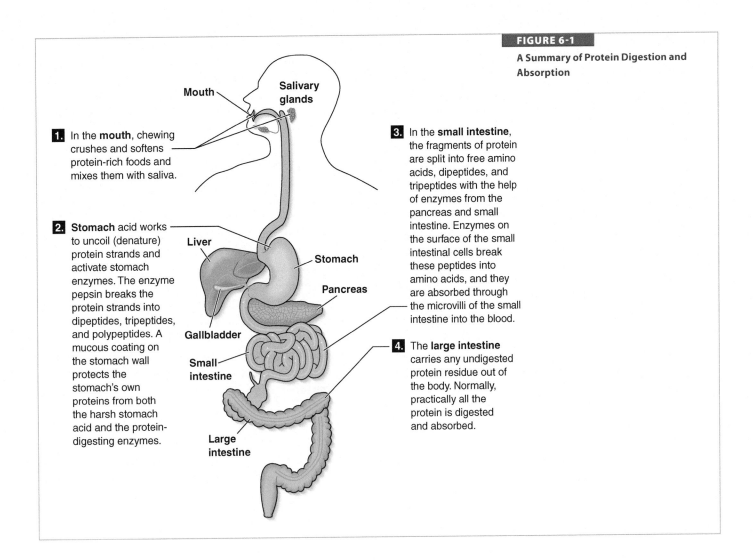

FIGURE 6-1

A Summary of Protein Digestion and Absorption

1. In the **mouth**, chewing crushes and softens protein-rich foods and mixes them with saliva.

2. **Stomach** acid works to uncoil (denature) protein strands and activate stomach enzymes. The enzyme pepsin breaks the protein strands into dipeptides, tripeptides, and polypeptides. A mucous coating on the stomach wall protects the stomach's own proteins from both the harsh stomach acid and the protein-digesting enzymes.

3. In the **small intestine**, the fragments of protein are split into free amino acids, dipeptides, and tripeptides with the help of enzymes from the pancreas and small intestine. Enzymes on the surface of the small intestinal cells break these peptides into amino acids, and they are absorbed through the microvilli of the small intestine into the blood.

4. The **large intestine** carries any undigested protein residue out of the body. Normally, practically all the protein is digested and absorbed.

Labels: Mouth, Salivary glands, Liver, Stomach, Pancreas, Gallbladder, Small intestine, Large intestine

Once they are circulating in the bloodstream, the amino acids are available to be taken up by any cell of the body. The cells can use them to make proteins, either for the cell's own use or for secretion into the circulatory system for other uses.

If a *non*essential amino acid (that is, one the body can make for itself) is unavailable for a growing protein strand, the cell will make one and will continue attaching amino acids to the strand. If, however, an essential amino acid (one the body cannot make) is missing, the building of the protein will halt. The cell cannot hold partially completed proteins to complete them later, for example, the next day. Instead, it must dismantle the partial structures and return surplus amino acids to the circulation, making them available to other cells. If other cells do not soon pick up these amino acids and insert them into protein, the liver will remove their amine groups for the kidney to excrete. Other cells will then use the remaining fragments for other purposes. The nutritional need calling for the production of that particular protein will not be met.

Protein Quality of Foods

The role of protein in food, as already mentioned, is not to provide body proteins directly but to supply the amino acids from which the body can make its own proteins. Because body cells cannot store amino acids for future use, it follows that all the essential amino acids must be eaten as part of a balanced diet. To manufacture

FIGURE 6-2

How Two Plant Proteins Combine to Yield a Complete Protein

Two incomplete proteins (for example, legumes plus grains) can be combined to equal a complete protein (peanut butter sandwich). In this example, the peanut butter provides adequate amounts of the amino acid lysine but is lacking in methionine. The bread "complements" the peanut butter because it contains adequate methionine but is lacking in lysine. When combined as a sandwich, all essential amino acids are present.

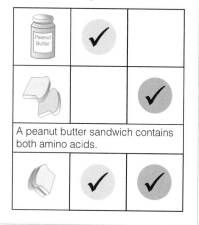

A peanut butter sandwich contains both amino acids.

complete proteins proteins containing all the essential amino acids in the right proportion relative to need. The *quality* of a food protein is judged by the proportions of essential amino acids that it contains relative to our needs. Animal and soy proteins are the highest in quality.

incomplete protein a protein lacking or low in one or more of the essential amino acids.

limiting amino acid a term given to the essential amino acid in shortest supply (relative to the body's need) in a food protein; it therefore *limits* the body's ability to make its own proteins.

complementary proteins two or more food proteins whose amino acid assortments complement each other in such a way that the essential amino acids limited in or missing from each are supplied by the others.

protein quality a measure of the essential amino acid content of a protein relative to the essential amino acid needs of the body.

biological value (BV) a measure of protein quality, assessed by determining how well a given food or food mixture supports nitrogen retention.

reference protein egg-white protein, the standard to which other proteins are compared to determine protein quality.

body proteins, then, all the needed amino acids must be available to the cells. Three important characteristics of dietary protein, therefore, are (1) that it should supply at least the nine essential amino acids, (2) that it should supply enough other amino acids to make nitrogen available for the synthesis of whatever nonessential amino acids the cell may need to make, and (3) that it should be accompanied by enough food energy (preferably from carbohydrate and fat) to prevent sacrifice of its own amino acids for energy.

This presents no problem to people who regularly eat **complete proteins**, such as those of meat, fish, poultry, cheese, eggs, milk, or many soybean products, as part of balanced meals.[2] The proteins of these foods contain ample amounts of all the essential amino acids relative to our bodies' need for them, and the rest of the diet provides protein-sparing energy and needed vitamins and minerals. An equally sound diet choice is to eat two or more **incomplete protein** foods from plants, each of which supplies the **limiting amino acid** in the other—also, of course, as part of a balanced diet. The *quality* of plant proteins (legumes, grains, and vegetables) having different limiting amino acids can therefore be balanced by combining different sources of plant proteins, either during a meal or over the course of a day, making sufficient amounts of all the essential amino acids available for protein synthesis. This strategy of using **complementary proteins** is shown in Figure 6-2. Note that by combining a grain (whole-wheat bread) that is low in lysine but high in methionine with a legume (peanut butter) that is low in methionine but high in lysine, all the essential amino acids are provided.

A person in good health can be expected to use dietary protein efficiently. However, malnutrition or infection can seriously impair digestion (by reducing enzyme secretion), absorption (by causing degeneration of the absorptive surface of the small intestine or losses from diarrhea), and the cells' use of protein (by forcing amino acids to meet other needs). In addition, infections cause increased production of antibodies, which are made of protein. Thus, malnutrition or infection can greatly increase protein needs while making it hard to meet them.[3]

People usually eat many foods containing protein. Each food has its own characteristic amino acid balance, and a mixture of foods almost invariably supplies plenty of each individual amino acid. However, when food energy intake is limited, this is not the case (as discussed in the section "Protein-Energy Malnutrition," later in the chapter). Also, even when food-energy intake is abundant, if the selection of foods available is severely limited, protein intake may not be adequate. The primary food source of protein must be taken into account because its quality is of great importance.

Researchers have studied many different individual foods as protein sources and have developed many different methods of evaluating the **protein quality** of foods. Protein quality is determined by two factors—the protein's digestibility and its amino acid composition. One method of evaluating protein quality judges how easily the body can absorb the protein. In general, amino acids from animal and soy proteins are the most easily absorbed (90 to 100 percent). Amino acids from other legumes are next best (80 to 90 percent); the absorption rates for those from grains and other plant foods vary (70 to 90 percent).

When amino acids are wasted, their amine groups (which contain their nitrogen) cannot be stored. Therefore, the efficiency of a protein can be assessed experimentally by measuring the net loss of nitrogen from the body. The higher the amount of nitrogen retained, the higher the quality of the protein. This is the basis for determining the **biological value (BV)** of proteins. A high-quality protein by this standard is egg-white protein, which has been designated the **reference protein** and given a score of 100. Other proteins are compared with it. The best guarantee of amino acid adequacy is to eat a variety of foods containing protein in the presence of adequate amounts of vitamins, minerals, and energy from carbohydrate and fat.

Recommended Protein Intakes

Recommended protein intakes can be stated in two ways: as a percentage of total calories, or as an absolute number (grams per day). The DRI committee recommends that protein provide 10 to 35 percent of total caloric intake.[4] The recommended protein allowance for a healthy adult is 0.8 gram per kilogram (or 2.2 pounds) of desirable body weight per day.

The recommendation for protein uses the desirable, not the actual, weight for a given height, because the desirable weight is proportional to the *lean* body mass of the average person. Lean body mass, not total weight, determines protein need. This is because fat tissue is composed largely of fat, which does not require much protein for maintenance.

The recommendations for protein intake are based on the assumption that the protein source will be a combination of plant and animal proteins, that it will be consumed with adequate calories from carbohydrate and fat, and that other nutrients in the diet will be adequate. These protein recommendations apply only to healthy individuals with no unusual metabolic need for protein.

Protein and Health

Protein deficiency effects are well known because, together with energy deficiency, they are the world's main form of malnutrition. In contrast, the health effects of too much protein—and particularly the effects of proteins of different kinds—are far less well known. The following sections discuss protein deficiency, excess protein, and types of protein. The Nutrition Action feature in this chapter discusses the problem of protein-related food allergies in children and adults.

Protein-Energy Malnutrition   Protein deficiency and energy deficiency very often go hand in hand and are called **protein-energy malnutrition (PEM)**. The two diseases and their symptoms overlap all along the spectrum, but the extremes have names of their own. Protein deficiency is **kwashiorkor**, and energy deficiency is **marasmus**.[5]

Kwashiorkor is the Ghanaian name for "the evil spirit that infects the first child when the second child is born." In countries where kwashiorkor is prevalent, parents customarily give their newly weaned children watery cereal rather than the food eaten by the rest of the family. The child has been receiving the mother's breast milk, which contains high-quality protein designed to support growth. However, when a new baby is born, the first child is weaned and suddenly is fed only a weak drink with scant protein of very low quality. It is not surprising that the just-weaned child becomes sick when the new baby arrives.

The child who has been banished from its mother's breast faces this threat to life by engaging in as little activity as possible. Apathy is one of the earliest signs of protein deprivation. The body is collecting all its forces to meet the crisis and so cuts down on any expenditure of protein not needed for the heart, lungs, and brain. As the apathy increases, the child doesn't even cry for food. All growth ceases, and the child is no larger at age 4 than at age 2. New hair grows without the protein pigment that gives hair its color. The skin also loses its color, and open sores fail to heal. Digestive enzymes are in short supply, the digestive tract lining deteriorates, and absorption

Calculation Practice

To calculate the percentage of calories you derive from protein:

1. Use your total calories as the denominator (example: 1,900 cal).

2. Multiply your total protein intake in *grams* by 4 cal/g to obtain calories from protein as the numerator (example: 70 g protein + 4 cal/g = 280 cal).

3. Divide to obtain a decimal, multiply by 100, and round off (example: 280/1,900 × 100 = 15% cal from protein).

To calculate your recommended protein intake (RDA):

1. Find the desirable weight for a person your height (see Appendix A). Assume that this weight is appropriate for you.

2. Change pounds to kilograms (divide pounds by 2.2; 1 kilogram = 2.2 pounds).

3. Multiply kilograms by 0.8 g/kg.

Example (for a 5'8" male):

1. Desirable weight: about 150 lb.

2. 150 lb ÷ 2.2 lb = 68 kg (rounded off).

3. 68 kg × 0.8 g/kg = 54 g protein (rounded off).

Chapter 11 discusses the protein needs of athletes, and the Spotlight in Chapter 11 presents the pros and cons of using popular amino acid and other supplements.

protein-energy malnutrition (PEM) also called protein-calorie malnutrition (PCM); the world's most widespread malnutrition problem; includes both kwashiorkor and marasmus as well as the states in which they overlap.

kwashiorkor (kwash-ee-OR-core) a deficiency disease caused by inadequate protein in the presence of adequate food energy.

marasmus (muh-RAZ-mus) an energy deficiency disease; starvation.

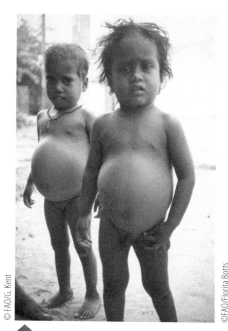

Kwashiorkor. These children have the characteristic edema and swollen belly often seen with kwashiorkor.

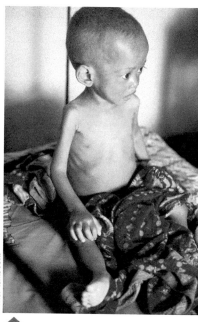

Marasmus. This child is suffering from the extreme emaciation of marasmus.

fails. The child can't assimilate what little food is eaten. Proteins and hormones that previously kept the fluids correctly distributed among the compartments of the body now are diminished, so that fluid leaks out of the blood (**edema**) and accumulates in the belly and legs. Blood proteins, including hemoglobin, are not synthesized, so the child becomes anemic, which increases the child's weakness and apathy. The kwashiorkor victim often develops a fatty liver, caused by a lack of the protein carriers that transport fat out of the liver. Antibodies to fight off invading bacteria are degraded to provide amino acids for other uses; hence, the child becomes an easy target for any infection. Then **dysentery**, an infection of the digestive tract that causes diarrhea, further depletes the body of nutrients, especially minerals. Measles, which might make a healthy child sick for a week or two, kills the child victim of kwashiorkor within 2 or 3 days. If the condition is caught in time, the starving child's life may be saved by careful nutrition therapy.

Children with *marasmus* suffer symptoms similar to those of children with kwashiorkor because both conditions cause loss of body protein tissue. However, there are differences between the two conditions. A marasmic child looks like a wizened little old person—just skin and bones. The child is often sick because his or her resistance to disease is low. All the muscles are wasted, including the heart muscle, and the heart is weak. Metabolism is so slow that body temperature is subnormal. There is little or no fat under the skin to insulate against cold. The experience of hospital workers with victims of this disease is that the victims' primary need is to be wrapped up and kept warm. The disease occurs most commonly in children from 6 months to 18 months of age. Because the brain normally grows to almost its full adult size within the first two years of life, marasmus impairs brain development and thus may have a permanent effect on a child's learning ability.

PEM is prevalent in Africa, Central America, South America, and Asia.[6] PEM has also been recognized in many undernourished hospital patients, including those with anorexia nervosa, **AIDS**, cancer, and other wasting conditions. The extent and severity of malnutrition worldwide is a political and economic problem. It is discussed further in the Spotlight feature in Chapter 13.

Too Much Protein Many of the world's people struggle to obtain enough food and enough protein to keep themselves alive, but in the developed countries, where protein is abundant, the problems of protein excess can be seen. Animals fed high-protein diets experience a protein overload effect, most notable in the enlargement of their livers and kidneys. In human beings, when protein intake is high, calcium excretion increases.[7] The higher a person's intake of animal-protein sources such as meat, the more likely it is that fruits, vegetables, and whole grains will be crowded out of the diet, creating deficiencies of other nutrients.

Although protein is essential to health, the body converts extra protein to energy (glucose), which is stored as body fat when energy needs are met. Despite the flood of new protein-packed snack bars and other products in the marketplace, there are no

edema (eh-DEEM-uh) swelling of body tissue caused by leakage of fluid from the blood vessels, seen in (among other conditions) protein deficiency.

dysentery (DISS-en-terry) an infection of the digestive tract that causes diarrhea.

AIDS (acquired immune deficiency syndrome) an immune system disorder caused by the human immunodeficiency virus (HIV).

known benefits from consuming excess protein. The recommended upper range for protein intake applies *when calorie intake is adequate.* Note the qualification "when calorie intake is adequate" in the preceding statement. Remember that your recommended protein intake can be stated as a percentage of calories in the diet or as a specific number of grams of dietary protein. The recommended protein intake for a 150-pound person is roughly 55 grams, or about 12 percent of their daily caloric intake. Fifty-five grams of protein is equal to 220 calories and equals 11 percent of a 2,000-calorie intake, which is reasonable for a 150-pound active person. If this person were to drastically reduce his or her caloric intake to, say, 800 calories a day, then 220 calories from protein is suddenly 28 percent of the total. However, it is still this person's recommended intake for protein, and a reasonable intake. It is the caloric intake that is unreasonable in this example. Similarly, if the person eats too many calories—say, 4,000—this protein intake represents only 6 percent of the total caloric intake, yet it is still a reasonable intake. It is the caloric intake that may be unreasonable.

Thus, it is important to be careful when judging protein intakes as a percentage of calories. Always ask what the absolute number of grams is, too, and compare it with the recommended protein intake in grams. As calorie intake decreases, it is necessary to increase the percentage of calories from protein so as to consume the RDA for protein. Recommendations stated as a percentage of calories are useful only when food energy intakes (calories) are within reason.

Protein in the Diet   Misconceived notions abound regarding protein in the diet; the most obvious of these is that more is better. American women eat about 60 to 65 grams of protein a day, notably higher than the recommended 46 grams a day. Young men average about 100 grams a day and drop to about 75 to 85 grams as older adults, still considerably higher than their recommended intake of 56 grams. Moreover, more than 65 percent of this protein comes from animal and dairy products (see Figure 6-3). Saturated fats supply half or more of the calories in some animal-protein foods. You can better balance your food choices by selecting one-third or less of your protein from animal sources and the rest from plants. (See the Eat Well Be Well feature later in this chapter). To limit your intake of saturated fat, consider the following tips when shopping for protein foods:

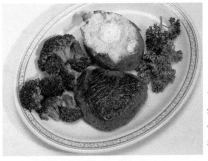

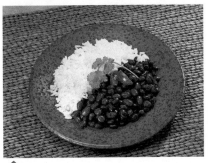

Both meals shown here supply an adequate assortment of amino acids needed for health.

- Dairy foods are excellent sources of protein, calcium, and other important nutrients. Look for fat-free and low-fat varieties for the recommended three servings each day. Look for low-fat cheeses that have less than 5 grams of fat per ounce, such as part-skim or fat-free ricotta or mozzarella, feta cheese, string cheese, or other reduced-calorie cheeses. These choices are lower in saturated fat and calories than their full-fat counterparts.

- Fish and shellfish—fresh, frozen, or canned in water—make excellent protein choices and are low in fat. Experts recommend that you eat at least two fish meals per week.

- Meat, chicken, and fish all provide excellent protein, as well as iron, zinc, and vitamin B$_{12}$. We are advised to choose low-fat varieties. Look for the leanest meats:

  - Flank steak, round steak, sirloin, tenderloin, or extra lean ground beef

  - Lean ham, Canadian bacon, pork tenderloin, and center-loin pork chops

  - Chicken, turkey, or game hens without the skin; fresh ground turkey breast or chicken breast meat

FIGURE 6-3

Protein Contributed by Food Groups in the Average American Diet

These foods provide 70% of the protein in the U.S. diet. The following foods also contribute at least 1% (in descending order): cold cuts (excluding ham), ready-to-eat cereal, white potatoes, sausage, flour and baking ingredients, ice cream, sherbet and frozen yogurt, nuts and seeds, cooked rice and other grains, and canned tuna.

SOURCE: Adapted from P. A. Cotton and coauthors, Dietary sources of nutrients among U.S. adults, 1994–1996, *Journal of the American Dietetic Association* 104 (2004): 921–930.

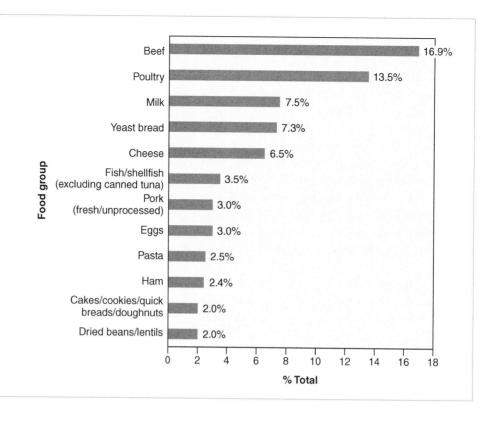

Food group	% Total
Beef	16.9%
Poultry	13.5%
Milk	7.5%
Yeast bread	7.3%
Cheese	6.5%
Fish/shellfish (excluding canned tuna)	3.5%
Pork (fresh/unprocessed)	3.0%
Eggs	3.0%
Pasta	2.5%
Ham	2.4%
Cakes/cookies/quick breads/doughnuts	2.0%
Dried beans/lentils	2.0%

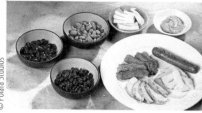

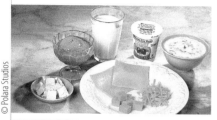

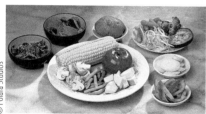

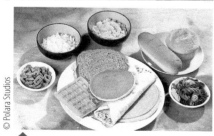

Foods that supply protein in abundance are shown here in the Dairy group and the Protein Foods group of the MyPlate food guide (top two photos). Servings of foods from the Vegetable group and the Grains group can also contribute protein to the diet (bottom two photos).

legumes (LEG-yoomz or leh-GYOOMZ) plants of the bean and pea family having roots with nodules containing bacteria that can trap nitrogen from the air in the soil and make it into compounds that become part of the seed. The seeds are rich in high-quality protein compared with those of most other plant foods.

- At the deli counter, select items with less than 1 gram of fat per ounce, such as lean ham, turkey or chicken breast, and lean roast beef.

- Nuts and nut butters are good sources of protein but are also high in fat. Look for nonhydrogenated varieties. A 1-tablespoon serving of peanut butter counts as 1 ounce of meat in the MyPlate food guide.

- Eggs are another excellent source of protein. Also look for egg substitutes, and substitute ¼ cup for one whole egg in recipes. One egg counts as 1 ounce of meat.

- Many interesting sources of protein are available. Try adding **legumes** to your meals using the tips in the Savvy Diner feature that follows. A ¼-cup serving counts as 1 ounce of meat in the MyPlate food guide.

As the vegetarian knows, one can easily design a perfectly acceptable diet around plant foods alone by choosing an appropriate variety. This chapter's Spotlight reviews the benefits of soy products, an excellent source of protein in the diet.

Adequate protein in the diet is easy to obtain. A breakfast of one egg, two slices of wheat bread, and a glass of milk provide nearly 20 grams of protein. This meets about 35 percent of an average man's recommended protein intake of 56 grams and about 43 percent of a woman's recommended protein intake of 46 grams. The Scorecard feature in this chapter shows you how to estimate your own protein intake.

The Vegetarian Diet

More and more people are following vegetarian diets. The reasons for becoming vegetarian vary widely.[8] Some people have health reasons, whereas others have religious, philosophical, or ethical reasons. Some believe that vegetarianism is ecologically sound, and others believe that it is less costly than the meat-eating alternative.

Legumes—dried beans, peas, and lentils—have been very highly praised in recent years.[9] The *Dietary Guidelines* recommend that Americans eat more beans. On the MyPlate food guide, legumes are the only food featured in two different categories, the Vegetables group and the Protein Foods group. Legumes are rich in the B vitamins and fiber. They are good sources of protein, iron, and zinc and are naturally low in fat and cholesterol-free. The Food and Drug Administration approved a health claim for bean packages and cans: "Diets including beans may reduce your risk of heart disease and certain cancers."[10] However, Americans typically eat only about half the recommended amount of legumes: one cup instead of the recommended 1.5 to 2 cups per week for a 2,000-calorie diet (see bean recommendations for other calorie levels at www.ChooseMyPlate.gov).

Here are three simple ways to increase your intake of this low-cost, easy-to-include group of foods:

1. Enjoy adding more legumes to your weekly meals. Include legumes in entrees (tacos), side dishes (baked beans), soups (split pea or lentil), and salads (chickpeas from the salad bar, or three-bean combos). Recipes can be prepared from dried beans (soaked, rinsed, and cooked) or more quickly from canned beans (rinsed to remove excess sodium). Thorough rinsing is recommended to remove the gas-causing sugar, known as *raffinose*, found in beans.

2. Explore the many varieties of legumes used in cooking—as noted in the Miniglossary.

3. Enjoy learning more about these nutritional powerhouses online. The following three sites can help:

   - *American Dry Bean Board:* www.americanbean.org/. Includes bean basics, photos, health tips, and 1,001 recipes.

   - *U.S. Dry Bean Council:* www.beansforhealth.com/. A more global focus, with many links and a useful bibliography.

   - *USA Dry Pea & Lentil Council:* www.pea-lentil.com/. Nutrition information, cooking instructions, and recipes.

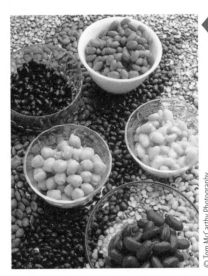

Legumes include such plant foods as the soybean, kidney bean, garbanzo bean, black bean, lentil, garden pea, black-eyed pea, and lima bean.

© Tom McCarthy Photography

Miniglossary of Legumes

black, Cuban, or turtle beans medium-size, black-skinned oval beans that have a rich, sweet taste. They are best served in Mexican and Latin American dishes or thick soups and stews.

black-eyed peas small, oval-shaped, creamy-white peas with a black spot. They have a vegetable flavor with mealy texture. Use in salads with rice and greens.

garbanzo beans or chickpeas large, round, tan-colored legumes that have a nutty flavor and crunchy texture. Use in soups and stews and puréed for dips.

Great Northern beans a medium-white, kidney-shaped bean. Enjoy the delicate flavor and firm texture in salads, soups, and main dishes.

kidney beans these familiar beans are large, red, and kidney shaped (the white variety is called *cannellini*). They have a bland taste and soft texture but tough skins. Use in chili, bean stews, and Mexican dishes (for red) or Italian dishes (for white).

lentils small, flat, and round legumes. Usually brown, lentils can also be green, pink, or red. They have a mild taste with firm texture. Best used when combined with grains or vegetables in salads, soups, or stews.

lima or butter beans limas are soft and mealy in texture. They are flat, oval shaped, and white tinged with green. The smaller variety has a milder taste. Use in soups and stews.

pinto beans medium-size, oval beans that are mottled beige and brown and have an earthy flavor. They are most often used in Mexican dishes, such as refried beans, stews, or dips.

red beans this versatile bean is a medium-size, dark-red oval. The taste and texture are similar to kidney beans. Use in soups and stews, and serve with rice.

soybeans you can find these creamy white ovals in numerous food products, such as tofu, flour, grits, and milk. They have a firm texture and bland flavor. See the Spotlight feature later in this chapter for a discussion of the possible health benefits derived from soy foods.

split peas green or yellow, these small, halved peas supply an earthy flavor with a mealy texture. They are best used in soups and with rice or grains.

white navy beans small, white, oval beans that are best used in soups and stews and as baked beans.

SOURCE: Adapted from K. Mangum, *Life's Simple Pleasures: Fine Vegetarian Cooking for Sharing and Celebration* (Boise, ID: Pacific Press, 1990), 149.

The ancient inhabitants of South America liked to eat a kind of paste made from peanuts. But modern peanut butter came into being around 1890 as the bright idea of a St. Louis physician, who thought it would be a good health food for elderly people. It was not linked with jelly until the 1920s.[11]

Many health organizations

now recommend a diet that emphasizes vegetables, fruits, legumes, and whole grains to protect against cancer, heart disease, stroke, diabetes, and obesity.[12] The key to getting enough, but not too much, protein seems to be to use a variety of plant-based foods and to de-emphasize meats.[13]

1 In the Kitchen.

- Small meat portions tend to work best when mixed into dishes with lots of vegetables and grains; try stir-fries, pastas, soups and stews, burritos, and main-dish salads. For example, cook a large pot of soup, stew, or chili. Minimize the amount of meat you use, and load up the pot with vegetables (fresh or frozen) and cooked beans.

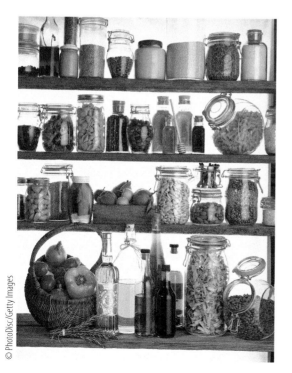

© PhotoDisc./Getty Images

- Go meatless one or more days each week. Experiment with recipes from health-minded cookbooks.
- Take a fresh look at your favorite recipes. Try to use less meat and add more vegetables. Instead of chicken and broccoli stir-fry, try stir-fried veggies with a little chicken.
- For quick, colorful, meals rich in nutrients and flavor, try various combinations of stir-fried vegetables on beds of steamed brown rice, whole-grain bulgur, or couscous.

2 In the Lunch Box.

- Get out of the peanut butter and jelly rut by filling sandwiches with water-packed tuna mixed with mandarin oranges, bean sprouts, and a bit of plain low-fat yogurt; chopped, cooked, skinless chicken combined with raw sliced vegetables and a little French dressing; cooked, mashed dried beans seasoned with chopped onion, garlic powder, rosemary, thyme, and pepper; or low-fat cottage cheese flavored with drained, chopped pineapple.
- Take a thermos filled with chili, vegetable soup, or a milk-based soup, such as cream of tomato prepared with nonfat milk, instead of a sandwich. Try cold lunches such as low-fat yogurt and fruit, brown rice with cubes of skinless poultry, or cooked pasta tossed with raw vegetables, low-fat cheese, and a bit of Italian dressing.

3 At the Table.

- When dining out, choose an ethnic restaurant with plant-based entrées on the menu. Consider Spanish paella, Asian stir-fries, Moroccan stew, Indian curries, or French ratatouille as your entrée. Or try Chinese, Vietnamese, or Thai take-out with lots of rice and vegetables.
- Twice a week, make seafood the protein on your plate.
- Eat more legumes as well as red, orange, and dark green vegetables, such as tomatoes, sweet potatoes, and broccoli.
- Make whole grains, vegetables, and legumes the main event of your meals. At least two-thirds of your meal should come from these plant-based foods and one-third or less from lean meat, poultry, fish, or low-fat dairy products.

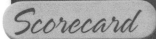

Scorecard — Estimate Your Protein Intake

The average American consumes much more than his or her recommended protein intake. How do you compare? First, figure your recommended protein intake (divide your weight in pounds by 2.2 and then multiply by 0.8). Next, write down everything you ate and drank yesterday. Using the values given below, estimate the grams of protein you ate from both animal and plant sources. If an item is not listed here, use Appendix D to determine the amount of protein it contains. How close are you to your recommended protein intake? What percentage of your protein comes from animal versus plant sources?

Recommended Protein Intake: _____ grams

Protein Foods	Amount	Grams of Protein in 1 Serving	Grams of Protein in Your Typical Diet
Animal Sources			
Hard cheese (e.g., cheddar)	1 oz	7	_____
Cottage cheese	½ c	14	_____
Milk	1 c	9	_____
Yogurt	1 c	12	_____
Egg	1 large	7	_____
Poultry	3 oz	21	_____
Ground beef, lean	3 oz	24	_____
Beef steak, lean	3 oz	26	_____
Pork chop, lean	3 oz	20	_____
Other	_____	_____	_____
		Animal Proteins Subtotal (grams):	_____
Plant Sources			
Vegetables	½ c	2	_____
Legumes, cooked	½ c	8	_____
Tofu	4 oz	9	_____
Cereals	1 c	2–6	_____
Bread	1 slice	2	_____
Tortilla	1	2	_____
Rice	½ c	3	_____
Pasta	½ c	3	_____
Peanut butter	1 tbsp	4	_____
Nuts	2 tbsp	3	_____
Seeds	2 tbsp	3	_____
Other	_____	_____	_____
		Plant Proteins Subtotal (grams):	_____

Day's Total Protein: _____ grams

In addition to the traditional types of vegetarians (see Table 6-2), some people eat seafood but not other meats, and some include chicken and other poultry but not red meat. Whatever the particular reasons for choosing a vegetarian diet, the vegetarian needs to be aware of its implications for nutrition and health.

Important goals for *any* diet planner include the following:

- Obtain neither too few nor too many calories—that is, to maintain a healthy weight

- Obtain adequate quantities of complete protein

TABLE 6-2   Types of Vegetarians

Semivegetarian Some but not all groups of animal-derived products, such as meat, poultry, fish, seafood, eggs, milk, and milk products, are included in this diet.

Lacto-vegetarian Milk and milk products are included in this diet, but meat, poultry, fish, seafood, and eggs are excluded.
   possible limiting nutrient: iron

Lacto-ovovegetarian Milk and milk products and eggs are included in this diet, but meat, poultry, fish, and seafood are excluded.
   possible limiting nutrient: iron

Ovovegetarian Eggs are included in this diet, but milk and milk products, meat, poultry, fish, and seafood are excluded.
   possible limiting nutrients: iron, vitamin D, calcium, riboflavin

Strict vegetarian/vegan All animal-derived foods, including meat, poultry, fish, seafood, eggs, milk, and milk products are excluded from this diet.
   possible limiting nutrients: iron, vitamin D, calcium, riboflavin, vitamin B_{12}, omega-3 fatty acids, high-quality protein

Macrobiotic diet Extremely restrictive diet based on metaphysical beliefs and consisting mostly of legumes, whole grains, and certain vegetables.
   when taken to extremes, includes only brown rice and water or herbal teas and can cause malnutrition and death

- Obtain the needed vitamins and minerals

- Limit intake of foods with added sugars or solid fats, especially saturated fat and *trans*-fat, and foods that are high in sodium

With guidance in meal planning, a vegetarian diet can be a healthful choice for individuals during all stages of the life cycle, including pregnancy, lactation, infancy, childhood, and adolescence.[14] An increasing variety of fortified foods such as soy and rice beverages, meat replacements, juices, and breakfast cereals are available that can add substantially to vegetarians' intakes of key nutrients such as calcium, iron, zinc, vitamin B_{12}, vitamin D, riboflavin, and omega-3 fatty acids.[15] In addition, vegetarians can use the special Vegetarian Food Pyramid (see Figure 6-4) to balance their diets.

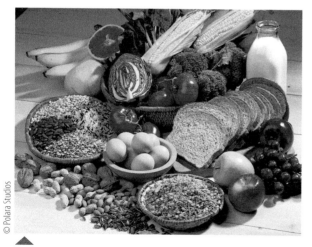

© Polara Studios

Well-planned, plant-based meals consisting of a variety of whole grains, legumes, nuts, vegetables, fruits—and for some vegetarians, eggs and dairy products—can offer sound nutrition and health benefits to vegetarians and nonvegetarians alike.

Proteins The vegetarian needs adequate amounts of all the essential amino acids. Because proteins from animals contain ample amounts of the essential amino acids, the lacto-ovovegetarian can get a head start on meeting protein needs by drinking recommended amounts of milk daily or by consuming the equivalent in milk products in the day's diet.

Adequate amounts of amino acids can be obtained from a plant-based diet when a varied diet is routinely consumed on a daily basis. Mixtures of proteins from whole grains, vegetables, beans, nuts, seeds, nut butters, peas, and soy products (tofu, tempeh, veggie burgers) eaten over the course of a day complement one another's amino acid profiles so that deficits in one are made up by the assets of another. Table 6-3 gives examples of how such mixtures of foods can be combined to form complete proteins.

Nutrition, Physical Activity, and Fitness

Energy for Physical Activity

Your body runs on water, oxygen, and food—primarily carbohydrate and fat. The chemical process that converts these substances to energy is called *metabolism*. Two interrelated energy-producing systems are at work in your body. One system, which depends on oxygen, is called **aerobic** metabolism. The other system functions without oxygen and is called **anaerobic** metabolism. Understanding how the two systems work is important because it explains why you would choose certain activities over others to strengthen your heart, why you eat what you do, and what factors influence your performance during sporting events.

Aerobic and Anaerobic Metabolism
At rest, your muscles burn mostly fat and some carbohydrate for energy. During exercise, though, the amount of energy the muscles use depends on the interplay between fuel availability and oxygen availability. To an exercising muscle, oxygen is everything. With ample oxygen, muscles can extract all available energy from carbohydrate and fat by means of aerobic metabolism. During moderate activity, your lungs and circulatory system have no trouble keeping up with the muscles' need for oxygen. You breathe deeply and easily, and your heart beats steadily—the activity is aerobic. Still, the heart and lungs can supply only so much oxygen only so fast.

When the muscles' exertion becomes great enough that their energy demand outstrips the oxygen supply, they must also rely on anaerobic metabolism for energy. Because the anaerobic metabolic pathway can only burn carbohydrate for fuel, it draws heavily on your limited body stores of carbohydrate. Nevertheless, this system provides an immediate energy source without requiring oxygen. Thanks to anaerobic metabolism, you can dash out of the way of an oncoming car or sprint ahead of your competitor at the finish line. Unfortunately, however, this energy-yielding system is extremely inefficient. Only 5 percent of carbohydrate's energy-producing potential is harnessed by this pathway.[10]

Because the anaerobic metabolic pathway only partially burns your carbohydrate, it also litters your muscle with lactic acid—partly broken-down portions of glucose. When lactic acid builds up in the muscles, it causes burning pain and can lead to muscle exhaustion within seconds if it is not drained away. An effective strategy for dealing with lactic acid buildup is to relax the muscles at every opportunity, allowing the circulating blood to carry it away and bring in oxygen to support aerobic metabolism. Fortunately, lactic acid is not a waste product. The blood delivers it to your liver, where it is converted back into glucose.

Objectives
- Describe the four components of fitness.
- Describe how nutrients are used during physical activity.

aerobic requiring oxygen.

anaerobic not requiring oxygen.

Get health. No labor, effort, nor exercise that can gain it must be grudged.

R. W. EMERSON (1803–1882, AMERICAN ESSAYIST AND POET)

Neither the aerobic nor the anaerobic metabolic pathway functions exclusively to supply energy to your body. The two work together, complementing and supporting each other. Keep in mind, however, that carbohydrate is absolutely essential for exercise. Without it, your muscles can't perform. When you exercise aerobically, muscles burn fat and extract energy from carbohydrate more efficiently in the presence of oxygen, thereby conserving your body's limited store of carbohydrate. Thus, you want to exercise at an intensity that allows your heart and lungs to keep pace with the oxygen needs of your working muscles.

Aerobic Exercise—Exercise for the Heart

To meet your body's increased oxygen needs during aerobic exercise, your heart must pump oxygen-rich blood to muscles at a faster pace than normal. This increased demand on the heart makes the heart stronger and increases its endurance. In addition, aerobic exercise improves the endurance of the lungs and the muscles along the arteries and in the walls of the digestive tract and, of course, the muscles directly involved in the activity. These all-over improvements are called **cardiovascular conditioning** or the **training effect**. In cardiovascular conditioning, the total blood volume increases so that the blood can carry more oxygen. The heart muscle becomes stronger and larger. Therefore, because each beat of the heart pumps more blood, it needs to pump less often. The muscles that work the lungs gain strength and endurance, and breathing becomes more efficient. Circulation through the body's arteries and veins improves. Blood moves easily, and the blood pressure falls. Muscles throughout the body become firmer. Figure 7-1 shows the major relationships among the heart, circulatory system, and lungs.

To make these gains in cardiovascular conditioning, you must elevate your heart rate (pulse). This elevated heart rate—called your **target heart rate**—must be considerably faster than the resting rate to push (overload) the heart but not so fast as to strain it. To achieve this goal, you must work up to the point at which you can exercise aerobically for at least 20 minutes or longer.

An informal pulse check can give you some indication of how conditioned your heart is to start with. As a rule of thumb, the average resting pulse rate for adults is around 70 beats per minute, but the rate can be higher or lower. Active people may have resting pulse rates of 50 or even lower.

For cardiovascular conditioning, you can calculate your target heart rate using your age as the starting point. The older you are, the lower your maximum target heart rate. As your heart becomes stronger, more intense activity will be required to reach the same target rate. For example, at first, walking at a pace of 3 miles per hour may cause you to reach your target heart rate. After 6 to 8 weeks of walking at this pace, you may notice that you no longer reach your target heart rate. That's because your heart is stronger. It now needs more of a challenge to beat faster. Increasing the intensity of your workout by walking faster can provide this challenge.

To calculate your target heart rate range, take the following steps:

1. *Estimate your maximum heart rate (MHR).* Subtract your age from 220. This provides an estimate of the absolute maximum heart rate possible for a person your age. You should never exercise at this rate, of course.
2. *Determine your target heart rate range.* Multiply your MHR by 55 percent and 90 percent to find your upper and lower limits (see margin example on page 146).

cardiovascular conditioning or **training effect** the effect of regular exercise on the cardiovascular system; includes improvements in heart, lung, and muscle function and increased blood volume; also called *cardiorespiratory endurance* or *cardiorespiratory training.*

target heart rate the heartbeat rate that will achieve a cardiovascular conditioning effect for a given person: fast enough to push the heart, but not so fast as to strain it.

When you can work out at your target heart rate for 20 to 60 minutes, you know that you have arrived at your cardiovascular fitness goal.

Fuels for Physical Activity

Your energy-producing pathways require oxygen and the two muscle fuels, glucose and fatty acids. As Figure 7-1 shows, the oxygen comes from the lungs, which pass it to the blood, which carries it to the muscles. Your muscles, and to some extent your liver, supply carbohydrate to your muscles from their carbohydrate supply (see Figure 7-2). The fatty acids come mostly from fat inside the muscles but partly from fat that is released from the body's fat stores, and the blood delivers these fatty acids to the muscles.

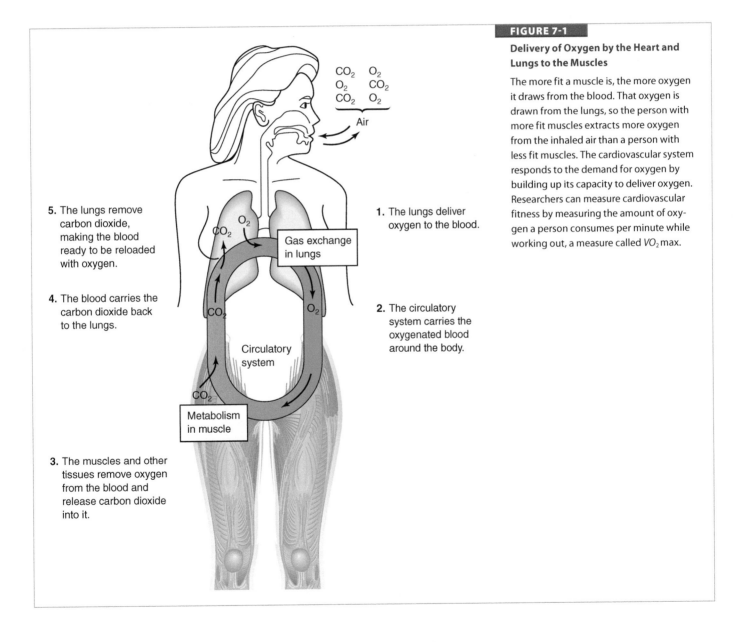

5. The lungs remove carbon dioxide, making the blood ready to be reloaded with oxygen.

4. The blood carries the carbon dioxide back to the lungs.

3. The muscles and other tissues remove oxygen from the blood and release carbon dioxide into it.

1. The lungs deliver oxygen to the blood.

2. The circulatory system carries the oxygenated blood around the body.

FIGURE 7-1

Delivery of Oxygen by the Heart and Lungs to the Muscles

The more fit a muscle is, the more oxygen it draws from the blood. That oxygen is drawn from the lungs, so the person with more fit muscles extracts more oxygen from the inhaled air than a person with less fit muscles. The cardiovascular system responds to the demand for oxygen by building up its capacity to deliver oxygen. Researchers can measure cardiovascular fitness by measuring the amount of oxygen a person consumes per minute while working out, a measure called VO_2 max.

How physically active are you?

For each question answered yes, give yourself the number of points indicated. Then total your points to determine your score.

A. VIGOROUS PHYSICAL ACTIVITY ROUTINES

1. I participate in active recreational sports such as tennis or racquetball for an hour or more:
   a. about once a week (2 points)
   b. about twice a week (4 points)
   c. three times a week (6 points)
   d. four times a week (8 points)
   e. not at all (0 points)

2. I participate in vigorous fitness activities like aerobic dancing, roller blading, jogging, or swimming (at least 20 minutes each session):
   a. about once a week (3 points)
   b. about twice a week (6 points)
   c. three times a week (9 points)
   d. four times a week (12 points)
   e. not at all (0 points)

B. OTHER PHYSICAL ACTIVITY ROUTINES

3. At least two times a week, I work out with weights for at least 10 minutes:
   a. two sessions a week (2 points)
   b. three sessions a week (3 points)
   c. four or more sessions a week (4 points)
   d. not at all (0 points)

4. At least two times a week, I perform floor workouts (sit-ups, push-ups) for at least 10 minutes:
   a. two sessions a week (2 points)
   b. three sessions a week (3 points)
   c. four or more sessions a week (4 points)
   d. not at all (0 points)

5. At least two times a week, I participate in yoga or perform stretching exercises for at least 10 minutes:
   a. two sessions a week (2 points)
   b. three sessions a week (3 points)
   c. four or more sessions a week (4 points)
   d. not at all (0 points)

C. OCCUPATION AND DAILY ACTIVITIES

6. I walk to and from school, work, and shopping (1/2 mile or more each way), two or three times a week or more. (1 point)

7. I climb stairs rather than using elevators or escalators, every other day or more. (1 point)

8. My school, job, or household routine involves physical activity that fits the following description:
   a. Most of my day is spent in desk work or light physical activity. (0 points)
   b. Most of my day is spent in farm activities, moderate physical activity, brisk walking, or comparable activities. (4 points)
   c. My typical day includes several hours of heavy physical activity (shoveling, lifting, etc.). (2 points per day)

D. LEISURE ACTIVITIES

9. I do several hours of gardening, lawn work, or similar hobby work each week. (1 point)

10. At least once a week, I dance vigorously (folk or line dancing) for an hour or more. (1 point)

11. In season, I play 9 to 18 holes of golf at least once a week, and I do not use a power cart. (2 points)

12. I walk for physical activity or recreation:
    a. 1–2 hours a week (1 point)
    b. 3–4 hours a week (2 points)
    c. 5 hours or more a week (3 points)
    d. not at all (0 points)

13. In addition to the above, I engage in other forms of physical activity:
    a. 1–2 hours a week (1 point)
    b. 3–4 hours a week (2 points)
    c. 5 hours or more a week (3 points)

SCORING

Record your point scores here.

Category	Score
A. Vigorous physical activity routines	_____
B. Other physical activity routines	_____
C. Occupation and daily activities	_____
D. Leisure activities	_____
Total:	_____

Evaluation of total score (circle one):

- Inactive (0–5 points)
- Moderately active (6–11 points)
- Active (12–20 points)
- Very active (21 points or over)

If your score categorizes you as inactive or only moderately active, think of activities that you could realistically engage in on a regular basis to raise your score to "active" (12 points).

SOURCE: Adapted with permission from Russell Pate (University of South Carolina, Human Performance Laboratory).

FIGURE 7-2

The Use of Glycogen and Body Fat for Energy* during Physical Activity

Training can increase the amount of glycogen a muscle can conserve during exercise. The more fit a muscle is, the more fat it can burn for energy when oxygen is present—sparing the valuable glycogen.

*In order to perform physical activity, the body generates ATP (adenosine triphosphate) from the breakdown of the energy nutrients (primarily carbohydrate and fat). ATP is the "energy molecule" used by all cells of the body. ATP is composed of the compound adenosine plus three phosphate groups attached to each other by high-energy bonds. Energy is released each time a phosphate group is split off from the ATP molecule. For example, ATP converts to ADP (adenosine diphosphate) + P when a phosphate bond is broken to release energy.

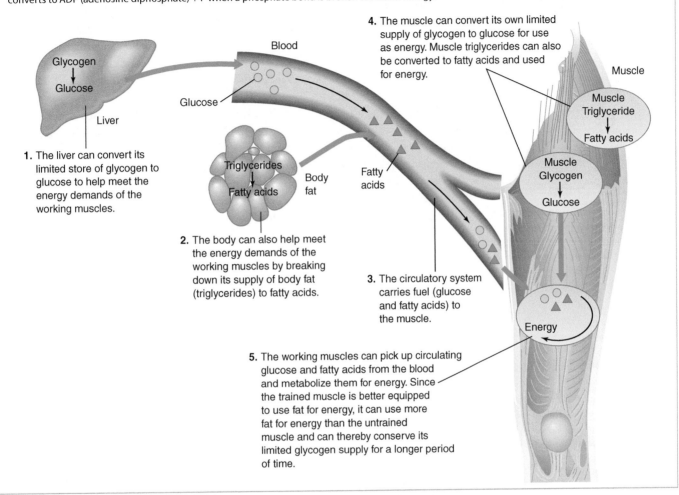

4. The muscle can convert its own limited supply of glycogen to glucose for use as energy. Muscle triglycerides can also be converted to fatty acids and used for energy.

1. The liver can convert its limited store of glycogen to glucose to help meet the energy demands of the working muscles.

2. The body can also help meet the energy demands of the working muscles by breaking down its supply of body fat (triglycerides) to fatty acids.

3. The circulatory system carries fuel (glucose and fatty acids) to the muscle.

5. The working muscles can pick up circulating glucose and fatty acids from the blood and metabolize them for energy. Since the trained muscle is better equipped to use fat for energy, it can use more fat for energy than the untrained muscle and can thereby conserve its limited glycogen supply for a longer period of time.

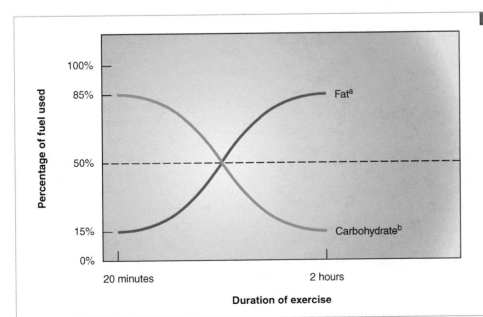

FIGURE 7-3

Fuel Use and Duration/Intensity of Physical Activity

For most people, fat isn't used much as a fuel for exercise until you've been working out aerobically for at least 20 minutes, and it is not used as a primary fuel until after 2 hours.

a The more moderate the intensity of activity (brisk walking, jogging, aerobic dancing), and the longer the duration, the greater the use of fat for fuel.
b The higher the intensity of activity (sprinting, hurdles, rowing), the greater the use of carbohydrate for fuel.

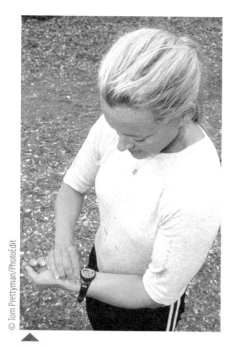

To take your pulse and monitor your heart rate during exercise, lightly press your middle and index fingers on the radial artery (on the thumb side of the wrist), as shown here. Count your pulse for 10 seconds, and then multiply by 6 to give beats per minute.

Example: Jennifer, age 25
Maximum heart rate: 220 – 25 = 195
Lower limit (55%) of target heart rate range:
0.55 × 195 = 107
Upper limit (90%) of target heart rate range:
0.90 × 195 = 176

Target heart rate range: 107 to 176 beats per minute. Therefore, when Jennifer exercises aerobically, her heart should beat at least as fast as 107 beats per minute but no faster than 176 beats per minute.

Glucose Use during Physical Activity

Glucose comes from carbohydrate-rich foods: breads, pasta, rice, legumes, fruits, vegetables, milk, and yogurt. Your body stores glucose in your liver and muscles in the form of glycogen, a long chain of glucose molecules linked together.

During physical activity, the body supplies glucose to the muscles from the stores of glycogen in the liver and in the muscles themselves. The longer the activity lasts or the more intense it is, the more glucose a person uses. Recall that activities done at an intensity that outstrips the ability of the heart and lungs to supply oxygen to working muscles relies primarily on glucose for fuel. Thus, activities such as sprinting quickly deplete the body's stores of glycogen. Other activities, such as jogging or brisk walking, in which the body can meet the muscles' oxygen demands, use glycogen more conservatively. Nonetheless, joggers and walkers still use glycogen, and eventually they can run out of it.

When a person begins exercising, for the first 20 minutes or so, about one-fifth of the body's total glycogen store is rapidly used.[11] If exercise continues beyond 20 minutes, glycogen use slows down (see Figure 7-3). To conserve the remaining glycogen supply, the body begins to rely more on fat for fuel. At some point, if exercise continues long enough, glycogen will run out almost completely. People who run out of muscle glycogen during an event (for example, before the finish line in a marathon) "hit the wall." They must slow down their pace because muscle glycogen is no longer available as fuel. Exercise can continue for a short time after that, only because the liver scrambles to produce the minimum amount of glucose needed to briefly forestall body shutdown. When blood sugars dip too low, the nervous system function comes almost to a halt, making exercise difficult, if not impossible, even though there is still plenty of fat left to burn.

Another factor that influences glycogen use during exercise is how well trained the person is. In the beginning stages of building a physical activity program, a person uses more glucose than a trained athlete. This is because their "untrained" muscles can quickly and easily extract energy from glucose. However, for muscles to easily extract energy from fat, the muscle cells must contain abundant fat-burning enzymes. With training, the muscles adapt and pack their cells with more fat-burning enzymes. Thus, trained muscles are able to use more fat and conserve their glucose.

The amount of glycogen that is present in the muscles before exercise also influences glycogen use. By following the diet prescription in Figure 7-4, athletes can provide their muscles with enough glycogen to support exercise. In low- to moderate-intensity activities (walking, bicycling, dancing), casual exercisers rarely deplete the glycogen in their stores. Carbohydrate loading—a practice that endurance athletes use to trick their muscles into storing extra glycogen—may not be beneficial for people who exercise less than 90 minutes per workout at a low intensity, although competitive athletes who exercise at a high intensity for more than 90 minutes at a time may benefit from carbohydrate loading. Muscles typically have enough glycogen to fuel 1½- to 2-hour bouts of activity.

An athlete who follows the glycogen-loading technique in preparation for an upcoming event will first exercise intensely without restricting carbohydrates and then gradually cut back on exercise the week

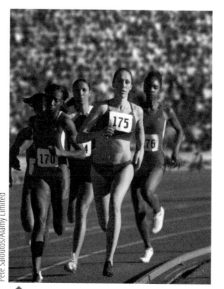

Anaerobic exercise. Glucose is the principal source of energy for activities of high intensity.

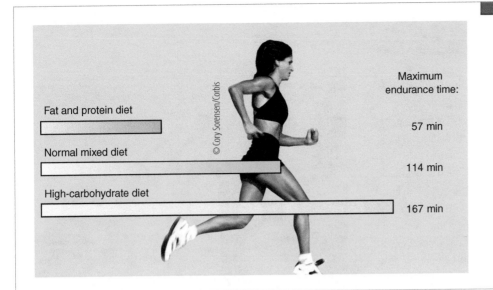

FIGURE 7-4

The Effect of Diet on Physical Endurance

A high-carbohydrate diet can increase an athlete's endurance. In this study, the fat and protein diet provided 94 percent of calories from fat and 6 percent from protein; the normal mixed diet provided 55 percent of calories from carbohydrate; and the high-carbohydrate diet provided 83 percent of calories from carbohydrate.

Maximum endurance time:

Fat and protein diet — 57 min

Normal mixed diet — 114 min

High-carbohydrate diet — 167 min

before the competition, rest completely the day before, and eat a very high-carbohydrate diet. Endurance athletes who follow this plan can keep going longer than their competitors without ill effects.[12] In a hot climate, extra glycogen offers an additional advantage. As glycogen breaks down, it releases water, which helps meet the athlete's fluid needs.

Fat Use during Physical Activity

When you exercise, the fat your muscles burn comes from the fatty deposits all over the body, especially from those with the greatest amounts of fat to spare. That is why physically fit people look trim all over: they reduce their fat stores all over the body, not just those overlaying the working muscles.

People who participate in endurance events know to build up their reserves of muscle glycogen before an event, so that they do not run out or "hit the wall" before the finish line.

A person with a desirable body weight may store 25 to 30 pounds of body fat but only about 1 pound of carbohydrate. Although your supply of fat is almost unlimited, the ability of your muscles to use fat for energy is not.

Recall that for a working muscle to burn fat, oxygen must be present. If you work out at a rate that allows your heart to supply ample oxygen to working muscles, the muscles will draw heavily on fat stores for fuel. When exercise intensity outstrips your oxygen supply, fat still contributes as much energy as ever, but glucose pitches in and is burned by the anaerobic pathway. Thus, the percentage of the total energy supplied by fat declines. Your breathing rate can signal which fuel is providing most of the energy. A rule of thumb for gauging exercise intensity for aerobic workouts is this: If you can't talk normally, you are incurring oxygen debt and are burning more glucose than fat; if you can sing, you aren't getting a cardiovascular workout or burning much of anything (so speed up).

Athletic training also controls the amount of fat used during an exercise period. Exercise training improves the body's ability to deliver fat to working muscles, and trained muscles have an increased ability to use the fat.

Much attention has been focused on the type of fuel used for varying exercise intensities and duration. Research shows that when athletes exercise at a moderate

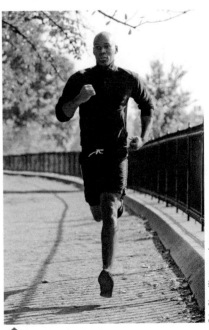

Aerobic activity. Fats are the main source of energy for activities of low to moderate intensity.

The word routine almost always accompanies *exercise plan* when the goal is to enhance health through physical activity. It should be no surprise that positive health effects cannot be realized with inconsistent physical activity. Sporadic binges of activity are of little or no benefit and often do more harm than good. But how do you find time and motivation to get fit and stay fit in today's hectic lifestyle? Many people are dying to tell you how, and they claim to have just the plan for you! Look at any late-night infomercial or shopping channel to see the many exercise gurus with videos, equipment, and supplements to allegedly keep you motivated and provide great results in a short amount of time. But just as fad diets come and go, the promised success with these gizmos and gadgets is usually unsustainable, and the equipment that works for one person may not work for another.

What's usually missing from these infomercials is the whole story. Although many products and programs promise to burn loads of fat in minimal time, they typically fail to mention that success with their product *must* be combined with a total fitness routine—which would mean that their product wasn't necessary in the first place! Don't be swayed by commercials that liberally use the phrase "scientific research." If their "scientific research" is not peer reviewed and published in a respected scientific journal, the results are most likely invalid or, at the very least, biased. Those who market these programs and products are skilled with their presentations, and their real goal is to separate you from your hard-earned money. If their product sounds too good to be true, it probably is!

Instead, pay attention to the guidelines in this text, do additional reading, consult experts, talk to your physician, and let education and common sense guide your fitness routine. Even though physical activity is not always easy, it is worthwhile and can change your life! In your physical activity program, consistency is the key, and no amount of gizmos or gadgets can replace that. Here are some tips for sustaining a physical activity program:

1. Check with your physician before starting any physical activity program or weight loss plan. Your doctor can assess your ability for a given level of activity and refer you to qualified professionals for assistance, such as physical therapists, exercise physiologists, dietitians, and/or certified personal trainers.
2. Find an exercise buddy. You can motivate each other. Use a gradual approach and set realistic goals. Don't jump out of bed tomorrow morning and expect to be able to run 10 miles.

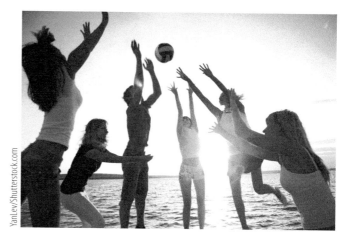

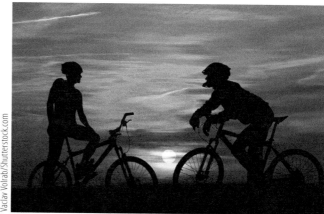

Make physical activity a habit. Choose an activity you enjoy.

Set a realistic smaller first goal and use it as motivation to set your next goal. Experiment a little to find the time that is right for you to exercise. Many people like to exercise in the morning before their day begins. If you try that and it doesn't work, don't give up. You might have more luck with a lunchtime routine or an after-work exercise schedule.

3. Don't overdo it, especially in the beginning! Listen to your body and let it set the pace while still challenging yourself. "No pain, no gain" is a myth that can be dangerous.
4. Don't focus on weight loss. Focus on your new energy level and how much better you feel as your clothes start to fit again!

intensity, they initially use more carbohydrate than fat for fuel.[13] Gradually, as exercise continues for more than 20 minutes, the fuel ratio shifts, and the athletes use more fat. For athletes participating in endurance sports, such as marathon runners and long-distance cyclists, who want to conserve their limited supply of carbohydrate, switching to a fat-burning energy system is crucial.

Protein Needs for Fitness

Fit people have more muscle than fat; exercise involves muscles; muscles are made largely of protein. It seems logical, then, that to become or stay fit, an athlete might need more protein. Although it's true that fat and glucose are the primary fuels for working muscles, 5 to 10 percent of energy needs for weight lifters and endurance-sport athletes comes from muscle protein. So, do athletes need more protein?

The athlete's body may use slightly more protein, especially during the early stages of training. Initial increases in muscle mass, numbers of red blood cells to carry oxygen, and amounts of aerobic enzymes in muscles to use fuel efficiently may elevate an athlete's protein needs. In addition, hormonal changes during exercise can temporarily slow the amount of protein the muscle makes and can encourage the muscle to break down its protein stores.[14] How much protein an athlete uses for fuel during hard exercise (endurance exercise and heavy weight lifting) depends on exercise intensity and duration, the athlete's fitness level, and the glycogen stores in the athlete's muscles. When glycogen stores are well stocked, however, protein contributes only 5 percent of fuel needs.

The important factor here is that, although muscle protein breakdown dominates during heavy exercise, muscle *growth* escalates after exercise. The muscles use the available amino acids to repair and build, and the net effect of these changes is muscle protein buildup. Consistent training enhances muscle protein buildup after exercise.

The American College of Sports Medicine recommends that endurance athletes consume 1.2 to 1.6 grams of protein per kilogram of desirable body weight.[15] Athletes who are involved in prolonged heavy resistance training may need even more protein (see Table 7-1).

Many people wonder if eating even more protein will help build muscles. Unfortunately, muscles don't respond to excess protein by simply accepting it. Instead, they respond to the hormones that regulate them and to the demands put upon them. Thus, the way to make muscle cells grow is to put a demand on them—that is, to make them work. They will respond by taking up nutrients—amino acids included—so that they can grow.

TABLE 7-1	Protein Recommendations for Athletes
	Recommendations (g/kg/day)
RDA for adults	0.8
Endurance athletes	1.2–1.4
Resistance training (bodybuilders, strength athletes)	1.2–1.7

SOURCE: Position of the American Dietetic Association, Dietitians of Canada, and the American College of Sports Medicine: Nutrition and athletic performance, *Journal of the American Dietetic Association* 109 (2009): 509–27.

Fluids and Physical Activity

The water in your blood—known as *plasma volume*, or just *plasma*—serves a function similar to the function of the water in your car's radiator. This particular function of water is critical to humans during physical activity because, as the blood continually circulates throughout your body, it picks up the tremendous amount of heat generated by your working muscles. The plasma then transports this heat to your skin, through which it is expelled from the body primarily by evaporation of sweat. You can think of sweating as your body's air-conditioning system. As sweat evaporates from your skin, it expels large amounts of heat, helping to keep your body cool. However, sweating cools your body only when the sweat evaporates from your skin. If the sweat simply rolls down your face or down your back, body heat is not released. On a humid day, for example, the air is already saturated with water, impairing the evaporation of sweat. Hot, humid days, then, are doubly dangerous because you continue to sweat and lose precious body water, but your body temperature doesn't fall.

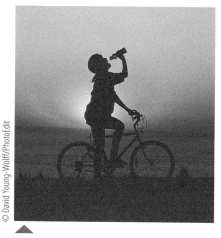

Plan to drink fluids before, during, and after exercise.

Signs of hyponatremia:

- Severe headache
- Nausea, vomiting
- Muscle cramps
- Bloating
- Confusion
- Seizure

Signs of dehydration and heat stroke include:

- Very high body temperature (104° Fahrenheit or higher)
- Hot, dry, red skin
- Sudden cessation of sweating
- Deep breathing and fast pulse
- Blurred vision
- Confusion, delirium, hallucinations
- Convulsions
- Loss of consciousness

To prevent heat stroke, drink plenty of fluid before, during, and after physical activity; avoid overexercising in hot weather; and stop exercising at any sign of heat exhaustion.

Signs of heat exhaustion include:

- Cool, clammy, pale skin
- Dizziness
- Dry mouth
- Fatigue/weakness
- Headache
- Muscle cramps
- Nausea
- Sweating
- Weak and rapid pulse

heat stroke an acute and dangerous reaction to heat buildup in the body, requiring emergency medical attention; also called sun stroke.

hyponatremia (HIGH-poe-na-TREE-mee-ah) a decreased concentration of sodium in the blood.

aerobic requiring oxygen.

anaerobic not requiring oxygen.

When exercising on humid days, it is extremely important to pay particular attention to your fluid needs.

Thus, as your body heats up because of the energy released during exercise, it loses water by sweating. How much sweat you lose depends on the intensity and duration of the activity. The more intense the activity, the more heat you generate and the more you sweat. If you don't replace this lost water, your plasma volume will decrease. In its attempt to maintain plasma volume, your body will pull water from your muscles and organs. As water is pulled from muscles, cramps may occur, along with premature fatigue and a noticeable decline in performance.

When plasma levels are low (meaning that blood volume is lower), your heart is forced to beat faster to supply sufficient oxygen to your muscles. Finally, because less plasma is circulating to transport the heat to your skin, the heat builds up, and your body's internal temperature continues to rise. All these changes force your body to work at a higher intensity, leading to early exhaustion. A water loss equal to 2 percent of body weight can reduce muscular work capacity by 20 to 30 percent.

Replenishing fluid lost during exercise is easy, yet many athletes and fitness enthusiasts either don't drink enough or don't drink at all.[16] Ignoring body fluid needs can hinder performance and increase risk of heat-related injury.[17]

The amount of fluid needed to prevent dehydration and **heat stroke** can be surprising. Athletes can lose two or more quarts of fluid during every hour of heavy exercise, and they must rehydrate *before*, *during*, and *after* exercise to replace the lost fluid. Even casual exercisers must drink some fluids while exercising. Thirst is an unreliable indicator of how much to drink: It signals too late, after fluid stores are depleted.[18] Table 7-2 presents one schedule of hydration. To know how much water is needed to replenish fluid losses after a workout, weigh yourself before and after: The difference is all water. One pound equals roughly 2 cups of fluid.

Endurance athletes need to be sure to replace both the water *and* sodium lost in heavy sweating during prolonged events (e.g., marathons) in order to avoid the dangerous condition known as **hyponatremia**. The symptoms of hyponatremia resemble dehydration to some extent and are listed in the margin.

Water and Fluid Replacement Drinks

For fitness enthusiasts, the choice between water and a sports drink is primarily a matter of personal taste and desired performance abilities. In contrast, for endurance events (continuous exercise for longer than 60 minutes), mounting evidence indicates that consuming a properly balanced sports drink during exercise will enhance energy status and endurance and help maintain plasma volume levels better than drinking water does.[19]

How the body manages water and carbohydrate use during exercise determines how well it performs. Sports drinks are designed to enhance the body's use of carbohydrate and water (see Table 7-3). The carbohydrate in a sports beverage serves three

TABLE 7-2	Schedule of Hydration Before, During, and After Exercise*
When to Drink	**Amount of Fluid**
2 hours before exercise	2–3 cups
15 minutes before exercise	1–2 cups
Every 15 minutes during exercise	½–2 cups
After exercise	2 cups fluid for each pound of body weight lost

*These guidelines are for exercise lasting less than 1 hour. During intense exercise lasting more than 1 hour, the consumption of approximately 1 liter of sports drink per hour (containing 4–8 percent carbohydrate per liter) is recommended to maintain oxidation of carbohydrates and delay fatigue.

SOURCE: American College of Sports Medicine, Position Stand, Exercise and Fluid Replacement, *Medicine & Science in Sports & Exercise* 39 (2007): 377–90.

Sports Drink	Calories/Cup	Carbohydrate Percentage	Sodium (mg)
All Sport	70	9.0	55
Gatorade Thirst Quencher	50	6.0	110
Isostar	70	8.0	150
Met-Rx	75	8.0	125
Accelerade	60	7.0	127
PowerAde	72	8.0	55

TABLE 7-3   Fluid Replacement Drinks

purposes during exercise: (1) It becomes an energy source for working muscles, (2) it helps maintain blood glucose at an optimum level, and (3) it helps increase the rate of water absorption from the small intestine, helping better maintain plasma volume. In addition, the drink can supply water and minerals lost through sweating.[20]

There are many factors to consider when choosing a sports drink. The ideal beverage should leave the digestive tract rapidly and enter circulation, where it is needed. Carbohydrate solutions don't all empty from the stomach at the same rate. The drink should contain at least 4 percent but no more than 8 percent carbohydrate by volume. Drinks containing more than 10 percent carbohydrate, such as sodas, fruit juice, Kool-Aid types of drinks, and some sports drinks, take longer to absorb. Some can cause cramps, nausea, bloating, and diarrhea. Drinks with less than 4 percent carbohydrate may not offer an endurance-enhancing effect. Drinks using a blend of glucose polymers—short chains of carbohydrate—and fructose leave the stomach at the same rate as water, speeding the availability of the carbohydrate and water to working muscles.[21]

Sodium is another important factor to consider when exercising.[22] Because most people consume enough salt in their regular diet to replace the sodium they lose during exercise, it's not essential for a fluid replacement drink to provide large amounts of sodium. In fact, too much sodium can delay muscles' receipt of water.

Research shows that about 50 milligrams of sodium per cup will help stimulate water absorption from your gut. Other studies have found that people who drink a beverage with some sodium tend to drink more of it. If the drink tastes good, athletes and exercisers will want to drink it and thereby meet their fluid needs.

For people who are exercising to lose weight, however, drinking a full quart of a sports drink may in fact simply resupply the amount of calories they expended during a 40-minute aerobic class or 30 minutes of swimming or biking. For these people, plain water is a better choice.

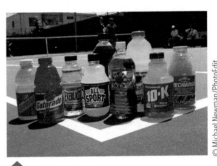

Sports drinks can enhance fluid and energy status during endurance events.

Vitamins and Minerals for Physical Activity

Your muscles burn food and oxygen to make energy. How well they burn these fuels depends, however, on your supply of vitamins and minerals. Without small amounts of these potent substances, your muscles' ability to work is compromised.

The Vitamins   Vitamins are the links and regulators of energy-producing and muscle-building pathways. Without them, your muscles' ability to convert food energy to body energy is hindered, and muscle protein formation is slowed. Table 7-4 lists a few vitamins and minerals and their exercise-supporting functions.

The B vitamins are of special interest to athletes and exercisers because they govern the energy-producing reactions of metabolism. Needs for these vitamins increase proportionally with energy expenditure. A person who expends 4,000 calories per day needs twice as much of the B vitamins as someone who expends 2,000 calories.

TABLE 7-4	Exercise-Related Functions of Vitamins and Minerals
Vitamin or Mineral	**Function**
Thiamin, riboflavin, pantothenic acid, niacin, magnesium	Energy-releasing reactions
Vitamin B_6, zinc	Building of muscle protein
Folate, vitamin B_{12}, copper	Building of red blood cells to carry oxygen
Biotin	Fat and glycogen synthesis
Vitamin C	Collagen formation for joint and other tissue integrity; antioxidant ability may reduce oxidative tissue damage
Vitamin E	Protect cell membranes from oxidative damage
Iron	Transport of oxygen in blood and in muscle tissue
Calcium, vitamin D, vitamin A, phosphorus	Building of bone structure; muscle contractions; nerve transmissions
Sodium, potassium, chloride	Maintenance of fluid balance; transmission of nerve impulses for muscle contraction
Chromium	Assistance in insulin's glucose-storage function
Magnesium	Cardiac and other muscle contraction

Note: This is just a sampling. All vitamins and minerals play indispensable roles in exercise.

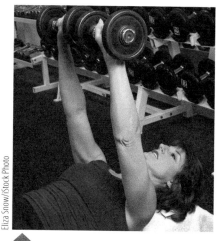

Eliza Snow/iStock Photo

Muscles grow in response to work, not to eating protein. Several vitamins regulate the muscle-building pathways.

sports anemia a temporary condition of low blood hemoglobin level, associated with the early stage of athletic training.

A well-balanced diet that meets athletes' energy needs and that features complex carbohydrate-rich foods will ensure B vitamin intakes proportional to energy intake.

Researchers are presently studying the protective effects of antioxidants on recovery from exercise and performance. Because the body uses oxygen at a higher rate during exercise, the generation of free radicals and the potential for exercise-induced tissue damage increase in the body. Although more research is needed, preliminary studies support a role for the antioxidant nutrients, which may enhance recovery from exercise by reducing exercise-induced oxidative injury.[23] Meeting the recommendation of eating five or more fruits and vegetables per day will help athletes meet recommended intakes for the antioxidant nutrients.

The Minerals   Iron is a core component of the body's oxygen taxi service: hemoglobin and myoglobin. A lack of oxygen compromises the muscles' ability to perform. Iron deficiency has not been reported as a problem for fitness enthusiasts who exercise moderately.[24] Male and female endurance athletes, though, may be prone to developing mild iron deficiency, diagnosed by low blood ferritin levels (a measure of the body's store of iron). Menstruating female athletes are at particular risk: growth and menstruation combined with strenuous training can take a toll on a woman's iron stores.[25]

A combination of factors increases an athlete's chances of depleting his or her iron stores. Inadequate dietary intakes of iron-rich foods combined with iron losses due to physical activity can compromise iron status. Physical activity may cause increased iron losses in sweat, feces, and urine, plus increased destruction of red blood cells that occurs during exercise. (Chapter 8 contains numerous suggestions for obtaining sufficient iron from foods.)

Sometimes iron deficiencies can be corrected only with iron supplements. If you are concerned about your iron level, see a physician. Iron supplements should not be taken without medical supervision. High iron intakes can induce deficiencies of trace minerals, such as copper and zinc, and can produce an iron overload in some people.

An apparent anemia—sometimes called **sports anemia**—also can occur in athletes. This condition does not reflect a reduction in the blood's iron supply, but rather indicates an increase in the blood plasma volume.[26] This occurs because athletic training causes the kidneys to conserve sodium and water. In other words, the extra blood volume dilutes the concentration of iron, thereby making it seem as if the blood does not contain enough of the mineral. Sports anemia is considered a temporary state and probably reflects a normal adaptation to physical training.

The Bones and Exercise　　Bones absorb great stresses during exercise, and like the muscles, they respond by growing thicker and stronger. Weight-bearing activities—running, walking, dancing, rope skipping, or activities such as strength training in which significant muscular force can be generated against the long bones of the body—encourage bone development. A bone that is not strong enough to withstand the strain of an athletic exertion can break, causing what has become known as a **stress fracture**. When a person suffers such a break, there are three probable causes. The first is unbalanced muscle development, which allows strong muscles to pull against the bone opposed only by weaker, undeveloped muscles, thereby leaving the bone susceptible to fractures. The second cause of stress fractures is bone weakness caused by inadequate calcium intake. A possible third cause, which occurs in women who have ceased menstruating, is when reduced estrogen concentration leads to bone mineral loss and therefore to fragile bones.

Balanced muscle development can protect the bones from undue stresses. Each set of muscles pulling against bone should be kept in check by an equally strong set of opposing muscles. Thus, when you work one set of muscles in training, you should also work the opposing muscles. For example, if you work your back and leg muscles (by jogging or walking, for example), also work your abdominal muscles, too (do sit-ups). Bones, like muscles, take time to develop strength. To avoid the likelihood of stress fractures, give your bones and muscles plenty of time to build up to one level of performance before moving up to the next level. Maintaining adequate calcium intake throughout life may be one of the primary defenses against developing weak bones.

Some women who exercise strenuously cease to menstruate, a condition called **amenorrhea**. Such women have lower than normal amounts of estrogen, a hormone essential for maintaining the integrity of the bones. With low estrogen levels, the mineral structures of the bones are rapidly dismantled, weakening the skeleton. Women who have athletic amenorrhea are at risk for stress fractures now and adult bone loss later in life.[27] To reverse the condition, they should not stop exercising altogether, because reasonable amounts of exercise may be a key defense against bone depletion. They should, however, seek evaluation from a health care provider who specializes in sports medicine to find the cause of and receive treatment for their amenorrhea.

Eating disorders are sometimes related to athletic amenorrhea, and a logical part of diagnosis is to look carefully at the woman's diet. It could be that a diet too low in calories, coupled with low body fat stores and strenuous activity, sets the stage for amenorrhea to develop. In such cases, calcium intakes between 1,000 and 1,300 milligrams per day may help protect the bones.

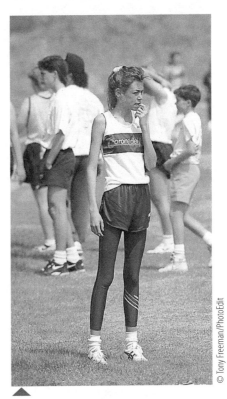

The condition characterized by the potentially fatal combination of disordered eating, amenorrhea, and low bone density is referred to as the female athlete triad.

stress fracture bone damage or breakage caused by stress on bone surfaces during exercise.

amenorrhea cessation of menstruation associated with strenuous athletic training.

The best nutrition prescription for peak performance is a well-balanced diet. Although no eating plan meets every athlete's needs, certain components are common to all well-balanced diets. The athlete's diet should account for increased energy needs, vitamin and mineral needs, the relative efficiency of various foods as fuels, and current knowledge about long-term health. An eating plan that supplies 60 percent of calories from complex carbohydrate, 15 percent of calories from protein, and 25 percent of calories from fat supplies a proper fuel mix to the muscles of athletes and fitness enthusiasts and will also maintain health.[28] Two critical nutrition periods for the athlete are the training diet and the pre-competition diet.

Planning the Diet

- A diet rich in complex carbohydrate and low in fat provides the best balance of nutrients for health and also the best support for physical activity. The following table shows some sample balanced eating plans for athletes who wish to increase their carbohydrate intake along with their calories.

- Choose foods to provide nutrients as well as calories—extra milk for calcium and riboflavin, many vegetables for B vitamins, meat or alternates for iron and other vitamins and minerals, and whole grains for magnesium and chromium. The photos on page 155 show examples of high-carbohydrate meals for the athlete.

- An athlete may be able to eat more food by consuming it in six or eight meals each day rather than in three or four meals. Large snacks of milkshakes, dried fruits, peanut butter sandwiches, or cheese and crackers can add substantial calories and nutrients.

The Pre-Game Meal

- The best choices for the meal before a competitive event are foods that are high in carbohydrate and low in fat, protein, and fiber. Fat and protein slow the stomach's emptying, and the waste products generated during protein metabolism require that too much water be excreted with them.

- Fiber intake is not desirable immediately before physical exertion, because it stays in the digestive tract too long and draws water out of the blood.

- A high-carbohydrate meal supports blood glucose levels during competition. Olympic training tables are laden with foods such as breads, whole-grain cereals, pasta, rice, potatoes, and fruit juices.

- For pre-game meals and snacks, choose foods such as grape juice, apricot nectar, pineapple juice, Jell-O, sherbet, popsicles, raisins, apricots, figs, dates, jams and toast, pancakes with syrup, honey, pasta, baked white or sweet potatoes, steamed vegetables, low-fat frozen yogurt, angel food or sponge cake with fresh fruit, and graham crackers.

- Stay away from higher-fat foods such as meats, cheese, nuts, gravies, cream, French fries, muffins, croissants, biscuits, butter, potato chips, pies, and ice cream.

- Include plenty of fluids—two or more 8-ounce glasses of water or juice per meal—to ensure adequate hydration.

- Any meal should be finished at least 2 to 4 hours before the event, because digestion requires routing the blood supply to the digestive tract to pick up nutrients. By the time the contest begins, the circulating blood should be freed from that task and, instead, should be available for carrying oxygen and fuel to the muscles.

High-Carbohydrate Eating Patterns for Various Energy Levels

Use the number of servings indicated to arrive at the specified energy levels.[a]

Food Group	Calorie Level					
	1,500	2,000	2,500	3,000	3,500	4,000
Dairy	3	3	4	4	4	4
Fruits	5	6	7	9	10	12
Vegetables	3	3	3	5	6	7
Grains	7	11	16	18	20	24
Oils[b]	2	3	5	6	8	10
Protein Foods[c]	5	5	5	5	6	6
Percentage of carbohydrate	58	58	63	64	60	62

[a] Refer to Table 2-6 in Chapter 2 for serving sizes.
[b] A serving of fat is equivalent to 1 tsp butter, margarine, or oil.
[c] Meat servings are given as total ounces of meat; a typical serving includes 2 to 3 ounces.

Sample Meals for High-Carbohydrate Intakes for the Exercise Enthusiast at Two Calorie Levels

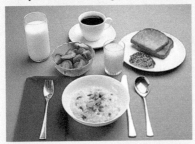

Breakfast
1 c coffee
8 oz low-fat milk
2 pieces whole-wheat
  toast
4 tsp jelly
½ c strawberries
½ c orange juice
1 c oatmeal and raisins
  with 2 tsp brown
  sugar

Breakfast
1 c coffee
½ c strawberries
8 oz nonfat milk
1 c oatmeal and raisins

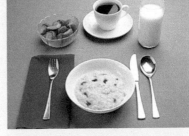

Morning Snack
4 tsp trail mix

Morning Snack
4 tsp trail mix

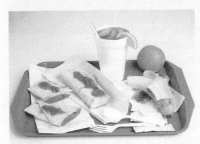

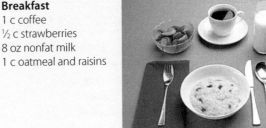

Lunch
12 oz iced tea with
  sugar
1 orange
1 banana
2 beef and bean
  burritos

Lunch
12 oz iced tea with
  sugar
1 orange
1 beef and bean burrito

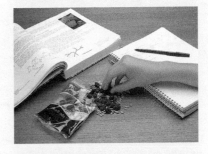

Afternoon Snack
A smoothie made from
  12 oz nonfat milk,
  1 frozen banana
1 apple
4 rye wafers with 1 oz
  low-fat cheese

Dinner
½ c sherbet
1 c spinach salad with
  1 tbsp dressing
8 oz nonfat milk
¼ tomato
1 c broccoli
½ c noodles with pars-
  ley and 2 tsp butter
4 oz salmon

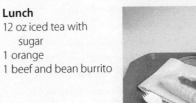

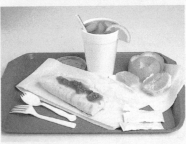

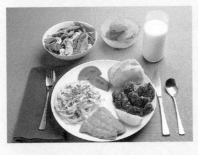

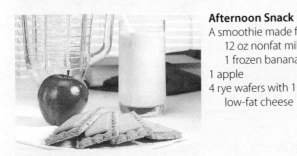

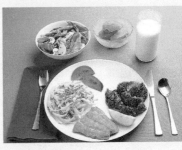

Dinner
8 oz low-fat milk
1 c sherbet
1 c spinach salad with
  1 tbsp dressing
1 dinner roll with 2 tsp
  butter
¼ tomato
1 c broccoli
4 oz salmon
¾ c noodles with pars-
  ley and 2 tsp butter

All © Felicia Martinez/PhotoEdit

Total Calories: 3,119
61% cal from carbohydrates, 24% cal from fat, 15% cal from protein

Total Calories: 1,759
57% cal from carbohydrates, 24% cal from fat, 19% cal from protein

Competitors in the ancient Greek Olympiad reportedly used mushrooms and herbs.[29] Since then, virtually every food has at one time or another been touted as the "magic bullet" that will enhance performance. Athletes have been known to swallow everything from bee pollen to brewer's yeast to kelp to wheat germ in their quest to gain the competitive edge. Although the idea of using pills and potions to achieve peak performance (to run faster or jump higher) may be seductive, scientific evidence supporting such claims is sorely lacking.[30]

Can nutritional supplements enhance the benefits I achieve from my everyday workouts?

Most so-called **ergogenic aids**—that is, substances that increase the ability to exercise harder—are costly versions of vitamins, minerals, sugar, and other substances that can be provided easily by a balanced diet.[31] Table 7-5 describes some of the many substances currently promoted as ergogenic aids.

For example, bee pollen is simply a mixture of protein, carbohydrate, a bit of fat, and a few vitamins and minerals.[32] Though touted by one manufacturer as a "natural and balanced source of extra energy" appreciated by "athletes worldwide," it has been tested at Louisiana State University among both runners and swimmers and found to confer no benefit whatsoever on an athlete's training or performance abilities.[33] The same goes for chromium picolinate, promoted by some to increase lean body mass and delay fatigue due to its role in glucose utilization. Although chromium is necessary for muscle function by transferring glucose from the blood to the muscle cells, true chromium deficiencies are rare to nonexistent. To date, there is no evidence that chromium supplements improve athletic performance in healthy individuals who do not have a chromium deficiency.[34]

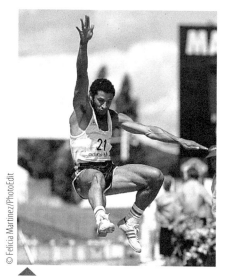

Athletes rank as prime targets of amino acid supplement manufacturers, whose products promote false hopes.

Surveys have found that more than 50 percent of athletes use a vitamin or mineral supplement, although no evidence exists that doing so improves performance.[35] More than 40 years of research has provided no strong evidence that popping vitamins and minerals increases energy or athletic prowess of adequately nourished people. Except for iron, vitamin and mineral deficiencies are rare among athletes. Because most athletes eat more food than nonathletes eat to meet their increased energy demands, the extra food intake usually provides the additional vitamins, minerals, and other beneficial substances they need, if they choose a well-balanced diet.

Of course, when athletes firmly hold that one or another ergogenic aid does indeed improve performance, convincing them otherwise can be extremely difficult. One reason for this is their profound belief that a particular substance can actually produce a psychological benefit. This phenomenon is known as the **placebo effect**.

I see many claims about amino acids and athletic ability. Can I improve my performance by using amino acid supplements?

Athletes rank as prime targets for amino acid supplement manufacturers. Pick up any copy of one of the bodybuilding magazines, and you'll probably see ads for supplements packed with "free-form," "predigested," and "peptide-bond" amino acids touted as optimum sources of protein for athletes. Scientific-sounding names notwithstanding, such products have never been proven to increase muscle size or enhance athletic prowess. Consider that one comparison of U.S. Marine officer candidates given protein supplements with another set of trainees who received a placebo indicated that the groups performed equally well before, during, and after the program.[36] (Refer to the Spotlight feature in Chapter 1 for some tips on how to spot fraudulent nutritional products.)

An additional important fact is that your body can't store extra amino acids, whether they come from food you eat or from supplements. Your body converts the excess into fat. This conversion generates urea, which increases your body's need for water. Increased urination of urea can lead to dehydration, which impedes training and performance.

What risks are associated with amino acid supplements?

The FDA recently asked a panel of experts to review the safety of amino acids currently available in the marketplace. The panel's conclusions underscore the need for better regulation of these supplements. For instance, the panel found that the labels of most amino acid supplements failed to carry vital information such as suggested doses, shelf life, and contraindications for use of the product. In addition, the panel identified certain groups of people who may be at particularly high risk for suffering health problems as a result of swallowing amino acid supplements. Children and teenagers, for example, may not grow properly if they take amino acid pills or powders. That's because young, underdeveloped

TABLE 7-5   A Sampling of Popular Ergogenic Aids[a,b]

Ergogenic Aids with Unproven Claims

Amino acids (for example, arginine, ornithine, glycine) nonessential amino acids falsely promoted to increase muscle mass and strength by stimulating growth hormone and insulin. Individual amino acids do not significantly increase muscle mass or growth hormone. Weight lifting and endurance training do.

Anabolic steroids synthetic male hormones (related to testosterone) that stimulate growth of body tissues, with many adverse effects (see the footnote on page 158).

Bee pollen mixture of bee saliva, plant nectar, and pollen touted falsely to enhance athletic performance. May cause allergic reactions in people with sensitivity to bee stings and honey allergies.

Carnitine a compound synthesized in the body from two amino acids (lysine and methionine) and required in fat metabolism. Falsely claimed to increase the use of fatty acids and spare glycogen during exercise, delay fatigue, and decrease body fat. The body produces sufficient amounts on its own. No evidence that supplementation in healthy people improves energy or enhances fat loss.

Chromium picolinate Chromium is an essential component of the glucose tolerance factor, which facilitates the action of insulin in the body. Picolinate is a natural derivative of the amino acid tryptophan. Falsely promoted to increase muscle mass, decrease body fat, enhance energy, and promote weight loss. Choose instead a diet rich in whole, unprocessed foods.

Coenzyme Q10 a lipid made by the body and used by cells in energy metabolism; falsely touted to increase exercise performance and stamina in athletes; potential antioxidant role. May increase oxygen use and stamina in patients with heart disease, but no significant effect is seen in healthy athletes.

DHEA (dehydroepiandrosterone) a precursor of the hormones testosterone and estrogen; falsely promoted to increase production of testosterone, build muscle, burn fat, and delay the effects of aging. Long-term effects unknown; self-supplementation not recommended.

Ginseng a collective term used to describe several species of plants, belonging to the genus Panax, that contain bioactive compounds in their roots. Falsely touted to enhance exercise endurance and boost energy. There is a lack of well-controlled research; what little has been done has yielded inconclusive evidence for the benefits of ginseng. The potential for adverse drug–herb or herb–herb interactions with ginseng exists.[a]

Pyruvate a three-carbon compound derived from the breakdown of glucose for energy in the body. Falsely promoted to increase fat burning and endurance. Side effects include intestinal gas and diarrhea, which could interfere with performance.

Ergogenic Aids with Some (Not All) Scientific Support for Claims

Creatine A nitrogen-containing substance made by the body that combines with phosphate to form the high-energy compound creatine phosphate (CP). CP is stored and used by muscle for ATP production. Some (not all) studies show that creatine may increase CP content in muscles and improve short-term (< 30 seconds) strenuous exercise performance (for instance, sprinting, weight lifting). Long-term effects are unknown.

Caffeine a stimulant that increases blood levels of epinephrine. Caffeine is promoted for improved endurance and utilization of fatty acids during exercise. Consuming 2 to 3 cups of coffee (equal to 3 to 6 milligrams of caffeine per kilogram body weight) 1 hour before exercise may improve endurance performance. High caffeine consumption may cause dehydration, headache, nausea, muscle tremors, and fast heart rate.

HMB (beta-hydroxy-beta-methylbutyrate) a metabolite of the branched-chain amino acid leucine that is promoted to increase muscle mass and strength by preventing muscle damage or speeding up muscle repair during resistance training. More research on long-term safety and effectiveness is needed.

Phosphate salt a salt with claims for improved endurance. Found to increase a substance in red blood cells (diphosphoglycerate) and enhance the cell's ability to deliver oxygen to muscle cells and reduce levels of disabling lactic acid in elite athletes. However, more research on safety and efficacy of phosphate loading is needed. Excess can cause loss of bone calcium.

Sodium bicarbonate baking soda is touted to buffer lactic acid in the body and thereby reduce pain and improve maximal-level anaerobic performance. High sodium load may cause diarrhea in users. Effects of repeated ingestion are unknown.

(Continued)

[a] See also Table 7-16 in Chapter 7 for information on herbal supplements.
[b] For more information, see M. Dunford and M. Smith, Dietary supplements and ergogenic aids, in M. Dunford (ed.), *Sports Nutrition: A Practice Manual for Professionals*, 4th ed. (Chicago: American Dietetic Association, 2006), pp. 116–41; S. A. Sarubin, *The Health Professional's Guide to Popular Dietary Supplements*, 3rd ed. (Chicago: American Dietetic Association, 2006).

bodies may metabolize amino acids differently than adult bodies, possibly leaving young people more vulnerable to harmful effects of excess amino acids.

The panel also found that much of the advertising and product label information about the effectiveness of amino acid supplements is based on anecdotes rather than grounded in careful, scientific research. In fact, the lack of data to support the usefulness of many amino acid supplements has been a concern for years.

Health risks aside, consumers should also note that special protein supplements are typically very expensive. Foods, in contrast, supply ample amounts of protein at a fraction of the cost. One glass of milk, a serving of rice and beans, or a 3-ounce portion of chicken, for example, provides a generous helping of all nine essential amino acids for less than half the price of a dose of most amino acid tablets, liquids, or powders.

What about arginine and other amino acid products advertised for weight control? Do these products work?

Arginine is an amino acid that has been promoted as "causing weight loss overnight" by stimulating secretion of a substance called *human growth hormone*, which in turn supposedly promotes weight loss. Although it's true that arginine can prompt the release of the hormone, it does so only when people take whopping doses that are unlikely to be found in supplements. Furthermore, even if a person were to take enough arginine to prompt a surge of the hormone in the body, he or she wouldn't automatically shed pounds. Human growth hormone has not been found to cause weight loss. Thus, claims that arginine "burns fat" are spurious at best. An FDA advisory panel on over-the-counter weight loss products investigated arginine along with 11 other amino acids touted as diet aids—cystine, histidine, isoleucine, leucine, L-lysine, methionine, phenylalanine, threonine, tryptophan, tyrosine, and valine—and found no basis for the claims about the effectiveness of any of these products in controlling weight.

Can anabolic steroids help me increase the size and strength of my muscles?

Psychological impact aside, pill popping may be harmful in some cases. Swallowing supplements known as **anabolic steroids**—synthetic hormones that appear to help build muscle—can be dangerous.

A popular practice particularly among weight lifters and bodybuilders, steroid abuse often begins around the age of 18 years.[37] Although steroids may help increase muscular size and strength in some people, they can also bring about numerous side effects, including acne, liver abnormalities, temporary infertility, and offensive outbursts often referred to as "roid rages."*

*Side effects of steroids include acne, anxiety, blood clots, blood poisoning, cancer, diarrhea, dizziness, fatigue, heart disease, hypertension, irreversible baldness in women, jaundice, kidney damage, liver damage, male pattern baldness, mood swings, nausea, oily skin, prostate enlargement, psychotic depression, shrunken testicles, sterility (reversible), stroke, stunted growth in adolescents, swelling of feet or lower legs, and yellowing of the eyes or skin.

Among adults, many effects of steroid use are reversible. Unfortunately, adolescents aren't so lucky. Several studies show that adolescent steroid users may suffer the serious consequences of premature skeletal maturation, decreased spermatogenesis, and elevated risk of injury.[38]

Along with being unhealthful, steroid use is considered unethical by domestic and international sports organizations such as the American College of Sports Medicine and the International Olympic Committee. As a case in point, track star Ben Johnson lost his Olympic gold medal for the 100-meter sprint in 1988 after officials discovered he had been using steroids.[39]

What about energy drinks? They seem perfect for athletic performance!

Carbohydrates, vitamins, minerals, and hydration all in one bottle . . . sounds too good to be true! Well, for the athlete who uses "energy drinks" for an extra edge, it probably is.[40] For the past 10 years, energy drinks have increased in variety and market share of beverage sales across the United States. Their formulation of high amounts of caffeine, simple carbohydrates, and mixtures of vitamins and minerals has caused many people to use them as a "pick me up" to get through their day. In particular, manufacturers target athletes because of their desire to gain an advantage over the competition. Unfortunately, however, energy drinks are not properly formulated to increase athletic performance.

Caffeine Thought of as the central ingredient in almost all "energy drinks," caffeine is a central nervous system stimulant that has been shown to increase athletic ability slightly when consumed in moderate amounts. However, higher doses are considered "doping" in most athletic organizations, and they cause unwanted side effects such as light-headedness and twitchiness, along with laxative and diuretic effects. Even though energy drinks do not all have exactly the same ingredients, nearly all contain high concentrations of caffeine.[41]

Carbohydrates Although carbohydrates are the preferred source of fuel for athletes, high levels of carbohydrates in an energy drink pose undesirable side effects. One problem is that absorption of water is slowed considerably, putting the athlete's hydration status at risk. Furthermore, like caffeine, simple carbohydrate ingestion immediately before physical exertion might cause gastrointestinal distress and create a laxative effect.

Vitamins and minerals There is little chance that an athlete who consumes a normal diet will be at risk for vitamin or mineral deficiency. Accordingly, adding nutrients to beverages has never been proven to markedly increase athletic performance. A daily multivitamin and a balanced diet are far less costly than relying on fortified energy drinks as a source of vitamins and minerals.

Other ingredients It is important to realize that these drinks sometimes include additional ingredients such as amino acids and herbal supplements. Even though they may be catchy items to list on the label, few, if any, have been proven to increase athletic performance. In fact, herbal ingredients may increase the risk of serious drug–nutrient interactions if the athlete is also taking medication.[42]

What questions should I ask if I'm considering consuming energy drinks?[43]

- Does the drink contain herbal ingredients that will affect a medication I am currently taking?
- Does any research back up the claimed or proposed benefits of this beverage?
- Does the beverage label include a Nutrition Facts panel? If not, avoid this product!
- Can I do anything else to positively affect my energy level when training? (For example, am I eating a balanced diet, getting enough rest and hydration, and training for the proper length of time?)
- Is the cost of the product really worth what I am getting?
- How high is the caffeine level? Will it cause me to fail a doping test?

Some athletes use caffeine or alcohol instead of popping pills to promote athletic prowess. Can these substances improve my athletic performance?

Many exercisers drink caffeine-containing beverages such as coffee, tea, or cola to enhance performance and endurance. Caffeine apparently stimulates the release of fats into the blood that the body can then use instead of glycogen as a source of energy. Thus, the glycogen is "spared," or saved, for later use, and the amount of time an exerciser can endure physical activity before running out of fuel is prolonged.

The glycogen-sparing effect of caffeine, however, is beneficial only for athletes who exercise for more than 1½ to 2 hours at a time. As noted earlier, the muscles generally store enough glycogen to fuel as much as 90 minutes of activity. Moreover, even endurance athletes can experience certain downsides to consuming caffeine. Because caffeine is a diuretic, it promotes frequent urination and fluid loss that can lead to dehydration. In addition, caffeine can induce rapid heart rate and jitters, which can interfere with performance. Athletes would also do well to remember that caffeine is a drug that neither the American College of Sports Medicine nor the International Olympic Committee condones for use among athletes.

Along with caffeinated beverages, alcoholic drinks are often touted as choice fluids for athletes. Beer, for example, is sometimes portrayed as the perfect carbohydrate-containing complement to both before- and after-competition meals. Despite such images, alcoholic drinks rank as poor sources of fluid and energy, for several reasons. For one, alcohol is a diuretic that can bring about fluid loss and dehydration. More importantly, the amount of alcohol in just one beer or glass of wine depresses the nervous system, thereby slowing an athlete's reaction time and interfering with reflexes and coordination. Also, one can of beer provides only 50 carbohydrate calories. The rest of the calories come from alcohol, which must be metabolized by your liver, not your muscles. The American College

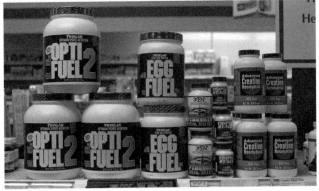

An endless array of ergogenic aids are marketed to athletes and other sports enthusiasts. Although big on claims, few are based on scientific evidence.

of Sports Medicine and the American Dietetic Association both conclude that use of alcohol hinders performance. (Chapter 9 presents a detailed explanation of how alcohol affects the body.)

The special supplements discussed here are just a sampling of the many "magic" pills and potions promoted to athletes. A nutritious diet and regular physical activity enhance performance far better than these products that are supposed to help you gain the competitive edge. If you're in doubt about a particular product you see touted as an ergogenic aid, ask yourself some of the following questions:

1. Is the promised action of the product based on magical thinking? ("Develop a trim body with no exercise.")
2. Does the promotion claim that "doctors agree" or "research has determined," without clarification? (Which doctors? What research?)
3. Does the promoter use scare tactics to pressure you into buying the product? ("It's the only one available without poisons.")
4. Is the product advertised as having a multitude of different beneficial effects? ("Makes bigger muscles; gives that pumped-up feeling; improves digestion, coordination, and breathing.")
5. Is the product available only from the sponsor by mail order and with payment in advance?
6. Does the promoter use many case histories or testimonials from grateful users?

Every yes answer is a point against the claimant—a warning signal that you are dealing with misinformation. Three or more points is a sure sign of quackery.

Miniglossary

ergogenic aids anything that helps increase the capacity to work or exercise (ergo = work; genic = give rise to).

placebo effect an improvement in a person's sense of well-being or physical health in response to the use of a placebo (a substance having no medicinal properties or medicinal effects).

anabolic steroids synthetic male hormones with a chemical structure similar to that of cholesterol; such hormones have wide-ranging effects on body functioning.

Nutrition on the Web

www.cengage.com/nutrition/boyle/personalnutrition8e
Go to the site to check for the latest updates to chapter topics or to access links to related websites.

www.nal.usda.gov/fnic
The Food and Nutrition Information Center (FNIC) provides credible and accurate information. Under Browse by Subject:

- Select Lifecycle Nutrition, scroll down, and click on Fitness, Sports and Sports Nutrition.
- Select Dietary Supplements, scroll down, and click on Ergogenic Aids.

www.cdc.gov/nccdphp/sgr/sgr.htm
The Centers for Disease Control website contains the Surgeon General's Report on Physical Activity and Health and other links related to health and physical activity.

www.fitness.gov
The President's Council on Fitness, Sports, and Nutrition website contains information about healthy eating, fitness, physical activity, and sports.

www.smallstep.gov
Select the Get Active tab at this government website to access practical fitness resources including an interactive activity tracker.

www.sportsci.org
This website for *Sportscience* allows access to information about sport research.

www.acsm.org
Click on the News tab to access research and publications from the American College of Sports Medicine (ACSM) website.

www.shapeup.org/fitness
This website provides practical advice on fitness and nutrition.

www.cdc.gov/nccdphp/dnpa
The Centers for Disease Control (CDC) website contains information on topics pertaining to fitness.

www.nhlbi.nih.gov/health/public/heart/obesity/lose_wt/index.htm
The National Heart Lung and Blood Institute website provides Aim for a Healthy Weight.

www.gssiweb.com
The Gatorade Sports Science Institute provides updates on exercise science, dietary supplements, sports drinks, and eating disorders in athletes.

www.ods.od.nih.gov/Health_Information/IBIDS.aspx
Search the International Bibliographic Information on Dietary Supplements (IBIDS) database for individual ingredients found in ergogenic aids.

www.ncahf.org
The National Council Against Health Fraud website offers current information on ergogenic aids and nutrition fads.

www.fda.gov/ForConsumers/ConsumerUpdates/ucm244206.htm
The Food and Drug Administration website provides resources to protect against health fraud.

www.mayoclinic.com
The Mayo Clinic maintains this website, and it provides a variety of health information. Click on the Healthy Living tab and then select Fitness.

www.acefitness.org
The American Council on Exercise provides fact sheets, an online newsletter, and an information resource center.

www.kidshealth.org
This website provides information about nutrition and fitness for children and teens. Choose the Parents Site (for Parents) and then click on the Nutrition and Fitness link.

Diet Analysis+ in Action

Go to the Track Activity portion of your Diet Analysis+ profile. If you haven't already done so, fill in at least one day's activity. Now go to the Energy Balance report for the day on which you tracked your actual activity. Did you consume more, fewer, or the same number of calories as you burned? If you want to burn more calories, look at the Scorecard activity in this chapter (you will find it on p. 144) for ideas about various types of activities. Choose one of those activities and include it in your activity profile for a second day of tracking. Look again at the Energy Balance report to see how your calorie intake matched up with your calorie expenditure. After doing this exercise, what changes might you make in your weekly activity to expend more calories? What changes would you have to make in your schedule to accommodate this level of activity?

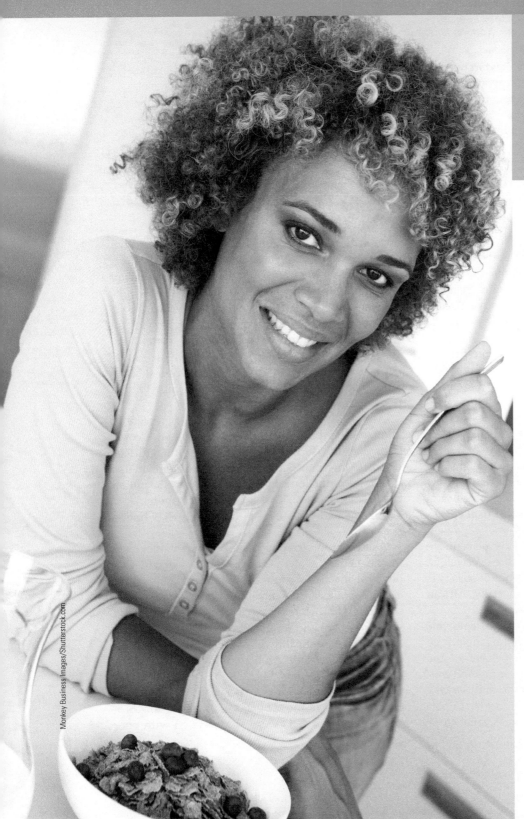

Weight Management

"Physical activity is the cornerstone of a sound weight management program. Thus, if you are unwilling to increase daily physical activity, do not attempt to lose weight because most likely you won't be able to keep it off."

Objectives

▶ **Recognize** myths and fallacies regarding weight management.

▶ **Understand** the physiology of weight control.

▶ **Become** familiar with the effects of diet and exercise on resting metabolic rate.

▶ **Recognize** the role of a lifetime exercise program in a successful weight management program.

▶ **Learn** to write and implement weight reduction and weight maintenance programs.

▶ **Identify** behavior modification techniques that help a person adhere to a lifetime weight maintenance program.

CENGAGE brain.com

Visit **www.cengagebrain.com** to access course materials and companion resources for this text including quiz questions designed to check your understanding of the chapter contents, activities, labs, and more! See the preface on page xiii for more information.

Real Life Story | Megan's Weight Struggles

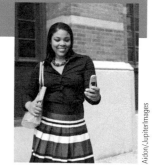

Similar to most students, I gained several pounds of weight my first year in college. I dieted several times but ended up regaining the weight, and then some more! I put off taking my fitness class because I wanted to lose the weight first and get in shape before I took the class. My roommate, however, took the class the spring semester and I couldn't help but notice how she had lost weight and looked so much better. After finding out more details about the course, I made an appointment with the course instructor and decided to enroll during the fall semester. That fall, we assessed my body composition and determined that I had 9 pounds to lose to get to 138 pounds and be at 23 percent body fat. With the aid of the instructor, we agreed on a 1,500-calorie diet, along with 45 minutes of walking/jogging five times per week

and 45 minutes of strength training twice per week. I also had to report every Monday morning to my instructor for a weigh-in and to turn in my weekly food and activity logs. I signed a contract with the instructor that I would adhere to the program as prescribed. I also talked to my roommates so they would understand what my goal was for the next 15 weeks. At the end of the semester, I had lost 10 pounds but actually came in at 22.7 percent body fat at 140 pounds. In essence, because of all my physical activity I had gained about 3 pounds of lean tissue along with 12 pounds of actual fat loss.

A good physical fitness program will include achieving and maintaining recommended body weight as a major objective. Two terms commonly used in reference to the condition of weighing more than recommended are **overweight** and **obesity**. Obesity levels are established at a point at which excess body fat can lead to significant health problems.

Obesity is a health hazard of epidemic proportions in most developed countries around the world. According to the World Health Organization, an estimated 35 percent of the adult population in industrialized nations is obese. Obesity has been established at a body mass index (BMI) of 30 or higher.

The number of people who are overweight and obese in the United States has increased dramatically in the past two decades, a direct result of physical inactivity and poor dietary habits. More than 68 percent of U.S. adults age 20 and older are overweight (have a BMI greater than 25), and 34 percent are obese.[1] More than 120 million people are overweight, and 30 million are obese. The prevalence of obesity is even higher in ethnic groups, especially African Americans and Hispanic Americans.

As illustrated in Figure 8.1, the obesity epidemic continues to escalate. Before 1990, not a single state reported an obesity rate above 15 percent of the state's total population (includes both adults and children). By the year 2009, only Colorado and the District of Columbia had an obesity rate below 20 percent, and 33 states had an obesity rate equal to or

greater than 25 percent, including nine states with a rate above 30 percent.

In the past decade alone, the average weight of American adults increased by about 15 pounds. Further, as the nation continues to evolve into a more mechanized and automated society (relying on escalators, elevators, remote controls, computers, electronic mail, cell phones, and automatic-sensor doors), the amount of required daily physical activity continues to decrease. We are being lulled into a high-risk sedentary lifestyle.

About 44 percent of all women and 29 percent of all men are on a diet at any given moment. People spend about $40 billion yearly attempting to lose weight. More than $10 billion goes to memberships in weight reduction centers and another $30 billion to diet food sales. The total cost attributable to obesity-related disease is approximately $117 billion per year.

As the second leading cause of preventable death in the United States, excessive body weight and physical inactivity cause more than 112,000 deaths each year.[2] Obesity is currently more prevalent than smoking (19 percent), poverty (14 percent), and problem drinking (6 percent).[3] Obesity, cigarette smoking, and unhealthy lifestyle habits are the most critical public health problems that we face in the 21st century.

The American Heart Association has identified obesity as one of the six major risk factors for coronary heart disease. Obesity is associated with poor

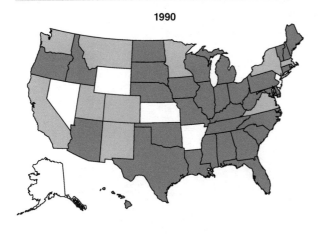

1990

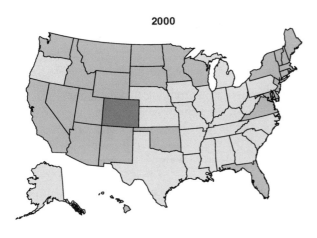

2000

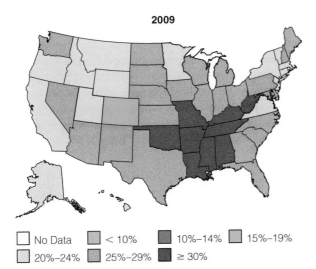

2009

| | No Data | | < 10% | | 10%–14% | | 15%–19% |
| | 20%–24% | | 25%–29% | | ≥ 30% |

Figure 8.1 Incidence of obesity in the United States (based on BMI > 30 or 30 pounds overweight), 1990, 2000, and 2009.

SOURCE: *Obesity Trends Among U.S. Adults Between 1985 and 2009* (Atlanta, GA: Centers for Disease Control and Prevention, 2011).

health status and is a risk factor for hypertension, congestive heart failure, high blood lipids, atherosclerosis, stroke, thromboembolitic disease, varicose veins, type 2 diabetes, osteoarthritis, gallbladder disease, sleep apnea, asthma, ruptured intervertebral disks, and arthritis. Estimates also indicate that 14 percent of all cancer deaths in men and 20 percent in women are related to current overweight and obesity patterns in the United States.[4] Furthermore, obesity is implicated in psychological maladjustment and a higher accidental death rate. Extremely obese people have worse mental health related to quality of life.

Overweight and obesity are not the same thing. Many overweight people (people who weigh about 10 to 20 pounds over the recommended weight) are not obese. Although a few pounds of excess weight may not be harmful to most people, this is not always the case. People with excessive body fat who have type 2 diabetes and other cardiovascular risk factors (elevated blood lipids, high blood pressure, physical inactivity, and poor eating habits) benefit from losing weight. People who have a few extra pounds of weight but are otherwise healthy and physically active, exercise regularly, and eat a healthy diet may not be at higher risk for disease and early death. Such is not the case, however, with obese individuals.

Research indicates that individuals who are 30 or more pounds overweight during middle age (30 to 49 years of age) lose about 7 years of life, whereas being 10 to 30 pounds overweight decreases the lifespan by about 3 years.[5] These decreases are similar to those seen with tobacco use. Severe obesity (BMI greater than 45) at a young age, nonetheless, may cut up to 20 years off one's life.[6]

Although the loss of years of life is significant, the decreased life expectancy doesn't even begin to address the loss in quality of life and increased illness and disability throughout the years. Even a modest reduction of 2 to 3 percent can reduce the risk for chronic diseases including heart disease, high blood pressure, high cholesterol, and diabetes.[7]

Key Terms

Overweight Excess body weight when compared to a given standard such as height or recommended percent body fat.

Obesity A chronic disease characterized by an excessively high amount of body fat (about 20 percent above recommended weight or a BMI at 30 or above).

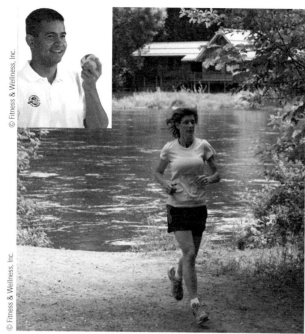
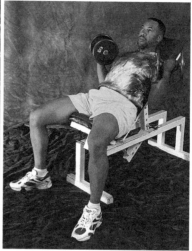

Achieving and maintaining a high physical fitness percent body fat requires a lifetime commitment to regular physical activity, exercise, and proper nutrition.

A primary objective of overall physical fitness and enhanced quality of life is to attain recommended body composition. Individuals at recommended body weight are able to participate in a wide variety of moderate to vigorous activities without functional limitations. These people have the freedom to enjoy most of life's recreational activities and reach their fullest potential. Excessive body weight does not afford an individual the fitness level to enjoy vigorous lifetime activities such as basketball, soccer, racquetball, surfing, mountain cycling, and mountain climbing. Maintaining high fitness and recommended body weight gives a person a degree of independence throughout life that the majority of people in developed nations no longer enjoy.

Critical Thinking

Do you consider yourself overweight? • If so, how long have you had a weight problem, what attempts have you made to lose weight, and what has worked best for you?

Tolerable Weight

Many people want to lose weight so they will look better. That's a noteworthy goal. The problem, however, is that they often have a distorted image of what they would really look like if they were to reduce to what they think is their ideal weight. Hereditary factors play a big role, and only a small fraction of the population has the genes for a "perfect body." **Tolerable weight** is a more realistic goal. This is a realistic standard that is not "ideal" but is "acceptable." It is likely to be closer to the health fitness standard than the physical fitness standard for many people.

The media have a great influence on people's perception of what constitutes ideal body weight. Most people rely on fashion, fitness, and beauty magazines to determine what they should look like. The "ideal" body shapes, physiques, and proportions shown in these magazines are rare and are achieved through airbrushing and medical reconstruction.[8] Many individuals, primarily young women, go to extremes in an attempt to achieve these unrealistic body shapes. Failure to attain a "perfect body" often leads to eating disorders.

When people set their own target weight, they should be realistic. Attaining the "high physical fitness" percent body fat standard shown in Table 2.11 (page 52) is extremely difficult for some. It is even more difficult to maintain, unless the person makes a commitment to a vigorous lifetime exercise program and permanent dietary changes. Few people are willing to do that. The "moderate" percent body fat category is more realistic for many people.

A question you should ask yourself is: Am I happy with my weight? Part of enjoying a higher quality of life is being happy with yourself. If you are not, you either need to do something about it or learn to live with it.

If your percent of body fat is higher than the health fitness standard shown in Table 2.11, page 52 (or a BMI above 25), you should try to reach and stay in this category, for health reasons. This is the category that seems to pose no detriment to health.

If you have achieved the health fitness standard but would like to be more fit, ask yourself a second question: How badly do I want it? Enough to implement lifetime exercise and dietary changes? If you are not willing to change, you should stop worrying about your weight and deem the health fitness standard tolerable for you.

Fad Dieting

Few people who begin a traditional weight loss program (without exercise) are able to lose the desired weight. Worse, less than 5 percent of this group is able to keep the weight off for a significant time. Traditional diets have failed in helping people keep the weight off because few diet programs incorporate lifetime changes in food selection and overall increases in daily physical activity and exercise as the keys to successful weight loss and maintenance.

Fad diets continue to deceive people. Capitalizing on hopes that the latest diet to hit the market will really work this time, fad diets continue to appeal to people of all shapes and sizes. These diets may work for a while, but their success is usually short-lived. Most of these diets are low in calories and deprive the body of certain nutrients, generating a metabolic imbalance that can be detrimental to health. With many of these diets, a large amount of weight loss is in the form of water and protein, not fat.

On a crash diet, close to half of the weight loss is in lean (protein) tissue (see Figure 8.2). When the body uses protein instead of a combination of fats and carbohydrates as a source of energy, the individual loses weight as much as 10 times faster. This is because a gram of protein produces less than half the amount of energy as fat does. In the case of muscle protein, one-fifth of protein is mixed with four-fifths of water. Each pound of muscle yields only one-tenth the amount of energy as a pound of fat. As a result, most of the weight loss is in the form of water, which on the scale, of course, looks good.

Among the popular diets on the market in recent years were the low-carbohydrate/high-protein

How to Recognize Fad Diets

Fad diets have characteristics in common. These diets typically

- are nutritionally unbalanced.
- rely primarily on a single food (for example, grapefruit).
- are based on testimonials.
- were developed according to "confidential research."
- are based on a "scientific breakthrough."
- promote rapid and "painless" weight loss.
- promise miraculous results.
- restrict food selection.
- are based on pseudo claims that excessive weight is related to a specific condition such as insulin resistance, combinations or timing of nutrient intake, food allergies, hormone imbalances, certain foods (fruits, for example).
- require the use of selected products.
- use liquid formulas instead of foods.
- misrepresent salespeople as individuals qualified to provide nutrition counseling.
- fail to provide information on risks associated with weight loss and of the diet use.
- do not involve physical activity.
- do not encourage healthy behavioral changes.
- are not supported by the scientific community or national health organizations.
- fail to provide information for weight maintenance upon completion of diet phase.

(LCHP) diet plans. Although variations exist among them, in general, "low-carb" diets limit the intake of carbohydrate-rich foods. Examples of these diets are the Atkins Diet, the Zone, Protein Power, the Scarsdale Diet, the Carb Addict's Diet, and Sugar Busters.

Rapid weight loss occurs during LCHP diets because the low carbohydrate intake forces the liver to produce glucose. The source for most of this glucose is body proteins. As mentioned, protein is mostly water; thus, weight is lost rapidly. When a person terminates the diet, the body rebuilds some of the protein tissue and the person quickly regains some weight.

Key Terms

Tolerable weight A realistic body weight that is close to the health fitness percent body fat standard.

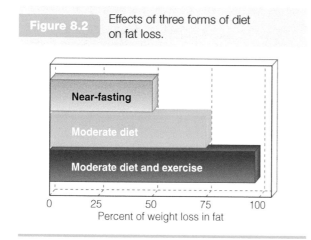

Adapted from *Alive Man: The Physiology of Physical Activity,* by R. J. Shephard (Springfield, IL: Charles C. Thomas, 1975): 484–488.

Research studies indicated that individuals on an LCHP (Atkins) diet lose slightly more weight in the first few months than those on a low-fat diet.[9] The effectiveness of the diet, however, seemed to dwindle over time. In one of the studies, at 12 months into the diet, participants in the LCHP diet had regained more weight than those on the low-fat diet plan.

Years of research will be required to determine the extent to which long-term adherence to LCHP diets increases the risk for heart disease, cancer, and kidney or bone damage. LCHP diets are contrary to the nutrition advice of most national leading health organizations (which recommend a diet low in animal fat and saturated fat and high in complex carbohydrates). Without fruits, vegetables, and whole grains, high-protein diets lack many vitamins, minerals, phytonutrients, and fiber—all dietary factors that protect against an array of ailments and diseases.

The major risk associated with long-term adherence to LCHP diets might be the increased risk of heart disease because high-protein foods are also high in fat content. Low carbohydrate intake also produces loss of vitamin B, calcium, and potassium. Side effects commonly associated with these diets are weakness, nausea, bad breath, constipation, irritability, light-headedness, and fatigue. Potential bone loss can further accentuate the risk for osteoporosis. Long-term adherence to an LCHP diet also can increase the risk for cancer. If you choose to go on an LCHP diet for longer than a few weeks, let your physician know so that he or she may monitor your blood lipids, bone density, and kidney function.

Some diets allow only certain specialized foods. If people would realize that no "magic" foods provide all the necessary nutrients, that a person has to eat a variety of foods to be well nourished, the diet industry would not be as successful. Most of these diets create a nutritional deficiency, which can be detrimental to health. Some people eventually get tired of eating the same thing day in and day out and start eating less—which results in weight loss. If they achieve the lower weight without making permanent dietary changes, however, they gain back the weight quickly if they return to their old eating habits.

A few diets recommend exercise along with caloric restrictions—the best method for weight reduction, of course. People who adhere to these programs will succeed, so the diet has achieved its purpose. Unfortunately, if the people do not change their food selection and activity level permanently, they gain back the weight once they discontinue dieting and exercise.

Principles of Weight Management

Traditional concepts related to weight control have centered on three assumptions:

1. Balancing food intake against output allows a person to achieve recommended weight.
2. Fat people just eat too much.
3. The human body doesn't care how much (or little) fat is stored.

Although these statements contain some truth, they still are open to much debate and research. We now know that the causes of obesity are complex and combine genetic, behavior, and lifestyle factors.

Energy-Balancing Equation

In keeping with the **energy-balancing equation**, if caloric intake exceeds output, the person gains weight; when caloric output is more than intake, the individual loses weight. Each pound of fat represents 3,500 calories. Therefore, theoretically, to increase body fat (weight) by 1 pound, a person would have to consume an excess of 3,500 calories. Equally, to lose 1 pound, the individual would have to decrease caloric intake by 3,500 calories. This principle seems straightforward, but the human body is not quite that simple.

The genetic instinct to survive tells the body that fat storage is vital, and, therefore, the body's weight-regulating mechanism or **setpoint** sets an acceptable fat level for each person. This setpoint remains somewhat constant or may climb gradually because of poor lifestyle habits.

Diet and Metabolism

Under strict calorie reduction (fewer than 800 calories per day), the body makes compensatory metabolic adjustments in an effort to maintain its fat storage. The **basal metabolic rate (BMR)** may drop dramatically against a consistent negative caloric balance, and the person may be on a plateau for days or even weeks without losing much weight. When the dieter goes back to the normal or even below-normal caloric intake, at which the weight may have been stable for a long time, he or she quickly regains the fat lost as the body strives to restore a comfortable fat level.

These findings were substantiated by research conducted at Rockefeller University in New York,[10] which showed that the body resists maintaining altered weight. Obese and lifetime nonobese individuals were used in the investigation. Following a 10 percent weight loss, in an attempt to regain the lost weight, the body compensated by burning up to 15 percent fewer calories than expected for the new reduced weight (after accounting for the 10 percent loss). The effects were similar in the obese and nonobese participants. These results imply that after a 10 percent weight loss, a person would have to eat less or exercise more to account for the estimated deficit of about 200 to 300 daily calories.

In this same study, when the participants were allowed to increase their weight to 10 percent above their "normal" body weight (pre–weight loss), the body burned 10 percent to 15 percent more calories than expected. This indicates an attempt by the body to waste energy and return to the preset weight. The study provides another indication that the body is highly resistant to weight changes unless the person incorporates additional lifestyle changes to ensure successful weight management. (Methods to manage weight will be discussed later in this chapter.)

This research shows why most dieters regain the weight they lose through dietary means alone. Let's use a practical illustration: Jim would like to lose some body fat and assumes that he has reached a stable body weight at an average daily caloric intake of 2,500 calories (no weight gain or loss at this daily intake). In an attempt to lose weight rapidly, he now goes on a strict low-calorie diet (or, even worse, a near-fasting diet). Immediately the body activates its survival mechanism and readjusts its metabolism to a lower caloric balance.

After a few weeks of dieting at under 800 calories per day, the body now can maintain its normal functions at 2,000 calories per day. Having lost the desired weight, Jim terminates the diet but realizes the original intake of 2,500 calories per day will have to be lower to maintain the new lower weight. To adjust to the new lower body weight, he restricts his intake to about 2,200 calories per day. Jim is surprised to find that even at this lower daily intake (300 fewer calories), his weight comes back at a rate of about 1 pound every 2 to 3 weeks. After the diet ends, this new lowered metabolic rate may take several months to kick back up to its normal level.

From this explanation, individuals clearly should not go on very low calorie diets. Doing so will decrease the resting metabolic rate and also will deprive the body of basic daily nutrients required for normal function. Very low calorie diets should be used only in conjunction with dietary supplements and under proper medical supervision. Furthermore, research indicates that people who go on very low calorie diets are not as effective in keeping the weight off once they terminate the diet.

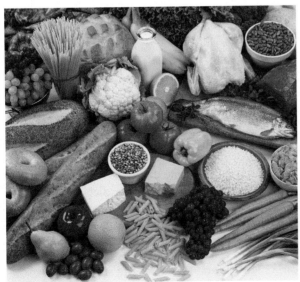

© 2001 PhotoDisc, Inc.

A wide variety of foods is required to maintain a well-nourished body.

Key Terms

Energy-balancing equation A body weight formula stating that when caloric intake equals caloric output, weight remains unchanged.

Setpoint Body weight and body fat percentage unique to each person that is regulated by genetic and environmental factors.

Basal metabolic rate (BMR) Lowest level of caloric intake necessary to sustain life.

Recommendation

A daily caloric intake of approximately 1,500 calories provides the necessary nutrients if they are distributed properly over the basic food groups (meeting the daily recommended amounts from each group). Of course, the individual will have to learn which foods meet the requirements and yet are low in fat and sugar. Diets below 1,500 daily calories may require a multivitamin supplement to obtain the daily nutrient requirements.

Under no circumstances should a person go on a diet that calls for a level of 1,200 calories or less for petite women or 1,500 calories or less for men. Weight (fat) is gained over months and years, not overnight. Likewise, weight loss should be gradual, not abrupt. At 1,200 calories per day, you may require a multivitamin nutrient supplement. Your health care professional should be consulted regarding such a supplement.

Furthermore, when a person tries to lose weight by dietary restrictions alone, **lean body mass** (muscle protein, along with vital organ protein) decreases. The amount of lean body mass lost depends entirely on the caloric limitation. When a person goes on a near-fasting diet, up to half of the weight lost can be lean body mass and the other half, actual fat loss. If the diet is combined with exercise, close to 100 percent of the weight loss is in the form of fat, and lean tissue actually may increase (see Figure 8.2). Loss of lean body mass is not good because it weakens the organs and muscles and slows the metabolism.

Reduction in lean body mass is common in people on severely restricted diets. No diet with caloric intakes below 1,500 calories will prevent loss of lean body mass. Even at this intake level, some loss is inevitable unless the diet is combined with exercise. Although many diets claim they do not alter the lean component, the simple truth is that, regardless of what nutrients may be added to the diet, caloric restrictions always prompt a loss of lean tissue.

Too many people go on low-calorie diets again and again. Every time they do, the metabolic rate slows as more lean tissue is lost. People in their 40s and older who weigh the same as they did when they were 20 often think they are at recommended body weight. During this span of 20 years or more, however, they may have dieted too many times without exercising. Shortly after terminating each diet, they regain the weight, but much of that gain is in fat. Maybe at age 20 they weighed 150 pounds, of which only 15 percent was fat. Now, at age 40, even though they still weigh 150 pounds, they might be

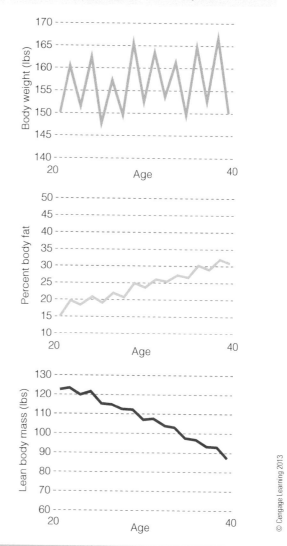

Figure 8.3 Effects of constant dieting without exercise on body weight, percent body fat, and lean body mass.

© Cengage Learning 2013

30 percent fat (see Figure 8.3, and also Figure 2.2, page 45). At recommended body weight, they wonder why they are eating so little and still having trouble staying at that weight.

Further, data indicate that diets high in fat and refined carbohydrates, near-fasting diets, and perhaps even artificial sweeteners, keep people from losing weight and, in reality, contribute to fat gain. The only practical and sensible way to lose fat weight is to combine exercise and a sensible diet high in complex carbohydrates and low in fat and sugar.

Because of the effects of proper food management on body weight, most of the successful dieter's effort should be spent in retraining eating habits, increasing the intake of complex carbohydrates and high-fiber foods, and decreasing the consumption of refined carbohydrates (sugars) and fats. This change in eating habits will bring about a decrease in total daily caloric intake. One gram of carbohydrates provides only 4 calories as contrasted with 9 calories per gram of fat. Thus, you could eat twice the volume of food (by weight) when substituting carbohydrates for fat. Some fat, however, is recommended in the diet—preferably polyunsaturated and monounsaturated fats. These so-called good fats do more than help protect the heart; they help delay hunger pangs.

A "diet" cannot be viewed as a temporary tool to aid in weight loss but, instead, as a permanent change in eating behaviors to ensure weight management and better health. The role of increased physical activity also must be considered because successful weight loss and recommended body composition seldom are attainable without a moderate reduction in caloric intake combined with a regular exercise program.

Sleep and Weight Management

Adequate sleep is a key component that enhances health and extends life. New evidence shows that sleep is also important to adequate weight management. Sleep deprivation appears to be conducive to weight gain and may interfere with the body's capability to lose weight.

Current obesity and sleep deprivation data point toward a possible correlation between excessive body weight and sleep deprivation. About 68 percent of the U.S. population is overweight or obese, and according to the National Sleep Foundation, 63 percent of Americans report that they do not get eight hours of sleep per night. The question must be raised: Is there a connection? Let's examine some of the data.

One of the most recent studies examining this issue showed that individuals who get fewer than six hours of sleep per night have a higher average BMI (28.3) compared to those who average eight hours per night (24.5).[11] Another study on more than 68,000 women between the ages of 30 and 55 found that those who got five or fewer hours of sleep per night were 30 percent more likely to gain 30 or more pounds compared to women who got eight hours per night.[12]

Researchers believe that lack of sleep disrupts normal body hormonal balances. Ghrelin and leptin are two hormones that play a critical role in weight gain and weight loss. Ghrelin, produced primarily in the stomach, stimulates appetite; that is, the more ghrelin the body produces, the more you want to eat. Leptin, produced by fat cells, on the other hand, lets the brain know when you are full; the more leptin you produce, the less you want to eat.

Sleep deprivation has now been shown to elevate ghrelin levels and decrease leptin levels, potentially leading to weight gain or keeping you from losing weight.[13] Data comparing these hormone levels in five-hour versus eight-hour sleepers found that the short sleepers had a 14.9 percent increase in ghrelin levels and a 15.5 percent decrease in leptin levels. The short sleepers also had a 3.6 percent higher BMI than the regular sleepers.[14]

Based on all these studies, the data appear to indicate that sleep deprivation has a negative impact on weight loss or maintenance. Thus, an important component to a well-designed weight management program should be a good night's rest (eight hours of sleep).

Monitoring Body Weight

A most critical component to lifetime weight management is to regularly monitor your body weight. Get into the habit of weighing yourself, preferably at the same time of day and under the same conditions, for instance, in the morning just as you get out of bed. Depending on your body size, activity patterns, rehydration level, and dietary intake on any given day, your weight will fluctuate by a pound or more from one day to the next. You do not want to be obsessed with body weight, which can potentially lead to an eating disorder, but monitoring your *recommended body weight* (and that is the key: *"healthy" recommended body weight*) on a regular basis allows you to make immediate adjustments in food intake and physical activity if your weight increases and stays there for several days. *Do not adapt and accept the higher weight as your new stable weight.* Understand that it is a lot easier to make sensible short-term dietary and activity changes to lose 1 or 2 pounds of weight rather than having to make drastic long-term changes to lose 10, 20, 50, or more pounds that you allowed yourself to gain over the course of several months or years. Whenever feasi-

Lean body mass Nonfat component of the human body.

ble, you also want to do periodic assessments of body composition using experienced technicians and valid techniques.

Exercise and Weight Management

A more effective way to tilt the energy-balancing equation in your favor is by burning calories through physical activity. Research indicates that exercise accentuates weight loss while on a negative caloric balance (diet) as long as you do not replenish the calories expended during exercise.

Exercise also seems to exert control over how much a person weighs. On average, the typical adult American gains 1 to 2 pounds of weight per year. A 1-pound weight gain per year represents a simple energy surplus of less than 10 calories per day ($10 \times 365 = 3,650$). In many cases, most of the additional weight accumulated in middle age comes from people becoming less physically active.

Exercise enhances the rate of weight loss and is vital in maintaining the weight loss. Not only will exercise maintain lean tissue, but advocates of the setpoint theory say that exercise resets the fat thermostat to a new, lower level.

A few individuals will lose weight by participating in 30 minutes of exercise per day, but most people need 60 to 90 minutes of daily physical activity for proper weight management (the 30 minutes of exercise are included as part of the 60 to 90 minutes of physical activity).

Although 30 minutes of moderate-intensity activity per day provides substantial health benefits, the Institute of Medicine of the National Academy of Sciences recommends that people trying to manage their weight accumulate 60 minutes of moderate-intensity physical activity most days of the week.[15] The evidence shows that people who maintain recommended weight typically accumulate an hour or more of daily physical activity.

As illustrated in Figure 8.4, greater weight loss can be achieved by increasing the amount of weekly physical activity. Of even greater significance, however, only the individuals who remain physically active for more than 60 minutes per day are able to keep the weight off.

Further, data from the National Weight Control Registry (http://www.nwcr.ws/) indicates that individuals who have lost at least 30 pounds and kept them off for a minimum of 6 years typically accumulate 90 minutes of daily activity. Those who are less

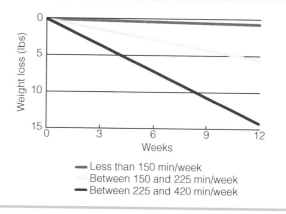

Figure 8.4   Approximate decrease in body weight based on total weekly minutes of physical activity (PA) without caloric restrictions.

— Less than 150 min/week
  Between 150 and 225 min/week
— Between 225 and 420 min/week

Adapted from American College of Sports Medicine, "Position Stand: Appropriate Physical Activity Intervention Strategies for Weight Loss and Prevention of Weight Gain for Adults," *Medicine & Science in Sports & Exercise* 41 (2009): 459–471.

active gradually regain the lost weight. Individuals who completely stop physical activity regain almost 100 percent of the weight within 18 months of discontinuing the weight loss program. Thus, if weight management is *not* a consideration, 30 minutes of daily activity provides health benefits. *To prevent weight gain, 60 minutes of daily activity are recommended; to maintain substantial weight loss, 90 minutes may be required.*

A combination of aerobic and strength-training exercises works best in weight loss programs. Aerobic exercise is the best to offset the setpoint, and the continuity and duration of these types of activities cause many calories to be burned in the process. Unfortunately, of those individuals who are attempting to lose weight, only a small percentage decrease caloric intake and exercise the recommended 30 minutes on most days of the week.

Strength training is critical in helping maintain lean body mass. Although the increase in BMR (basal metabolic rate) through increased muscle mass is currently being debated in the literature and merits further research, data indicate that each additional pound of muscle tissue raises the BMR in the range of 6 to 35 calories per day.[16] The latter figure is based on calculations that an increase of 3 to 3.5 pounds of lean tissue through strength training increased basal metabolic rate by about 105 to 120 calories per day.[17]

Most likely, the benefit of strength training goes beyond the new muscle tissue itself. Maybe a pound of muscle tissue requires only 6 calories per day to sustain itself, but as all muscles undergo strength training, they undergo increased protein synthesis to build and repair themselves, resulting in increased energy expenditure of 1 to 1.5 calories per pound in all trained muscle tissue. Such an increase would explain the 105 to 120 calorie-BMR increase in some research studies.

To examine the effects of a small increase in BMR on long-term body weight, let's use a very conservative estimate of an additional 50 calories per day as a result of a regular strength-training program. An increase of 50 calories represents an additional 18,250 calories per year (50 × 365), or the equivalent of 5.2 pounds of fat (18,250 ÷ 3,500). This increase in BMR would more than offset the typical adult weight gain of 1 to 2 pounds per year.

This figure of 18,250 calories per year does not include the actual energy cost of the strength-training workout. If we use an energy expenditure of only 150 calories per strength-training session, done twice per week, over a year's time it would represent 15,600 calories (150 × 2 × 52) or the equivalent of another 4.5 pounds of fat (15,600 ÷ 3,500).

In addition, although the amounts seem small, the previous calculations do not account for the increase in metabolic rate following the strength-training workout (the time it takes the body to return to its pre-workout resting rate—about 2 hours). Depending on the intensity and length of training, this recovery energy expenditure ranges from 20 to 100 calories following each strength-training workout.[18] All these "apparently small" changes make a big difference in the long run.

Although size (inches) and percent body fat both decrease when sedentary individuals begin an exercise program, body weight often remains the same or might even increase during the first couple of weeks after beginning the program. Exercise helps to increase muscle tissue, connective tissue, blood volume (as much as 500 mL, or the equivalent of 1 pound, following the first week of aerobic exercise), enzymes and other structures within the cell, and glycogen (which binds water). All of these changes lead to a higher functional capacity of the human body. With exercise, most of the weight loss becomes apparent after a few weeks of training, when the lean component has stabilized.

The Myth of Spot-Reducing

Research has revealed the fallacy of spot-reducing or losing cellulite, as some people call the fat deposits that bulge out in certain areas of the body. Cellulite is caused by the herniation of subcutaneous fat within fibrous connective tissue, giving it a padded appearance. Merely doing several sets of sit-ups daily will not get rid of fat in the midsection of the body. When fat comes off, it does so throughout the entire body, not just in the exercised area. Although the greatest proportion of fat may come off the

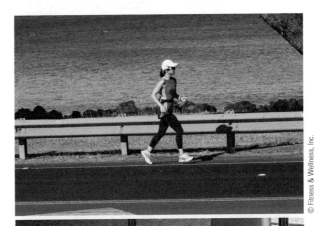

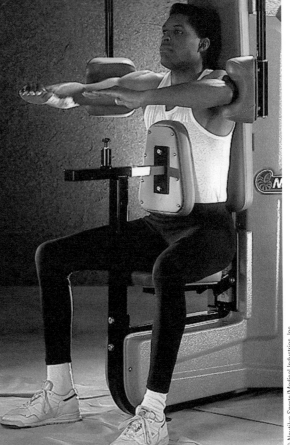

Regular participation in a combined lifetime aerobic and strength-training exercise program is the key to successful weight management.

© Fitness & Wellness, Inc.

© Nautilus Sports/Medical Industries, Inc.

Weight Maintenance Benefits of Lifetime Aerobic Exercise

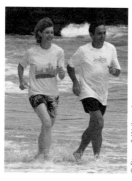

The authors of this book have been jogging together a minimum of 15 miles per week (3 miles/5 times per week) for the past 35 years. Without considering the additional energy expenditure from their regular strength-training program and their many other sport and recreational activities, the energy cost of this regular jogging program over 35 years has been approximately 2,730,000 calories (15 miles × 100 calories/mile × 52 weeks × 35 years), or the equivalent of 780 pounds of fat (2,730,000 ÷ 3,500). In essence, without this 30-minute workout 5 times per week, the authors would weigh 922 and 896 pounds, respectively!

Try It Ask yourself whether a regular aerobic exercise program is part of your long-term gratification and health enhancement program. If the answer is no, are you ready to change your behavior? Use the Behavior Change Planner to help you answer the question.

biggest fat deposits, the caloric output of a few sets of sit-ups has almost no effect on reducing total body fat. A person has to exercise regularly for extended periods of time to really see results.

The Role of Exercise Intensity and Duration in Weight Management

A hotly debated and controversial current topic is the exercise volume required for adequate weight management. Depending on the degree of the initial weight problem and the person's fitness level, there appears to be a difference in the volume of exercise that is most conducive toward adequate weight loss, weight loss maintenance, and weight management.

We have known for years that compared with vigorous intensity, a greater proportion of calories burned during light-intensity exercise are derived from fat. The lower the intensity of exercise, the higher the percentage of fat utilization as an energy source. During light-intensity exercise, up to 50 percent of the calories burned may be derived from fat (the other 50 percent from glucose [carbohydrates]). With vigorous exercise, only 30 to 40 percent of the caloric expenditure comes from fat. Overall, however, you can burn twice as many calories during vigorous-intensity exercise and, subsequently, more fat as well.

Let's look at a practical illustration. If you exercised for 30 to 40 minutes at light intensity and burned 200 calories, about 100 of those calories (50 percent) would come from fat. If you exercised at a vigorous intensity during those same 30 to 40 minutes, you could burn 400 calories, with 120 to 160 of the calories (30 to 40 percent) coming from fat. Thus, even though it is true that the percentage of fat used is greater during light-intensity exercise, the overall amount of fat used is still less during light-intensity exercise. Plus, if you were to exercise at a light intensity, you would have to do so twice as long to burn the same amount of calories. Another benefit is that the metabolic rate remains at a slightly higher level longer after vigorous-intensity exercise, so you continue to burn a few extra calories following exercise.

The previous discussion does not mean that light-intensity exercise is ineffective. Light-intensity exercise provides substantial health benefits, including a decrease in premature morbidity among overweight individuals. Additionally, beginners are more willing to participate and stay with light-intensity programs. The risk of injury when starting out is quite low with this type of a program. Light-intensity exercise does promote weight loss.

In terms of overall weight loss, there is controversy regarding the optimal exercise dose. Initial research indicated that vigorous-intensity exercise triggered more fat loss than light- to moderate-intensity exercise. Research conducted in the 1990s at Laval University in Quebec, Canada, using both men and women participants, showed that subjects who performed a high-intensity interval-training (HIIT) program lost more body fat than participants in a light- to moderate-intensity continuous aerobic endurance group.[19] Even more surprising, this finding occurred despite the fact that the vigorous-intensity group burned fewer total calories per exercise session. The researchers concluded that the "results reinforce the notion that for a given level of energy expenditure, vigorous exercise favors negative energy and lipid balance to a greater extent than exercise of low- to moderate-intensity. Moreover, the metabolic adaptations taking place in the skeletal muscle in response to the HIIT program appear to favor the process of lipid oxidation." If time constraints do not allow much time for exercise, to increase energy expenditure, a vigorous 20- to 30-minute exercise program is recommended.

Recently, it has been suggested that *when attempting to lose weight,* particularly for women, lengthy exercise sessions may not be helpful because they actually trigger greater food consumption following exercise, whereas shorter exercise sessions do not lead to a greater caloric intake. Thus, some people think that the potential weight reduction effect of lengthy exercise sessions may be attenuated because people end up eating more food when they exercise.

A recent 2009 study had postmenopausal women exercise at 50 percent of their maximal aerobic capacity for about 20 minutes, 40 minutes, or 60 minutes three to four times per week.[20] On average, the groups lost 3, 4.6, and, 3.3 pounds of weight, respectively. The data indicated that the 20- and 40-minute groups lost weight closely to what had been predicted, whereas the 60-minute group lost significantly less than predicted. The researchers concluded that 60 minutes of exercise led this group of women to compensate with greater food intake, possibly triggered by an increase in ghrelin levels. All three groups, nonetheless, exhibited a significant decrease in waist circumference, independent of total weight lost. Researchers theorize that the biological mechanism to maintain fat stores in women is stronger than in men.

On the other hand, a 2010 study of more than 34,000 women who were followed for 13 years, starting at an average age of 54, found that on average the women gained 6 pounds of weight; but a small group of them who reported 60 minutes of almost daily exercise at a moderate intensity closely maintained their body weight.[21] The exercise routine of the latter group was not something new to them, but rather exercise that they had been doing for years. While the best exercise dose for optimal weight loss may not be a precise science, the research is quite clear that regular exercise is the best predictor of long-term weight maintenance. The data also indicate that even as little as 80 weekly minutes of aerobic or strength-training exercise prevents regain of the harmful visceral fat.

The take-home message from these studies is that when trying to lose weight, initial lengthy exercise sessions (longer than 60 minutes) may not be the best approach to weight loss, *unless* you carefully monitor daily caloric intake and avoid caloric compensation. The data show that people who carefully monitor caloric intake, instead of "guesstimating" energy intake, are by far more successful with weight loss.

Caloric compensation in response to extensive exercise in overweight individuals may be related to a low initial fitness level and the already low caloric intake. Overall, inactive people tend to eat fewer calories, and a lengthy exercise session may very well trigger a greater appetite due to the large negative caloric balance. Research confirms that energy deficit, and not exercise, is the most significant regulator of the hormonal responses seen in previously inactive individuals who begin an exercise program.[22] In active/fit individuals, lengthy exercise sessions are not at all counterproductive. If such was the case, health clubs and jogging trails would be full of overweight and obese people.

New research is beginning to look into the role of increasing light-intensity ambulation (walking) and standing activities (doing some of the work on your feet instead of sitting the entire time) on weight loss. In essence, the individual will increase light-intensity physical activity throughout the day. Light-intensity activities do not seem to trigger the increase in ghrelin levels seen in previously inactive individuals who undertake long moderate- or vigorous-intensity exercise sessions. The difference in energy expenditure from increasing light-intensity activities throughout the day can represent several hundred calories. As you achieve a higher fitness level, you can combine light-intensity activities performed throughout the day with moderate-and/or vigorous-intensity exercise.

The most important reason why physical activity and exercise are so vital for weight loss maintenance is because sedentary living expends no additional energy (calories) over the resting metabolic rate. With limited physical activity throughout the day, sedentary people cannot afford to eat very many calories, perhaps only 1,000 to 1,200 calories per day. And such a low level of energy intake is not sufficient to keep the person from constantly feeling hungry. The only choice they now have is to go hungry every day, an impossible task to sustain. After terminating the diet, in just a few short days energy intake climbs, with an end result of weight regain. Thus, the only logical way to increase caloric intake and maintain weight loss is by burning more calories through exercise and incorporating physical activity throughout daily living.

If you wish to engage in vigorous-intensity exercise to either maintain lost weight or for adequate weight management, a word of caution is in order: Be sure that it is medically safe for you to participate in such activities and that you build up gradually to that level. If you are cleared to participate in vigorous-intensity exercise, do not attempt to do too much too quickly because you may incur injuries and become discouraged. You must allow your body a proper conditioning period of 8 to 12 weeks or even longer.

Also keep in mind that vigorous intensity does not mean high impact. High-impact activities are the most common cause of exercise-related injuries. Additional information on proper exercise prescription is presented in Chapter 3. And remember, when on a weight loss program, *always* carefully monitor your daily caloric intake to avoid food overconsumption.

In addition to exercise and food management, sensible adjustments in caloric intake are recommended. Most research finds that a negative caloric balance is required to lose weight. Perhaps the only exception is with people who are eating too few calories. A nutrient analysis often reveals that "faithful" dieters are not consuming enough calories. These people actually need to increase their daily caloric intake (combined with an exercise program) to get their metabolism to kick back up to a normal level.

Designing Your Own Weight Loss Program

Estimating Your Caloric Intake

With Activity 8.1 (pages 181–182) and Tables 8.1 and 8.2, you can estimate your daily energy (caloric) requirement. Because this is only an estimated value, individual adjustments related to many of the factors discussed in this chapter may be necessary to establish a more precise value. Nevertheless, the estimated value does offer a beginning guideline for weight control or reduction.

The **estimated energy requirement (EER)** without additional planned activity and exercise is based on age, total body weight, height, and gender. Individuals who hold jobs that require a lot of walking or heavy manual labor burn more calories during the day than those who have sedentary jobs (such as working behind a desk). To estimate your EER, refer to Table 8.1. For example, the EER computation for a

Table 8.1	Estimated Energy Requirement (EER) Based on Age, Body Weight, and Height (includes activities of independent living only and no moderate physical activity or exercise)

Men: EER = 662 − (9.53 × Age) + (15.91 × BW) + (539 × HT)

Women: EER = 354 − (6.91 × Age) + (9.36 × BW) + (726 × HT)

BW = body weight in kilograms (divide BW in pounds by 2.2046), HT = height in meters (multiply HT in inches by .0254).

SOURCE: National Academy of Sciences, Institute of Medicine, *Dietary Reference Intakes for Energy, Carbohydrates, Fiber, Fat, Protein and Amino Acids (Macronutrients)* (Washington, DC: National Academy Press, 2002).

20-year-old man, 71 inches tall, who weighs 160 pounds, would be as follows:

1. Body weight in kilograms = 72.6 kg (160 lbs ÷ 2.2046)

   Height in meters = 1.8 m (71 × .0254)

2. EER = 662 − (9.53 × Age) + (15.91 × BW) + (539 × Ht)

   EER = 662 − (9.53 × 20) + (15.91 × 72.6) + (539 × 1.8)

   EER = 662 − 190.6 + 1,155 + 970

   EER = 2,596

Thus, the EER to maintain body weight for this individual would be 2,596 calories per day.

The second step is to determine the average number of calories this man burns daily as a result of exercise. To get this number, he must figure out the total number of minutes he exercises weekly and then figure the daily average exercise time. For instance, if he cycles at 10 miles per hour five times a week, 60 minutes each time, he exercises 300 minutes per week (5 × 60). The average daily exercise time is 42 minutes (300 ÷ 7, rounded off to the lowest unit).

Next, from Table 8.2, find the energy requirement for the activity (or activities) he has chosen for the exercise program. In the case of cycling (10 miles per hour), the requirement is .05 calories per pound of body weight per minute of activity (cal/lb/min). With a body weight of 160 pounds, this man would burn 8 calories each minute (body weight × .05, or 160 × .05). In 42 minutes, he burns approximately 336 calories (42 × 8).

The third step is to obtain the estimated total caloric requirement, with exercise, needed to maintain

Table 8.2	Caloric Expenditure of Selected Physical Activities				
Activity*	**Cal/lb/min**	**Activity***	**Cal/lb/min**	**Activity***	**Cal/lb/min**
Aerobics		Gymnastics		Stationary Cycling	
Moderate	0.065	Light	0.030	Moderate	0.055
Vigorous	0.095	Heavy	0.056	Vigorous	0.070
Step Aerobics	0.070	Handball	0.064	Strength Training	0.050
Archery	0.030	Hiking	0.040	Swimming (crawl)	
Badminton		Judo/Karate	0.086	20 yds/min	0.031
Recreation	0.038	Racquetball	0.065	25 yds/min	0.040
Competition	0.065	Rope Jumping	0.060	45 yds/min	0.057
Baseball	0.031	Rowing (vigorous)	0.090	50 yds/min	0.070
Basketball		Running (on a level surface)		Table Tennis	0.030
Moderate	0.046	11.0 min/mile	0.070	Tennis	
Competition	0.063	8.5 min/mile	0.090	Moderate	0.045
Bowling	0.030	7.0 min/mile	0.102	Competition	0.064
Calisthenics	0.033	6.0 min/mile	0.114	Volleyball	0.030
Cycling (on a level surface)		Deep water**	0.100	Walking	
5.5 mph	0.033	Skating (moderate)	0.038	4.5 mph	0.045
10.0 mph	0.050	Skiing		Shallow pool	0.090
13.0 mph	0.071	Downhill	0.060	Water Aerobics	
Dance		Level (5 mph)	0.078	Moderate	0.050
Moderate	0.030	Soccer	0.059	Vigorous	0.070
Vigorous	0.055	Stairmaster		Wrestling	0.085
Golf	0.030	Moderate	0.070		
		Vigorous	0.090		

*Values are for actual time engaged in the activity.   ** Treading water

Adapted from:

    P. E. Allsen, J. M. Harrison, and B. Vance, *Fitness for Life: An Individualized Approach* (Dubuqe, IA: Wm. C. Brown, 1989).

    C. A. Bucher and W. E. Prentice, *Fitness for College and Life* (St. Louis: Times Mirror/Mosby College Publishing, 1989).

    C. F. Consolazio, R. E. Johnson, and L. J. Pecora, *Physiological Measurements of Metabolic Functions in Man* (New York: McGraw-Hill, 1963).

    R. V. Hockey, *Physical Fitness: The Pathway to Healthy Living* (St. Louis: Times Mirror/Mosby College Publishing, 1989).

    W. W. K. Hoeger et al., Research conducted at Boise State University, 1986–1993.

body weight. To do this, add the typical daily requirement (without exercise) and the average calories burned through exercise. In our example, it is 2,932 calories (2,596 + 336).

Therefore, this man has to consume fewer than 2,932 calories daily to lose weight. Because of the many factors that play a role in weight control, this is only an estimated daily requirement. Furthermore, to lose weight, we cannot predict that he will lose exactly 1 pound of fat in 1 week if he cuts his daily intake by 500 calories (500 × 7 = 3,500 calories, or the equivalent of 1 pound of fat).

The daily energy requirement is only a target guideline for weight control. Periodic readjustments are necessary because individuals differ and the estimated daily cost changes as you lose weight and modify your exercise habits.

To determine the target caloric intake to lose weight, multiply your current weight by 5 and subtract this amount from the total daily energy require-

ment (2,932 in our example) with exercise. For our moderately active male example, this would mean consuming only 2,132 calories per day to lose weight (160 × 5 = 800 and 2,932 − 800 = 2,132 calories).

This final caloric intake to lose weight should not be below 1,500 calories for most people. If distributed properly over the various food groups, 1,500 calories appears to be the lowest caloric intake that still provides the necessary nutrients the body needs. A multivitamin complex is recommended for diets that call

Key Terms

Estimated energy requirement (EER) The average dietary energy (caloric) intake that is predicted to maintain energy balance in a healthy adult of defined age, gender, weight, height, and level of physical activity, consistent with good health.

for less than 1,500 calories. In terms of percentages of total calories, the daily distribution should be approximately 60 percent carbohydrates (mostly complex carbohydrates), less than 30 percent fat, and about 12 percent protein.

The time of day when food is consumed also may play a part in losing weight. When a person is attempting to lose weight, intake should consist of a minimum of 25 percent of the total daily calories for breakfast, 50 percent for lunch, and 25 percent or less at dinner. Breakfast, in particular, is a critical meal. Many people skip breakfast because it's the easiest meal to skip. Evidence, however, indicates that people who skip breakfast are hungrier later in the day and end up consuming more total daily calories than those who eat breakfast. Furthermore, regular breakfast eaters have less of a weight problem, lose weight more effectively, and have less difficulty maintaining lost weight.

If most of the daily calories are consumed during one meal (as in the typical evening meal), the body may perceive that something is wrong and will slow down the metabolism so it can store more calories in the form of fat. Also, eating most of the calories during one meal causes a person to go hungry the rest of the day, making it more difficult to adhere to the diet.

Monitoring Your Diet Through Daily Food Logs

To help you monitor and adhere to your diet plan, you may use the daily food intake record form in Activity 8.2, pages 183–186. First make a master copy so you can make copies as needed in the future. Guidelines are provided for 1,200-, 1,500-, 1,800-, and 2,000-calorie diet plans. These plans have been developed based on the MyPlate food plan and the Dietary Guidelines for Americans to meet the Recommended Dietary Allowances. The objective is to meet (not exceed) the number of servings allowed for each diet plan. Each time you eat a serving of any food, record it in the appropriate box. Evidence indicates that people who monitor daily caloric intake are more successful at weight loss than those who don't self-monitor.

To lose weight, you should use the diet plan that most closely approximates your target caloric intake. The plan is based on the following caloric allowances for these food groups:

- Grains: 80 calories per serving.
- Fruits: 60 calories per serving.
- Vegetables: 25 calories per serving.
- Dairy (use low-fat products): 120 calories per serving.
- Protein: Use low-fat (300 calories per serving) frozen entrees or an equivalent amount if you prepare your own main dish (see the following discussion).

As you start your diet plan, pay particular attention to food serving sizes. Take care with cup and glass sizes. A standard cup is 8 ounces, but most glasses nowadays contain between 12 and 16 ounces. If you drink 12 ounces of fruit juice, in essence you are getting two servings of fruit because a standard serving is ¾ cup of juice.

Read food labels carefully to compare the caloric value of the serving listed on the label with the caloric guidelines provided above. Here are some examples:

- One slice of standard whole-wheat bread has about 80 calories. A plain bagel may have 200 to 350 calories. Although it is low in fat, a 350-calorie bagel is equivalent to almost 4 servings in the grain group.

- The standard serving size listed on the food label for most cereals is 1 cup. As you read the nutrition information, however, you will find that for the same cup of cereal, one type of cereal has 120 calories and another cereal has 200 calories. Because a standard serving in the grain group is 80 calories, the first cereal would be 1½ servings and the second one 2½ servings.

- A medium-size fruit is usually considered to be 1 serving. A large fruit could provide as many as 2 or more servings.

- In the dairy group, 1 serving represents 120 calories. A cup of whole milk has about 160 calories, compared with a cup of skim milk, which contains 88 calories. A cup of whole milk, therefore, would provide 1⅓ servings in this food group.

Using Low-Fat Entrees

To be more accurate with caloric intake and to simplify meal preparation, use commercially prepared low-fat frozen entrees as the main dish for lunch and dinner meals (only one entree for the 1,200-calorie diet plan—see Activity 8.2, page 183). Look for entrees that provide about 300 calories and no more than 6 grams of fat per entree. These two entrees can be used as the protein group selections and will provide most of the daily requirement for the body. Along with each entree, supplement the meal with some of your servings from the other food groups.

This diet plan has been used successfully in weight loss research programs.[23] If you choose not to use these low-fat entrees, prepare a similar meal using 3 ounces (cooked) of lean meat, poultry, or fish with additional beans, vegetables, rice, or pasta that will provide 300 calories with fewer than 6 grams of fat per dish.

Analyze Your Intake

As you record your food choices, be sure to write the precise amount for each serving. If you choose to do so, you then can run a computerized nutrient analysis to verify your caloric intake and food distribution pattern (percent of total calories from carbohydrate, fat, and protein).

Behavior Modification and Adherence to a Lifetime Weight Management Program

Achieving and maintaining recommended body composition is by no means impossible, but it does require desire and commitment. If weight management is to become a priority in life, people must realize that they have to transform their behavior to some extent.

Modifying old habits and developing new, positive behaviors take time. Individuals who apply the management techniques provided in the Behavior Modification Planning box (pages 178–179) are more successful at changing detrimental behavior and adhering to a positive, lifetime weight control program. In developing a retraining program, people are not expected to use all of the strategies listed but should pick the ones that apply to them.

Critical Thinking

What behavioral strategies have you used to properly manage your body weight? • How do you think those strategies would work for others?

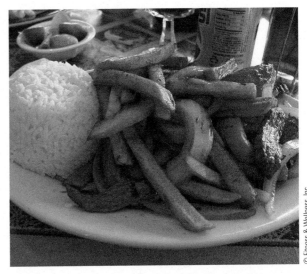

"Supersized" portion sizes at restaurants in the United States contribute to the growing epidemic of obesity.

During the weight loss process, surround yourself with people who have the same goals as you do (weight loss). Data released in 2007 showed that obesity can spread through "social networks."[24] That is, if your friends, siblings, or spouse gain weight, you are more likely to gain weight as well. People tend to accept a higher weight standard if someone they are close to or care about gains weight.

In the study, the social ties of more than 12,000 were examined over 32 years. The findings revealed that if a close friend becomes obese, your risk of becoming obese during the next two to four years increases 171 percent. The risk also increases 57 percent for casual friends, 40 percent for siblings, and 37 percent for the person's spouse. The reverse was also found to be true. When a person loses weight, the likelihood of friends, siblings, or spouse to lose weight is also enhanced.

Furthermore, the research found that gender plays a role in social networks. A male's weight has a greater effect on the weight of male friends and brothers than on female friends or sisters. Similarly, a woman's weight has a far greater influence on sisters and girlfriends than on brothers or male friends. Thus, if you are trying to lose weight, choose your friendships carefully: Do not surround yourself with people who either have a weight problem or are still gaining weight.

Weight Loss Strategies

1. *Make a commitment to change.* The first necessary ingredient is the desire to modify your behavior. You have to stop precontemplating or contemplating change and get going! You must accept that you have a problem and decide by yourself whether you really want to change. Sincere commitment increases your chances for success.

2. *Set realistic goals.* The weight problem developed over several years. Similarly, new lifetime eating and exercise habits take time to develop. A realistic long-term goal also will include short-term objectives that allow for regular evaluation and help maintain motivation and renewed commitment to attain the long-term goal.

3. *Weigh yourself regularly, preferably at the same time of day and under the same conditions.* Do not adapt and accept a higher body weight as a new stable weight. Make dietary and physical activity adjustments accordingly.

4. *Incorporate exercise into the program.* Choosing enjoyable activities, places, times, equipment, and people to work out with will help you adhere to an exercise program. (See Chapters 6, 7, 8, and 9.)

5. *Differentiate hunger and appetite.* Hunger is the actual physical need for food. Appetite is a desire for food, usually triggered by factors such as stress, habit, boredom, depression, availability of food, or just the thought of food itself. Developing and sticking to a regular meal pattern will help control hunger.

6. *Eat less fat.* Each gram of fat provides 9 calories, and protein and carbohydrates provide only 4. In essence, you can eat more food on a low-fat diet because you consume fewer calories with each meal. Most of your fat intake should come from unsaturated sources.

7. *Pay attention to calories.* Just because food is labeled "low-fat" does not mean you can eat as much as you want. When reading food labels—and when eating—don't just look at the fat content. Pay attention to calories as well. Many low-fat foods are high in calories.

8. *Cut unnecessary items from your diet.* Substituting water for a daily can of soda would cut 51,100 (140 × 365) calories yearly from the diet—the equivalent of 14.6 (51,000 ÷ 3,500) pounds of fat.

9. *Maintain a daily intake of calcium-rich foods,* especially low-fat or nonfat dairy products.

10. *Add foods to your diet that reduce cravings,* such as eggs; small amounts of red meat, fish, poultry, tofu, oils, fats; and nonstarchy vegetables such as lettuce, green beans, peppers, asparagus, broccoli, mushrooms, and Brussels sprouts. Also increasing the intake of low-glycemic carbohydrates with your meals helps you go longer before you feel hungry again.

11. *Avoid automatic eating.* Many people associate certain daily activities with eating, for example, cooking, watching television, or reading. Most foods consumed in these situations lack nutritional value or are high in sugar and fat.

12. *Stay busy.* People tend to eat more when they sit around and do nothing. Occupying the mind and body with activities not associated with eating helps take away the desire to eat. Some options are walking; cycling; playing sports; gardening; sewing; or visiting a library, a museum, or a park. You also might develop other skills and interests not associated with food.

13. *Plan meals and shop sensibly.* Always shop on a full stomach, because hungry shoppers tend to buy unhealthy foods impulsively—and then snack on the way home. Always use a shopping list, which should include whole-grain breads and cereals, fruits and vegetables, low-fat milk and dairy products, lean meats, fish, and poultry.

14. *Cook wisely:*
    - Use less fat and fewer refined foods in food preparation.
    - Trim all visible fat from meats and remove skin from poultry before cooking.
    - Skim the fat off gravies and soups.
    - Bake, broil, boil, or steam instead of frying.
    - Sparingly use butter, cream, mayonnaise, and salad dressings.
    - Avoid coconut oil, palm oil, and cocoa butter.
    - Prepare plenty of foods that contain fiber.
    - Include whole-grain breads and cereals, vegetables, and legumes in most meals.
    - Eat fruits for dessert.
    - Stay away from soda pop, fruit juices, and fruit-flavored drinks.
    - Use less sugar, and cut down on other refined carbohydrates, such as corn syrup, malt sugar, dextrose, and fructose.
    - Drink plenty of water—at least six glasses a day.

15. *Do not serve more food than you should eat.* Measure the food in portions and keep serving dishes away from the table. Do not force yourself or anyone else to "clean the plate" after they are satis-

continued

fied (including children after they already have had a healthy, nutritious serving).

16. *Try "junior size" instead of "super size."* People who are served larger portions eat more, whether they are hungry or not. Use smaller plates, bowls, cups, and glasses. Try eating half as much food as you commonly eat. Watch for portion sizes at restaurants as well: Supersized foods create supersized people.

17. *Eat out infrequently.* The more often people eat out, the more body fat they have. People who eat out six or more times per week consume an average of about 300 extra calories per day and 30 percent more fat than those who eat out less often.

18. *Eat slowly and at the table only.* Eating on the run promotes overeating because the body doesn't have enough time to "register" consumption and people overeat before the body perceives the fullness signal. Eating at the table encourages people to take time out to eat and deters snacking between meals. After eating, do not sit around the table but, rather, clean up and put away the food to avoid snacking.

19. *Avoid social binges.* Social gatherings tend to entice self-defeating behavior. Use visual imagery to plan ahead. Do not feel pressured to eat or drink and don't rationalize in these situations. Choose low-calorie foods and entertain yourself with other activities, such as dancing and talking.

20. *Do not place unhealthy foods within easy reach.* Ideally, avoid bringing high-calorie, high-sugar, or high-fat foods into the house. If they are there already, store them where they are hard to get to or see—perhaps the garage or basement.

21. *Avoid evening food raids.* Most people do really well during the day but then "lose it" at night. Take control. Stop and think. To avoid excessive nighttime snacking, stay busy after your evening meal. Go for a short walk; floss and brush your teeth, and get to bed earlier. Even better, close the kitchen after dinner and try not to eat anything 3 hours prior to going to sleep.

22. *Practice stress management techniques* (discussed in Chapter 7). Many people snack and increase their food consumption in stressful situations.

23. *Get support.* People who receive support from friends, relatives, and formal support groups are much more likely to lose and maintain weight loss than those without such support. The more support you receive, the better off you will be.

24. *Monitor changes and reward accomplishments.* Being able to exercise without interruption for 15, 20, 30, or 60 minutes; swimming a certain distance; running a mile—all these accomplishments deserve recognition. Create rewards that are not related to eating: new clothing, a tennis racquet, a bicycle, exercise shoes, or something else that is special and you would not have acquired otherwise.

25. *Prepare for slip-ups.* Most people will slip and occasionally splurge. Do not despair and give up. Reevaluate and continue with your efforts. An occasional slip won't make much difference in the long run.

26. *Think positive.* Avoid negative thoughts about how difficult changing past behaviors might be. Instead, think of the benefits you will reap, such as feeling, looking, and functioning better, plus enjoying better health and improving the quality of life. Avoid negative environments and unsupportive people.

Try It In your Online Journal or class notebook, answer the following questions: How many of the above strategies do you use to help you maintain recommended body weight? Do you feel that any of these strategies specifically help you manage body weight more effectively? If so, explain why.

You Can Do It!

The challenge of taking off excessive body fat and keeping it off for good has no simple solution. Weight management is accomplished through lifetime commitment to physical activity and proper food selection. When taking part in a weight reduction program, people have to decrease their caloric intake moderately and implement strategies to modify unhealthy eating behaviors.

Relapses into past negative behaviors are almost inevitable. Making mistakes is human and does not mean failure. Failure comes to those who give up and do not use previous experiences to build upon and, instead, develop skills that will prevent self-defeating behaviors in the future. Where there's a will, there's a way, and those who persist will reap the rewards.

Assess Your Behavior

CENGAGENOW Log on to www.cengagebrain.com to access CengageNOW and the Behavior Change Planner where you can track your progress in your exercise log and update your pedometer log if you are tracking your steps.

1. Are you satisfied with your current body composition and quality of life? If not, are you willing to do something about it. If so, what do you plan to do to reach your goal?

2. Are physical activity, aerobic exercise, and strength training a regular part of your lifetime weight management program?

3. Do you weigh yourself regularly and make adjustments in energy intake and physical activity habits if your weight starts to slip upward?

4. Do you exercise portion control, watch your overall fat intake, and plan ahead before you eat out or attend social functions that entice overeating?

Assess Your Knowledge

CENGAGENOW Evaluate how well you understand the concepts presented in this chapter using the chapter-specific quizzing available in the online materials at www.cengagebrain.com.

1. Obesity is defined as a body mass index equal to or above
   a. 10.
   b. 25.
   c. 30.
   d. 45.
   e. 50.

2. The yearly estimated number of deaths attributed to excessive body weight and physical inactivity in the United States is
   a. 28,000.
   b. 55,000.
   c. 93,000.
   d. 112,000.
   e. 350,000.

3. Obesity increases the risk for
   a. hypertension.
   b. congestive heart failure.
   c. atherosclerosis.
   d. type 2 diabetes.
   e. All are correct choices.

4. Tolerable weight is a body weight
   a. that is not ideal but one that you can live with.
   b. that will tolerate the increased risk of chronic diseases.
   c. with a BMI range between 25 and 30.
   d. that meets both ideal values for percent body fat and BMI.
   e. All are correct choices.

5. When the body uses protein instead of a combination of fats and carbohydrates as a source of energy,
   a. weight loss is very slow.
   b. a large amount of weight loss is in the form of water.
   c. muscle turns into fat.
   d. fat is lost very rapidly.
   e. fat cannot be lost.

6. One pound of fat represents
   a. 1,200 calories.
   b. 1,500 calories.
   c. 3,500 calories.
   d. 5,000 calories.
   e. None of the above choices is correct.

7. The mechanism that seems to regulate how much a person weighs is known as
   a. setpoint.
   b. weight factor.
   c. basal metabolic rate.
   d. metabolism.
   e. energy-balancing equation.

8. The key to successful weight management is
   a. frequent dieting.
   b. very low calorie diets when "normal" dieting doesn't work.
   c. a lifetime physical activity program.
   d. regular low-carbohydrate/high-protein meals.
   e. All are correct choices.

9. The daily amount of physical activity recommended for weight loss maintenance is
   a. 15 to 20 minutes.
   b. 20 to 30 minutes.
   c. 30 to 60 minutes.
   d. 60 to 90 minutes.
   e. Any amount is sufficient as long as it is done daily.

10. A daily energy expenditure of 300 calories through physical activity is the equivalent of approximately _____ pounds of fat per year.
    a. 12
    b. 15
    c. 22
    d. 27
    e. 31

Correct answers can be found on page 307.

Caloric Requirement: Computation Form

Name _____ Date _____

Course _____ Section _____

A. Current body weight   _____

B. Estimated energy requirement per day (use Table 8.1, page 174)   _____

C. Selected physical activity (e.g., jogging)*   _____

D. Number of exercise sessions per week   _____

E. Duration of exercise session (in minutes)   _____

F. Total weekly exercise time in minutes (D × E)   _____

G. Average daily exercise time in minutes (F ÷ 7)   _____

H. Caloric expenditure per pound per minute (cal/lb/min) of selected physical
   activity (use Table 8.2, page 175)   _____

I. Total calories burned per minute of exercise (A × H)   _____

J. Average daily calories burned as a result of the exercise program (G × I) _____

K. Total daily caloric requirement with exercise to maintain body weight (B + J) _____

L. Number of calories to subtract from daily requirement to achieve a
   negative caloric balance (multiply current body weight by 5)**   _____

M. Target caloric intake to lose weight (K − L)   _____

---

*If more than one physical activity is selected, you will need to estimate the average daily calories burned as a result of each additional
 activity (steps C through J) and add all of these figures to K above.

**This figure should never be below 1,200 calories for women or 1,500 calories for men. See Activity 8.2 for the 1,200-, 1,500-, 1,800-,
 and 2,000-calorie diet plans.

Caloric Requirement: Computation Form (continued)

1. How much effort are you willing to put into reaching your weight loss goal?

   _____

   _____

2. Indicate your feelings about participating in an exercise program.

   _____

   _____

3. Will you commit to be more physically active and to participate in a combined aerobic and strength-training program?
   Yes ☐ No ☐

   If your answer is "Yes," proceed to the next question; if you answered "No," please review Chapters 3 and 6 again.

4. Indicate your current number of daily steps: ☐

5. List aerobic activities you enjoy or may enjoy doing.

   _____

   _____

6. Select one or two aerobic activities in which you will participate regularly.

   ☐   ☐

7. List facilities available to you where you can carry out the aerobic and strength-training programs.

   _____

   _____

8. Indicate days and times you will set aside for your aerobic and strength-training program (accumulate 60 to 90 minutes of physical activity 6 to 7 days per week, including 3 to 5 weekly sessions of aerobic exercise lasting about 30 minutes each and 2 to 3 weekly strength-training sessions).

   Monday: _____

   Tuesday: _____

   Wednesday: _____

   Thursday: _____

   Friday: _____

   Saturday: _____

   Sunday: _____

9. Conclusion: Briefly describe whether you think you can meet the goals of your physical activity, aerobic, and strength-training programs. What obstacles will you have to overcome, and how will you overcome them?

   _____

   _____

   _____

Daily Food Intake Record: 1,800-Calorie Diet Plan

Name _____   Date _____

Course _____   Section _____

Instructions

The objective of the diet plan is to meet (not exceed) the number of servings allowed for the food groups listed. Each time you eat a particular food, record it in the space provided for each group along with the appropriate serving size. Be sure not to exceed the number of calories allowed per serving listed below. Instead of the meat and beans group, you are allowed to have two commercially available low-fat frozen entrees for two of your meals (these entrees should provide no more than 300 calories and less than 6 grams of fat). You can make additional copies of this form as needed.

Dairy: 2 servings

Grains: 8 servings

Fruits: 3 servings

Veggies: 5 servings

Protein: 2 low-fat frozen entrees

ChooseMyPlate.gov

Grains (80 calories/serving): 8 servings

1 _____   5 _____

2 _____   6 _____

3 _____   7 _____

4 _____   8 _____

Vegetables (25 calories/serving): 5 servings

1 _____   4 _____

2 _____   5 _____

3 _____

Fruits (60 calories/serving): 3 servings

1 _____

2 _____

3 _____

Dairy (120 calories/serving, use low-fat milk and low-fat milk products): 2 servings

1 _____

2 _____

Low-Fat Frozen Entrees (Protein) (300 calories and less than 6 grams of fat): 2 servings

1 _____

2 _____

Daily Food Intake Record: 2,000-Calorie Diet Plan

Name _____ Date _____

Course _____ Section _____

Instructions

The objective of the diet plan is to meet (not exceed) the number of servings allowed for the food groups listed. Each time you eat a particular food, record it in the space provided for each group along with the appropriate serving size. Be sure not to exceed the number of calories allowed per serving listed below. Instead of the meat and beans group, you are allowed to have two commercially available low-fat frozen entrees for two of your meals (these entrees should provide no more than 300 calories and less than 6 grams of fat). You can make additional copies of this form as needed.

Dairy: 2 servings
Grains: 10 servings
Fruits: 4 servings
Veggies: 5 servings
Protein: 2 low-fat frozen entrees

ChooseMyPlate.gov

Grains (80 calories/serving): 10 servings

1 _____ 6 _____

2 _____ 7 _____

3 _____ 8 _____

4 _____ 9 _____

5 _____ 10 _____

Vegetables (25 calories/serving): 5 servings

1 _____ 4 _____

2 _____ 5 _____

3 _____

Fruits (60 calories/serving): 4 servings

1 _____

2 _____

3 _____

4 _____

Dairy (120 calories/serving, use low-fat milk and low-fat milk products): 2 servings

1 _____

2 _____

Low-Fat Frozen Entrees (Protein) (300 calories and less than 6 grams of fat): 2 servings

1 _____

2 _____